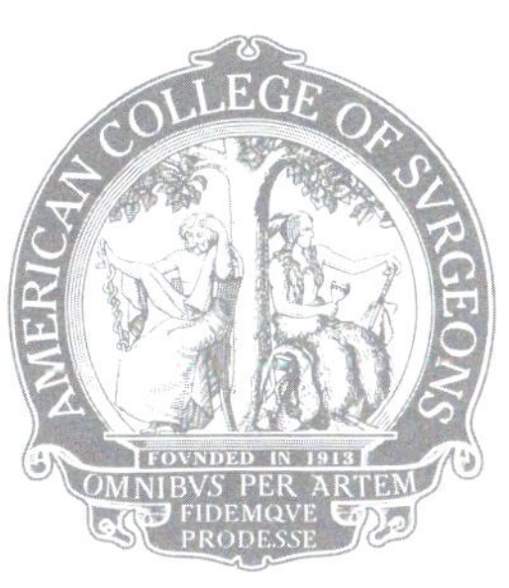

Optimal Resources for Surgical Education and Training

AMERICAN COLLEGE OF SURGEONS

ISBN 978-1-7369212-0-3

Dedication

J. David Richardson, MD, FACS, MAMSE, contributed many things during his remarkable career, but at the heart of what he did was a passion for surgical education. He looked out for the general surgeons, but also for young surgeons trying to make their way in the field at a time when surgery has changed so much. He advocated for this publicly in trauma and emergency surgery more than 30 years ago and, more recently, he advocated for a reevaluation of surgical training while he served as Chair of the Board of Regents and President of the American College of Surgeons (ACS). His advocacy led to an annual conference to bring the House of Surgery together to discuss and address surgical issues and the development of a transition to practice program. His advocacy for the rural surgeon and a broadly trained general surgeon is a direct reflection of the need for surgical education to be reevaluated.

Four years ago, it was determined that there needed to be a common template for defining the optimal resources and elements for a successful surgical training program. Though certainly the American Board of Surgery and the ACGME define specific elements, an overall comprehensive approach and guide did not exist. Dr. Richardson's help in creating the Editorial Oversight Committee and his constant vigilance to get surgical education right was, in many regards, responsible for changes in surgical education that have occurred in the last decade in the United States.

His untimely passing precluded his completion of his own foreword for this book, and as such, it seems appropriate to dedicate this work to Dr. Richardson and all those trainees whose lives he touched. As he looks down from above and raises an eyebrow, as he often did to get us to be true to our efforts, I hope he sees surgical education moving forward and achieving a level of excellence our patients expect and we have always tried to deliver.

—David B. Hoyt, MD, FACS
Executive Director, American College of Surgeons

Foreword

David B. Hoyt, MD, FACS
Executive Director
American College of Surgeons

Much of surgical education has followed the traditions of apprenticeship and hierarchical training established more than 100 years ago in the Halsted tradition. Prolonged time of exposure allowed for enough time to accomplish the complexity of learning surgical care of the patient. Changes have occurred, in particular in the last 25 years, that require us to redefine the specific goals and process by which surgical education is accomplished with a predictable outcome.

Optimal Resources for Surgical Education and Training was conceived to address the issue and create a resource that exists specifically to define the optimal way to train residents. Surgical education, like residency training in all of medicine in the United States, is distributed between the boards, the ACGME and RCs, and the professional societies, and each had a different perspective on defining expectations based on their set of responsibilities. After many attempts by ACS in the last decade to "Fix the Five," we realized that restarting the process by coming to agreement on the optimal resources for surgical training was needed.

To accomplish this goal, a Steering Committee and an Editorial Oversight Committee were created. I want to recognize and thank the members, including L.D. Britt, MD, MPH, DSc(Hon), FACS, FCCM, MAMSE, FRCSEng(Hon), FRCSEd(Hon), FWACS(Hon), FRCSI(Hon), FCS(SA)(Hon), FRCSGlasg(Hon); Lewis M. Flint, MD, FACS, MAMSE; Anna M. Ledgerwood, MD, FACS; J. David Richardson, MD, FACS, MAMSE; Ajit K. Sachdeva, MD, FACS, FRCSC, FSACME, MAMSE; Courtney M. Townsend, Jr., MD, FACS, FRCSEd(Hon); and Patrice Gabler Blair, MPH. They worked tirelessly to create an outline and author list. Over the last three years, 72 authors have collaborated to define all aspects of surgical training with a focus on general surgical training, realizing that the majority of features apply to all surgical training.

This work puts forth an attempt to define the best way to evaluate and think about surgical training going forward. Many of the chapters cannot cover the entire curricula but give examples of how a curriculum should be implemented and how specific procedures should be taught. Similarly, the broad domain of responsibility of a modern surgeon is covered in terms of professionalism, advocacy, financial health, diversity, and overall well-being. We hope this work will find an audience who sees it as a valuable contribution that becomes a template for implementation of surgical training going forward.

Ajit K. Sachdeva, MD, FACS, FRCSC, FSACME, MAMSE
Director, Division of Education
American College of Surgeons

Residency training in surgery has undergone monumental changes over the past several decades. The environment of health care in which surgery training is embedded has continued to evolve, new regulations and mandates have constantly impacted residency training, and advances in the science and practice of surgical education have progressed at an unprecedented pace. Surgery residency training has very unique characteristics as compared to training in other medical specialties because of the need to blend the requisite skills in the cognitive, clinical, technical, and non-technical domains, along with exemplary professionalism in providing care to patients. These characteristics of surgical training require special organizational structures, methods, and processes to prepare residents for surgical practice.

The need for a comprehensive, national resource that addresses critical elements in surgery residency training and is aimed at a variety of different constituents prompted the American College of Surgeons to embark on the exciting endeavor to create such a resource. This is fondly known as the "Gold Book" and is composed of 14 chapters on important topics. The "Gold Book" should be of great value to surgical leaders, surgical educators, and surgery residents. Also, key stakeholders, such as leaders of academic medical centers and hospital administrators, should find this resource helpful. The content of the "Gold Book" should facilitate transformational changes in surgery residency training that result in an enduring difference in the education of surgery residents and through their efforts in ensuring delivery of optimal patient care.

We are deeply indebted to Dr. David Hoyt, Executive Director of the American College of Surgeons, for making this vision a reality and bringing the major project to fruition. We are most grateful to the surgical leaders and educators who have contributed to this outstanding resource. We would also like to express our sincere thanks to the staff of the Division of Education and the Division of Integrated Communications who have supported this project with great fidelity, skill, and dedication. We hope you find this unique resource useful in your professional work and look forward to your feedback.

Lewis M. Flint, MD, FACS, MAMSE
Editor-in-Chief, *Selected Readings in General Surgery*
American College of Surgeons

Participation in the preparation of this manual has been an honor and a privilege for me. The experience was one of pleasure and sadness. Pleasure arose from being able to edit and occasionally improve content prepared by experts. Sadness came at the end of the journey when we lost Dr. J. David Richardson, the surgeon-leader who stimulated us to recognize the need for a single source of knowledge that would provide definitive guidance for educators responsible for the preparation of future surgeons. Graduate surgical education has definitely evolved since I became a residency program director in 1981. We have gone from a totally immersive training paradigm that existed in a relatively simple health care system to one that is more intellectually challenging, more stressful, and is required to function within a complex care delivery environment. The authors of chapters included in this guidebook have recognized the need to adapt educational approaches and have learned how to prepare excellent surgeons for future practice. I hope that readers will learn from and build upon the knowledge presented herein so that our tradition of clinical excellence can continue.

L. Scott Levin, MD, FACS, MAMSE
Chair
American College of Surgeons Board of Regents

The Gold Book is a ***compendium*** that defines the principles and practice of surgical education. William Stewart Halsted is credited with creating the "training program" in 1889. Halsted founded a residency training program that dramatically changed the way surgeons were trained. Before Halsted, surgical training was a haphazard series of preceptorships without a definite end. Halsted believed that surgical training should be accomplished in a set period of time, have a progressive increase in responsibility and operative experience, and have a final period of independent study. For the most part, surgical training has followed these guidelines, and one might assume little has changed in the last 142 years. What has changed is the evolution of surgical specialties, and specialties within specialties!

While the time-honored practice of general surgery is practiced by many who serve all with skill and fidelity, the trend in medicine has been continued diversification. Knowledge is expanding exponentially. The complexity of care is increasing due to an aging population and often limited access to health system resources. Evolving technology and constant bench-to-bedside discoveries challenge trainees and practitioners alike to keep up. The surgeon must be a lifelong learner.

Education is defined as the process of receiving or giving systematic instruction. Training is the action of teaching a person a particular skill or type of behavior. Both education and training go hand in hand. The surgical resident is much like a raw gemstone. Every facet must be polished so that it can sparkle and become something of value. This metaphor applies to surgical trainees. When the medical students select surgery as a career, they have expectations that they will be educated and trained. When the residency selection committee ranks medical students for the match, they expect that those who match into their programs will learn and acquire the skills to practice surgery after the training program or fellowship.

The Gold Book is a tome that guides both the teacher and the learner. Nothing is left to chance. Every aspect of education and training, including surgical technique, professionalism, and measurement of competency is outlined. It is the "checklist of checklists" for program directors and educators. This edition included general surgery modules on what must be learned by the resident. The majority of chapters are generic to all surgical training programs, and I believe this edition will serve as a guide for all surgical disciplines to add their "flavor and techniques" to the next rendition!

The book guides surgical departments with regard to what resources are required to educate and train the next generation adequately. Surgical checklists, shared decision-making, defining patient expectations, setting standards, improving quality, and attention to detail optimize the delivery of surgical care. These principles of care have evolved since the beginning of ACS. This book is another milestone in the legacy and history of the College. We strive to get it right. For both the educator and the student, they cannot go wrong in meeting their respective goals if they follow the writings of the wise and distinguished authors of this text.

Contributing Authors

Editors

David B. Hoyt, MD, FACS
Executive Director
American College of Surgeons

Ajit K. Sachdeva, MD, FACS, FRCSC, FSACME, MAMSE
Director, Division of Education
American College of Surgeons
Adjunct Professor of Surgery
Feinberg School of Medicine, Northwestern University

Lewis M. Flint, MD, FACS, MAMSE
Editor-in-Chief, *Selected Readings in General Surgery*
American College of Surgeons

J. David Richardson, MD, FACS, MAMSE
Berel L. Abrams, MD, Chair in Surgery; Professor and Vice Chairman for Academic Affairs,
The Hiram C. Polk Jr., MD Department of Surgery
University of Louisville School of Medicine
Chief of Surgery and Director of Emergency Surgical Services
University of Louisville Hospital

Mark Aeder, MD, MS, FACS
Associate Professor of Transplant and Hepatobiliary Surgery
Case Western Reserve University
Director of Surgical Quality and Transplant Quality
University Hospitals Cleveland Medical Center

Linda R. Archer, PhD
Vice Dean of Graduate Medical Education
Eastern Virginia Medical School

Patrick V. Bailey, MD, MLS, FACS
Medical Director, Advocacy, Division of Advocacy and Health Policy
American College of Surgeons

Barbara L. Bass, MD, FACS, MAMSE
Professor of Surgery
George Washington University
Vice President for Health Affairs; Dean
GW School of Medicine and Health Sciences
Chief Executive Officer
The GW Medical Faculty Associates

Karen J. Brasel, MD, MPH, FACS, MAMSE
Professor of Surgery; Assistant Dean for Graduate Medical Education; Residency Program Director, Surgery
Oregon Health & Science University School of Medicine

L.D. Britt, MD, MPH, DSc(Hon), FACS, FCCM, MAMSE, FRCSEng(Hon), FRCSEd(Hon), FWACS(Hon), FRCSI(Hon), FCS(SA)(Hon), FRCS(Glasg)(Hon)
Henry Ford Professor and Edward J. Brickhouse Chairman
Eastern Virginia Medical School

Molly Brittain, MEd
Director of Education
Eastern Virginia Medical School

Jo Buyske, MD, FACS, DABS
President and Chief Executive Officer
American Board of Surgery

C

William G. Cioffi, MD, FACS
J. Murray Beardsley Professor
and Chairman, Department of Surgery
Warren Alpert Medical School at Brown University
Surgeon-in-Chief
The Miriam Hospital and Rhode Island Hospital

Thomas H. Cogbill, MD, FACS
Emeritus Surgeon
Gundersen Health System

Christian Miguel de Virgilio, MD, FACS
Chair, Department of Surgery
Harbor-UCLA Medical Center
Co-Chair, College of Applied Anatomy, and Professor of Clinical Surgery
UCLA School of Medicine

Demetrios Demetriades, MD, PhD, FACS, MAMSE
Professor of Surgery
University of Southern California
Director of Trauma, Emergency Surgery, and Critical Care
LAC+USC Medical Center

Daniel L. Dent, MD, FACS
Professor, Department of Medical Education; Director, Competency Education and Assessment; Professor, Department of Surgery; Vice Chair for Education, Division of Trauma and Emergency Surgery
Joe R. and Teresa Lozano Long School of Medicine
UT Health San Antonio

Justin B. Dimick, MD, MPH, FACS
Frederick A. Coller Distinguished Professor of Surgery and Chair, Department of Surgery
University of Michigan Health System

Timothy J. Eberlein, MD, FACS, MAMSE
Bixby Professor and Chair, Department of Surgery; Spencer T. and Ann W. Olin Distinguished Professor; Director
Alvin J. Siteman Cancer Center
Senior Associate Dean for Cancer Programs and Surgeon-in-Chief
Barnes Jewish Hospital
Washington University School of Medicine in St. Louis

James S. Economou, MD, PhD, FACS
Beaumont Distinguished Professor of Surgery; Distinguished Professor of Microbiology, Immunology, and Molecular Genetics; Distinguished Professor of Molecular and Medical Pharmacology
University of California, Los Angeles

E. Christopher Ellison, MD, FACS, MAMSE
Robert M. Zollinger Professor of Surgery Emeritus, Department of Surgery
The Ohio State University College of Medicine

Paola Fata, MD
Associate Professor of Surgery; Director, Division of General Surgery
McGill University and McGill University Health Centre

David V. Feliciano, MD, FACS, MAMSE
Clinical Professor of Surgery
University of Maryland School of Medicine
Attending Surgeon Emeritus, Shock Trauma Center/Department of Surgery
University of Maryland Medical Center

Katherine L. Files, MBA
Internal and Corporate Communications Manager
Atrium Health Wake Forest Baptist

Julie A. Freischlag, MD, FACS, FRCSEd(Hon), DFSVS, MAMSE
Chief Executive Officer
Atrium Health Wake Forest Baptist
Dean
Wake Forest School of Medicine
Chief Academic Officer
Atrium Health

Gerald M. Fried, MD, FACS, FRCSC, FCAHS, MCS
Professor of Surgery; Associate Dean, Education Technology and Innovation; Director, Steinberg Centre for Simulation and Interactive Learning
McGill University Faculty of Medicine and Health Sciences

Mary T. Hawn, MD, MPH, FACS
Emile Holman Professor of Surgery and Chair
Stanford University

James C. Hebert, MD, FACS
Professor of Surgery Emeritus
University of Vermont Larner College of Medicine

Amy N. Hildreth, MD, FACS
Associate Professor and Associate Chair of Education, Department of Surgery; Program Director, General Surgery Residency
Wake Forest School of Medicine

Benjamin T. Jarman, MD, FACS
General Surgeon and General Surgery Residency Program Director
Gundersen Health System

Muneera R. Kapadia, MD, MME, FACS, FASCRS
Associate Professor of Surgery and Associate Vice Chair of Education
University of North Carolina School of Medicine

K. Craig Kent, MD, FACS, MAMSE
Chief Executive Officer
UVA Health
Executive Vice President for Health Affairs
University of Virginia

Melina R. Kibbe, MD, FACS, FAHA
Dean
University of Virginia School of Medicine
James Carroll Flippin Professor of Medical Science and Chief Health Affairs Officer
University of Virginia Health

Allan D. Kirk, MD, PhD, FACS, MAMSE
David C. Sabiston, Jr., Distinguished Professor and Chair, Department of Surgery; Professor of Pediatrics and Immunology
Duke University School of Medicine

Clifford Y. Ko, MD, MS, MSHS, FACS, FASCRS
Director, ACS Division of Research and Optimal Patient Care
American College of Surgeons
Professor and Vice Chair of Surgery
David Geffen School of Medicine, University of California, Los Angeles

James R. Korndorffer, Jr., MD, MHPE, FACS, MAMSE
Associate Professor of Surgery and Vice Chair of Education
Stanford University

Anna M. Ledgerwood, MD, FACS
Professor of Surgery
Wayne State University

Amy E. Liepert, MD, FACS
Medical Director, Acute Care Surgery, and Associate Professor of Surgery
University of California, San Diego

Keith D. Lillemoe, MD, FACS, MAMSE
Chief of Surgery and Surgeon-in-Chief
Massachusetts General Hospital
W. Gerald Austen Professor of Surgery
Harvard Medical School

Charles E. Lucas, MD, FACS
Professor of Surgery
Wayne State University

M

Charles D. Mabry, MD, FACS
Medical Director of Practice Management
Jefferson Regional Medical Center
Associate Professor, College of Medicine, Department of Surgery
University of Arkansas for Medical Sciences

Jeffrey B. Matthews, MD, FACS, MAMSE
Dallas B. Phemister Professor and Chair, Department of Surgery
The University of Chicago
Surgeon-in-Chief
The University of Chicago Medicine

James S. McCartney, MA
Writer/Editor
JSM Communications LLC

Mary H. McGrath, MD, MPH, FACS, MAMSE
Professor of Surgery Emerita, Division of Plastic Surgery
University of California, San Francisco

Kelly M. McMasters, MD, PhD, FACS
Ben A. Reid, Sr., MD, Professor and Chair
University of Louisville School of Medicine

John D. Mellinger, MD, FACS
J. Roland Folse, MD, Endowed Chair in Surgery; Professor and Vice Chair, Department of Surgery; Director, Leadership and Excellence, Center for Human and Organizational Potential
Southern Illinois University School of Medicine

J. Wayne Meredith, MD, FACS, MCCM, MAMSE
Richard T. Myers Professor and Chairman, Department of Surgery
Wake Forest School of Medicine

Fabrizio Michelassi, MD, FACS, MAMSE, ESA(Hon), SIC(Hon)
Lewis Atterbury Stimson Professor and Chairman, Department of Surgery
Weill Cornell Medical College
Surgeon-in-Chief
New York Presbyterian/Weill Cornell Medical Center

Susan Moffatt-Bruce, MD, PhD, FRCSC, MBA, FACS, MAMSE
Chief Executive Officer
Royal College of Physicians and Surgeons of Canada

Ernest E. "Gene" Moore, MD, FACS, MCCM, FACN, FISS, MAMSE
Director of Research
Ernest E. Moore Shock Trauma Center at Denver Health
Distinguished Professor of Surgery
University of Colorado Denver

O

Frank G. Opelka, MD, FACS
Medical Director, Quality and Health Policy, Division of Advocacy and Health Policy
American College of Surgeons
Professor of Surgery
The George Washington University

P

Carlos A. Pellegrini, MD, FACS, FRCSI(Hon), FRCS(Hon), FRCSEd(Hon), FWACS(Hon), MAMSE
Professor and Chair Emeritus
University of Washington
Chief Medical Officer
UW Medicine

Roy Phitayakorn, MD, MHPE (MEd), FACS
Director of Medical Student Education and Surgery Education Research
Massachusetts General Hospital
Associate Professor of Surgery
Harvard Medical School

John R. Potts III, MD, FACS, MAMSE
Partner
SVinPA Consulting

Taylor S. Riall, MD, PhD, FACS
Interim Chair, Department of Surgery, and Professor of Surgery
University of Arizona College of Medicine - Tucson

Michael F. Rotondo, MD, FACS
Professor of Surgery; Vice Dean for Clinical Affairs; Chief Executive Officer
University of Rochester Medical Faculty Group
Senior Vice President
University of Rochester Medical Center

S

Mohsen M. Shabahang, MD, PhD, FACS, MAMSE
Vice President, Chief Medical Officer
Wellspan Surgery Service Line

Christian Shalgian
Director, Division of Advocacy and Health Policy
American College of Surgeons

Douglas S. Smink, MD, MPH, FACS, MAMSE
Chief of Surgery
Brigham and Women's Faulkner Hospital
Vice Chair of Education, Department of Surgery
Brigham and Women's Hospital
Associate Professor of Surgery
Harvard Medical School

Brigitte K. Smith, MD, MHPE, FACS, FSVS
Vice Chair of Education, Department of Surgery; Program Director, Vascular Surgery Fellowship; Associate Professor of Vascular Surgery
University of Utah School of Medicine

Mitchell C. Sokolosky, MD
Associate Dean, Graduate Medical Education; ACGME Designated Institutional Official; Associate Professor, Emergency Medicine
Wake Forest School of Medicine

Nathaniel J. Soper, MD, FACS, MAMSE
Jean and Harlan Stone, MD, Chair of Surgery; Chairman, Department of Surgery
University of Arizona College of Medicine - Phoenix
Physician Executive Director, General Surgery
Banner - University Medical Center Phoenix

Steven C. Stain, MD, FACS, MAMSE
Chair, Department of Surgery
Lahey Hospital and Medical Center

Dimitrios Stefanidis, MD, PhD, FACS, FASMBS, FSSH
Professor of Surgery; Vice Chair of Education; Chief, Minimally Invasive and Bariatric Surgery; Surgical Director, IU ACS-AEI Skills Center, Department of Surgery
Indiana University School of Medicine

John F. Sweeney, MD, FACS
Joseph Brown Whitehead Professor and Chair, Department of Surgery
Emory University School of Medicine
Director, Surgical Services; Surgeon-in-Chief
Emory Healthcare

T

Gary L. Timmerman, MD, FACS, MAMSE
Professor and Chair, Department of Surgery
University of South Dakota Sanford School of Medicine
Medical Director, Undergraduate Medical Education, Sanford Medical Education
Sanford Health

Courtney M. Townsend, Jr., MD, FACS, FRCSEd(Hon)
Professor
Robertson-Poth Distinguished Chair in General Surgery
Department of Surgery
University of Texas Medical Branch

Patricia L. Turner, MD, MBA, FACS
Director, Division of Member Services
American College of Surgeons
Clinical Associate Professor of Surgery
The University of Chicago Medicine

Daniel J. Vargo, MD, FACS
Director, Utah Center for Innovation and Simulation in Education (UCISE), and Professor of Surgery
University of Utah School of Medicine

Selwyn M. Vickers, MD, FACS
James C. Lee, Jr., Endowed Chair; Professor of Surgery; Senior Vice President of Medicine; Dean
University of Alabama at Birmingham School of Medicine

W

Andrew L. Warshaw, MD, FACS, FRCSEd(Hon), MAMSE
Surgeon-in-Chief Emeritus
Massachusetts General Hospital
W. Gerald Austen Distinguished Professor of Surgery
Harvard Medical School

Ronald J. Weigel, MD, PhD, MBA, FACS
EA Crowell, Jr., Professor and Chair; Professor of Surgery, Surgical Oncology, and Endocrine Surgery; Professor of Anatomy and Cell Biology; Professor of Biochemistry and Molecular Biology; Professor of Molecular Physiology and Biophysics
University of Iowa Carver College of Medicine

John A. Weigelt, MD, DVM, MMA, FACS, MAMSE
Professor of Surgery
University of South Dakota

Table of Contents

AMERICAN C
SURGEONS A
OF SURGEON
COLLEGE OF
AMERICAN C
SURGEONS A
OF SURGEON
COLLEGE OF
AMERICAN C
SURGEONS A

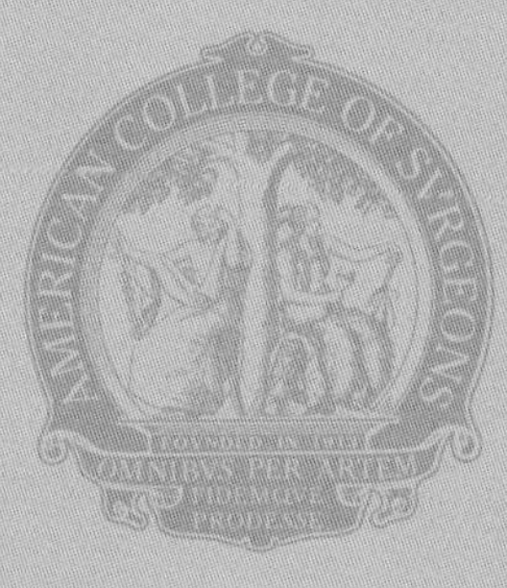

CHAPTER 1
Preamble

Lead Author
J. David Richardson, MD, FACS, MAMSE

Co-Authors
Jo Buyske, MD, FACS, DABS
Steven C. Stain, MD, FACS, MAMSE

CHAPTER 1
Preamble

Introduction

The complexities of modern surgical practice have posed challenges to our ability to efficiently educate all surgical trainees using the traditional paradigm that required long work hours and assumed that the acquisition of the necessary knowledge and skills to prepare the resident for independent practice would be achieved through conventional surgical rotations. Leaders of the American College of Surgeons (ACS), American Board of Surgery (ABS), and the Review Committee for Surgery (RC-S) have determined that we need a single, consensus-based, comprehensive resource that describes the elements of an effective surgical residency and provides guidance on how to design and implement them. This guidebook is designed to be that resource. The information contained herein can be used to help ensure that trainees acquire the knowledge and skills to independently practice their specialty upon completion of training. The book will also describe the responsibilities of each of the groups overseeing surgical education (Specialty Boards, Review Committees, and component societies and professional organizations).

We hope to provide useful perspectives that will help set the stage for this effort by reviewing a few important points in the history of surgical training in the United States. These are described in chronological order in the following list:

- The surgical training program that William Stewart Halsted founded in 1889 at the Johns Hopkins Hospital, Baltimore, MD, is recognized as one of the earliest examples of a structured, multilevel educational approach to prepare surgeons for general surgery practice.[1]
- The founding of the ACS in 1913 launched an organization with an enduring commitment to create standards for the highest-quality patient care and to educate health care professionals to ensure they have the knowledge and skills to provide the best possible care to patients.
- The American Board of Medical Specialties (ABMS) was formed in 1933 to establish independent surgical boards to certify individuals who have met a defined standard of surgical education, training, and knowledge.
- The "rectangular" surgical residency program at Massachusetts General Hospital in Boston, established in 1939, allowed trainees to attain increased graded responsibility and autonomy and, thereby, provided an important educational template for preparing surgeons for independent practice.[2]
- The Accreditation Council for Graduate Medical Education (ACGME), formed in 1981, oversees individual Review Committees (RCs) for each surgical specialty. The RCs set standards for accreditation of training programs and ensure that accredited programs adhere to those standards. Members of the RCs are nominated by the American Medical Association (AMA), relevant boards, and specialty societies.
- Other organizations that influence surgical training include professional organizations such as the Association for Surgical Education (ASE), the Association of Program Directors in Surgery (APDS), and societies representing the various surgical specialties.

Why Do We Need This Book?

The opportunity to enhance surgical education given the constraints that have emerged in the last 30 years challenging surgical training and readiness for practice is apparent. This issue is apparent within the field of general surgery in particular because:

- The discipline of general surgery is extremely broad.
- Many hospitals that provide general surgery residency training have increasingly focused on tertiary or quaternary "service lines," which may not prepare a trainee for commonly encountered surgical conditions.
- Societal and regulatory expectations for faculty oversight have diminished training opportunities for residents to learn to perform procedures and provide patient care independently.

- Duty-hour restrictions have reduced training time. The current structure of duty-hours has limited training hours overall and this often impacts evening and nighttime hours when many emergency conditions are evaluated and treated. The answer is not to roll back current duty-hour restrictions, but rather to make duty hours more flexible.

The trend toward surgical specialization within the field of general surgery and the creation of postresidency fellowships to provide focused training for surgeons also has affected the training of general surgery residents. For example, specialties such as cardiothoracic surgery, vascular surgery, and pediatric surgery all had their origins in general surgery. Fellowships in areas once considered parts of the "core" of general surgery (breast, endocrine, bariatric) have the potential to diminish the general surgery residency experience.

Certainly, many residents complete their general surgery training well prepared for independent practice without a need for additional fellowship training, but, unfortunately, some trainees completing residency are not prepared. Surgeons have recognized the need to improve surgical training over several years. Opinions collected through the ACS Board of Governors comprehensive survey of ACS Fellows[3] confirm this concern. The available data indicate that some young surgeons lack confidence in their ability to conduct independent practice after the requisite five-year training program.[4, 5] The opportunity to improve this through modification of the residency training program is the reason for taking on the challenge of preparing this manual.

The essential characteristics of general surgery have been described. For example, the ABS has crafted a useful definition of general surgery, which defines the scope of practice and the areas for which a certified general surgeon should have broad knowledge and experience. (Document available on the ABS website at *www.absurgery.org.)* These areas include conditions of the alimentary tract, the abdomen and its contents, breast and soft tissue, and the endocrine system. General surgeons also should demonstrate experience in surgical critical care and trauma management, as well as surgical oncology. The general surgeon should know the anatomic and physiologic principles necessary to surgically treat conditions that fall under the scope of these domains. This definition acknowledges that certain other areas, once within the broad purview of general surgery, have emerged as fields of specialization. For example, although general surgeons should have some understanding of vascular, pediatric, and thoracic surgery and a basic understanding of transplantation, comprehensive knowledge and management of these areas would require additional training.

Using these definitions, the ABS has developed assessment mechanisms to evaluate the knowledge and judgment of surgical residents through the qualifying (written) and the certifying (oral) examinations. The qualifying examination effectively assesses the knowledge base of a prospective certified surgeon, and the certifying examination assesses the candidate's ability to recognize a clinical problem, describe a treatment plan, evaluate surgical judgment, and confirm the ability to manage complications.

The oral exam uses various case scenarios to determine if the candidate has the knowledge, judgment, and skill to safely address the condition at hand. Thorough training of examiners, structured examiner feedback through observers, and reviews of examiner psychometric data enable them to assess residents in a short exam (generally 90 minutes). Recent studies have confirmed that passing the oral and written elements of ABS board certification are each independently correlated with a lower risk of losing a state medical license and other disciplinary actions, suggesting that both add independent value to the quality of the assessment.[6-8]

The ACGME, through the component review committees (for example, the RC-S) is a critical authority that has purview over the surgical residency training programs. Individual surgeons who have met the requirements of an ACGME-accredited training program can enter the examination process of the ABS. The RC-S requires that each approved program have curricula that include documented observations and feedback as well as clearly specified time requirements for educational experiences. To successfully complete training, residents must perform a minimum number of operative cases in each area of general surgery. Those residents who have demonstrated their knowledge base, good judgment, skills, and professionalism through a combination of evaluations will receive written affirmation of training completion.

The RC for Surgery assesses training programs using the following criteria:

- Does the program have appropriate educational resources?
- Is there a committed group of faculty to train the residents?
- Is there an adequate breadth and depth of surgical cases to ensure proper training?
- Is there adequate supervision of residents?
- Are measures in place to promote resident well-being?

Verification of these processes occurs during regularly scheduled onsite visits by members of the RC-S.

This separation of tasks between program accreditation and individual certification is a unique feature of training in the U.S., which draws a "bright line" between these two processes. It is worthy of note that in Canada and other countries, these authorities are vested in a single organization (such as The Royal College of Physicians and Surgeons of Canada).

Historically, the decision to separate program accreditation from individual certification was made to avoid conflicts of interest and to create a separation and balance of responsibility. Clearly, these two pillars should work in concert to support the best interests of resident education. For example, if the ABS requires an "experience" in solid organ transplantation for certification candidates, the RC-S must require approved programs to provide the needed experience and confirm an approved training program is able to offer it. This system sustains the alignment between the two organizations, reflected in the fact that ABS certifies surgeons trained in ACGME-accredited programs, and the RC measures programs in part by their trainees' success rate in passing the board exams.

Likewise, if one group has case-volume requirements, both groups should be consistent in their printed documents. Similarly, milestones should incorporate the resources necessary for trainees to meet those milestones (an RC-S issue) and be aligned with the requirements to be eligible for board certification (an ABS issue).

Another example of collaboration between national organizations is the Surgical Council on Resident Education (SCORE) curriculum, which was created by extensive collaboration between the ABS, ACS, APDS, ASE, the American Surgical Association, and the Society of American Gastrointestinal and Endoscopic Surgeons, with extensive consultation with the RC-S as well. Through this collaborative approach, surgical education is served best.

The third component of the training triumvirate is the educational institution and its component hospitals. In addition, the program directors (PDs), their professional societies, and the institutional graduate medical education committees (GMEC) provide oversight at the local program level. While the ACGME accredits these institutions through the RC and assures the common program requirements are met, training experiences between institutions can vary greatly. The focused program goals can also run the spectrum from training surgeons for academic practice and basic research so to be ready for specialty fellowship training, to training general surgeons for practice in a particular local environment (for example, community or rural surgery practice). These different foci have led to variability in current programs. This manual will define the essential baseline that all programs should achieve.

The ultimate responsibility for creating a proper training environment rests with the residency PD, who may be the chair of the department of surgery; the hospital's chief of surgery in a nonuniversity setting; or a surgeon appointed by the institution. The RC authorizes the PD to conduct resident training and codifies the required experience. The RC requires that PDs have "authority and accountability for the overall program" and adequate time to address the administrative and educational needs of the program, which can vary widely from program to program. PDs' educational backgrounds and the duration of their appointments can vary. The position is best served by a skilled, experienced educator or a more junior faculty member mentored by an experienced educator. PDs model their influence based on the requirements put forth by the ABS and the RC and this manual will try to emphasize these salient elements. The PD and the program faculty must continuously reexamine the educational functions and the progress of each trainee to identify gaps where improvement can occur. Organizations, such as the APDS, provide important assistance for residency programs by creating new models for residency training, sharing best practices, disseminating knowledge, gathering expert consensus, and influencing training. Through these efforts, these groups catalyze change. A central feature of the ACS' role is to convene these participant groups for productive discussion that will facilitate this catalytic process.

PDs have ultimate responsibility for the residency program and the training process because they are charged with attesting that their residents are well trained and possess adequate knowledge and skills to sit for the certifying examination. This responsibility requires appropriate authority over the program so that requisite sign-off can be done with appropriate confidence. There also must be the opportunity to identify someone in trouble so that learning deficiencies can be identified and matched with appropriate improvement interventions. Trainees not on track to meet expectations are ideally identified early in their training and are either remediated or asked to leave the program and pursue other opportunities. ABS and RC requirements help guide and support the PD in their decisions to remediate or terminate a resident.

Several factors can contribute to the failures of identifying an unsuccessful residency matriculation process. These include a delayed realization of the resident needing remediation; fear of developing a poor reputation among potential recruits; unrealistically hoping the resident will be remediated by additional training; and even fear of legal reprisals. One specific goal of this resource manual is to specify the evaluation process requirements to ensure that the attestation process is authentic and uncompromised.

The Role of Professional Organizations

Among the organizations directly involved with residency training, the specialty professional organizations (such as, the ACS) play a unique and vital role in supporting residency training through developing and disseminating innovative education and training programs, convening the various parties involved with residency training, and providing ongoing improvement opportunities to surgeons in practice.

Historically, the ACS created initial hospital accreditation when surgical training was first offered and this effort led to the formation of The Joint Commission in 1951. The commitment of the ACS to ensure the provision of quality patient care has been the foundation of ongoing efforts focused on the education of surgeons during all phases of their careers. The opportunity to convene stakeholders, develop consensus, and create a comprehensive guide to the optimal resources required to train general surgeons was recognized as an effort that was a natural byproduct of this tradition. The ACGME develops and promotes general program requirements for institutions and specific requirements for the programs themselves. This manual will help to identify the necessary resources and strategies to meet these requirements.

The ability of ACS to fill this essential and unique role is based on its experience in improving surgical quality and education. Quality has been the hallmark of the ACS since its founding in 1913. Among the many ACS quality initiatives are the development of hospital standards and an accreditation process that eventually led not only to the creation of The Joint Commission but also to the provision of verification programs for cancer treatment centers and trauma centers by the Commission on Cancer and the Committee on Trauma, respectively. The ACS National Surgical Quality Improvement Program (ACS NSQIP®), which the ACS adapted from a successful Department of Veterans' Affairs Hospitals program and expanded to hundreds of other hospitals, is another example of an accreditation program with specific standards.

Educational resources available to support residency education in the ACS Division of Education include:

- ACS Fundamentals of Surgery Curriculum® (ACS FSC)
- *Selected Readings in General Surgery (SRGS®)*
- *SESAP® 17*
- Surgical Palliative Care Guide
- ACS Multimedia Atlas Volumes: Hernia, Colorectal, Pancreas, and Liver
- ACS Entering Resident Readiness Assessment (ACS ERRA)
- ACS/APDS Surgery Resident Skills Curriculum
- Fundamentals of Laparoscopic Surgery (FLS)
- Ultrasound for Surgeons: The Basic Course
- Preventing Errors and Near Misses in Surgery: Strategies for Individuals and Teams
- Communicating with Patients about Surgical Errors and Adverse Outcomes
- Disclosing Surgical Errors: Vignettes for Discussion
- *Ethical Issues in Surgical Care*
- Professionalism in Surgery: Challenges and Choices
- ACS/ASE Medical Student Simulation-Based Surgical Skills Curriculum
- ACS/ASE Medical Student Core Curriculum
- ACS/APDS/ASE Resident Prep Curriculum
- Optimizing Perioperative Pain Management: An Evidenced-Based Approach
- Evidence-Based Decisions in Surgery (EBDS)
- *ACS Case Reviews in Surgery*
- Clinical Congress Program
- ACS Surgery Resident Objective Structured Clinical Examination (OSCE)
- Residents as Teachers and Leaders (RATL)

To provide excellent patient care, the verification of hospital resources is also essential. Quality programs, however, do not suffice to ensure high-quality care; the most important element is a well-trained, qualified surgeon who is committed to high-quality surgical education as a foundation of quality care.

Comprehensive surgical care depends on a broad complement of skilled surgeons providing access to care throughout the country. Although specialists provide many of the services traditionally provided by general surgeons, much of the nation is without basic general surgical coverage.[9-12] This challenge is true not only for rural areas, but also for many nonrural locales.

Access to surgical care is a significant issue because of the shortage of general surgeons in many areas of our country. Workforce studies have demonstrated problems with access to general surgery in many parts of the country (data available at *www.facs.org/advocacy/federal/surgworkforce).* Few of our surgical organizations are poised to address this issue. The RC-S focuses on whether a surgical program provides appropriate training, but, overall, does not address the broad, evolving health care needs of the country. Similarly, the ABS decides the appropriateness of certifications but does not consider the type of practice surgeons enter. The ACS contributes to identify and address this deficiency.

The ACS aspires to be a convener and leader of and catalyst for discussions on surgical training. We have convened surgeon-training bodies since 2016 in an annual meeting with representatives from all boards, academies, and RCs to survey the training landscape and facilitate collaboration. In 2012, we convened a joint meeting with the ACGME and boards to develop strategies to better prepare residents for surgical practice.[13]

This resource manual is an effort to continue and intensify efforts to ensure that general surgeons are better prepared to enter practice by facilitating collaboration between the ABS, RC, and professional organizations. The goal of consensus amongst all stakeholders should be our aim to create consistency in graduate surgical education as the essential element of sound surgical quality.

Conclusion

Together, the ACS, ABS, and the RC for Surgery, along with other organizations with stakes in the development of resident education, can address these well-documented and significant problems in surgical education through shared oversight, responsibility, and decision-making. As part of that solution, this manual creates a common vision of the goals of surgical training and clarifies and improves the training process through broader and increased stakeholder engagement. If we are to continue to provide quality care for our patients, we can and must act together to better prepare surgeons.

References

1. Halsted WS. The training of the surgeon. *Bull Johns Hopkins Hosp*. 1904;15:267-275.
2. Grillo HC. Edward D. Churchill and the "rectangular" surgical residency. *Surgery*. 2004;136(5):947-952. doi:10.1016/j.surg.2004.09.02
3. Napolitano LM, Savarise M, Paramo JC, et al. Are general surgery residents ready to practice? A survey of the American College of Surgeons Board of Governors and Young Fellows Association. *J Am Coll Surg*. 2014;218(5):1063-1072.e31. doi:10.1016/j.jamcollsurg.2014.02.001
4. Snyder RA, Terhune KP, Williams DB. Are today's surgical residency graduates less competent or just more cautious? *JAMA Surg*. 2014;149(5):411-412. doi:10.1001/jamasurg.2013.3784
5. Mattar SG, Alseidi AA, Jones DB, et al. General surgery residency inadequately prepares trainees for fellowship: results of a survey of fellowship program directors. *Ann Surg*. 2013;258(3):440-449. doi:10.1097/SLA.0b013e3182a191ca
6. Jones AT, Kopp JP, Malangoni MA. Recertification exam performance in general surgery is associated with subsequent loss of license actions. *Ann Surg*. 2020;272(6):1020-1024. doi:10.1097/SLA.0000000000003330
7. Jones AT, Kopp JP, Malangoni MA. Association between maintaining certification in general surgery and loss-of-license actions. *JAMA*. 2018;320(11):1195-1196. doi:10.1001/jama.2018.9550
8. Kopp JP, Ibanez B, Jones AT, et al. Association between American Board of Surgery initial certification and risk of receiving severe disciplinary actions against medical licenses. *JAMA Surg*. 2020;155(5):e200093. doi:10.1001/jamasurg.2020.0093
9. Khubchandani JA, Shen C, Ayturk D, Kiefe CI, Santry HP. Disparities in access to emergency general surgery care in the United States. *Surgery*. 2018;163(2):243-250. doi:10.1016/j.surg.2017.07.026
10. Misercola B, Sihler K, Douglas M, Ranney S, Dreifus J. Transfer of acute care surgery patients in a rural state: a concerning trend. *J Surg Res*. 2016;206(1):168-174. doi:10.1016/j.jss.2016.06.090
11. Sheldon GF. Access to care and the surgeon shortage: American Surgical Association forum. *Ann Surg*. 2010;252(4):582-590. doi:10.1097/SLA.0b013e3181f886b6
12. Thompson MJ, Lynge DC, Larson EH, Tachawachira P, Hart LG. Characterizing the general surgery workforce in rural America. *Arch Surg*. 2005;140(1):74-79. doi:10.1001/archsurg.140.1.74
13. Sachdeva AK, Flynn TC, Brigham TP, et al. Interventions to address challenges associated with the transition from residency training to independent surgical practice. *Surgery*. 2014;155(5):867-882. doi:10.1016/j surg.2013.12.027

AMERICAN CO
SURGEONS A
OF SURGEON
COLLEGE OF
AMERICAN CO
SURGEONS A
OF SURGEON
COLLEGE OF
AMERICAN CO
SURGEONS A

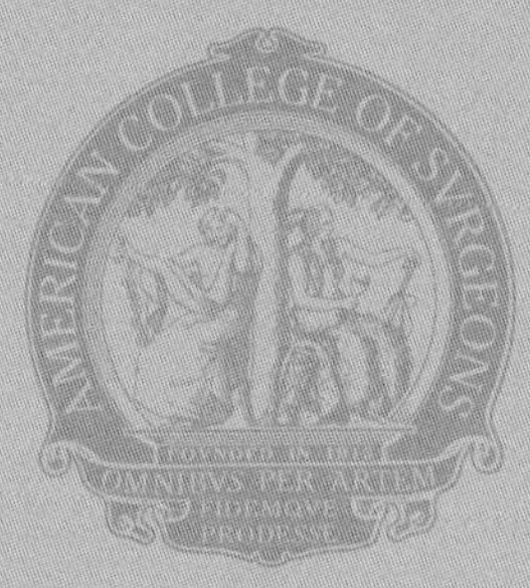

CHAPTER 2
Educational Underpinnings and Their Application to Surgery Resident Education

Lead Author
Ajit K. Sachdeva, MD, FACS, FRCSC, FSACME, MAMSE

Co-Authors
James R. Korndorffer, Jr., MD, MHPE, FACS, MAMSE
Roy Phitayakorn, MD, MHPE (MEd), FACS

CHAPTER 2

Educational Underpinnings and Their Application to Surgery Resident Education

Executive Summary

The underpinnings of a contemporary surgery residency training program should take into consideration the foundational educational principles of effective teaching and learning. As we evolve surgery residency training going forward, these foundational principles of teaching and learning should be considered and used in the design, implementation, and evaluation of the education and training programs.

Background

Surgery residency education is undergoing major transformation. The environment of surgical practice in which surgery residency training is embedded is constantly evolving as a result of the unprecedented pace of scientific advances, new technologies, and a sharp focus on outcomes of surgical care. These changes, as well as the ongoing advances in the science and practice of surgical education, continue to heavily influence the work of surgical educators. Residency training is a critical component of the continuum of professional development of surgeons, which spans decades—from the first day of medical school to the last day of surgical practice. During this career progression, many transitions need special attention.[1] These transitions are important because they may pose risks to the delivery of safe and effective patient care and create challenges for both surgeons and surgical trainees.

Longstanding concerns regarding the preparation of medical students for surgery residency training are corroborated by several research studies that have demonstrated major gaps in the clinical skills of entering surgery residents.[2] Also, the transitions from one level to the next during surgery residency training present many challenges that need to be addressed through a variety of interventions, including competency-based education and assessment, coupled with regular, specific feedback, to ensure that residents achieve the requisite levels of knowledge and skills. Furthermore, concerns regarding the preparation of residents for surgical practice are widespread and are supported by studies that have demonstrated gaps in the clinical, technical, and decision-making skills of surgeons entering practice.[3-5]

Members of the surgical faculty responsible for residency training face competing priorities resulting from the demands for increased revenue-producing clinical productivity and high expectations for ongoing scholarly contributions necessary to support their career advancement. In addition, surgeon educators at affiliated institutions who are not part of the full-time academic surgery departments need additional educational support and recognition to contribute effectively to surgery residency training.

Efforts to provide high-quality surgery residency training amid these challenges require novel approaches based on the underpinnings of educational theory and practice. Continuous improvement in the quality of surgery training necessitates evaluation of the outcomes of educational programs and introduction of further changes based on these data. This chapter outlines the educational underpinnings on which specific interventions should be built to achieve optimal outcomes.

Educational Framework

Surgical curricula, as well as surgery education and training programs, need to adopt a standardized educational framework to design and implement effective programs to address the specific needs of the learners. A widely accepted framework for this purpose includes the following six steps.[6]

- *Step One:* The first step involves identification of problems and assessment of the current needs in health care and the overarching needs of the learners. The educational program being planned should address the gap between where learners need to be and where they are in their development.

- *Step Two:* The second step involves targeted needs assessments of the groups of learners and their local environments and is accomplished through a number of strategies. These include thorough review of the pertinent literature, feedback from the performance assessments of previous learners who participated in the educational program, faculty expertise, and local resources. A comprehensive needs assessment plays an important role in motivating adult learners to pursue education and training by demonstrating the gap between the desired and existing levels of knowledge and performance. The needs assessment also sets the stage for the definition of clear goals and objectives for the education program. Recently, there has been a major change in the focus of education from the broad needs of groups of learners to the specific needs of individuals. This provides surgical educators unique opportunities for innovation.
- *Step Three:* The third step involves the definition of the broad goals of the educational program along with specific, measurable objectives. The objectives may focus on a range of competencies, including cognitive skills, technical skills, and other competency domains. The objectives, which need to be clear and actionable, are the basis of developing the educational content, selecting the learning methods, assessing the learners, and evaluating the effectiveness of the program. A useful anchor for the objectives is the American Board of Medical Specialties/ Accreditation Council for Graduate Medical Education (ABMS/ACGME) Competency Framework, which includes the six core competencies of medical and surgical knowledge, patient care and procedural skills, professionalism, interpersonal and communication skills, practice-based learning and improvement, and systems-based practice.[7,8]
- *Step Four:* The fourth step involves development and adoption of the curriculum and use of specific educational methods that will help to achieve the desired outcomes.
- *Step Five:* The fifth step involves development of strategies and approaches to successfully implement the educational program and to address any barriers. The methods used to implement the program should be rooted in sound educational theories and constructs. Appropriate resources needed to implement the program should be identified and provided to surgical educators. Faculty members need to be offered ongoing training in both contemporary teaching and assessment methods through targeted faculty development efforts. An effective faculty development program should use experiential learning, provide specific feedback, stress peer and collegial relationships, adhere to principles of contemporary education, and use diverse educational methods.[9] Faculty development programs should also take into consideration the role of context, impact of motivation and experience, value of extended programs, and use of peer coaching and mentorship.[9] The department and institutional leaders should visibly recognize and tangibly support faculty in their efforts to provide the best education to residents.
- *Step Six:* The sixth step involves the assessments of learners and the provision of specific feedback to the learners based on the results. The assessments may be formative or summative. Also, the effectiveness and outcomes of the educational program must be evaluated through various strategies. The training program should be evaluated using methods that go beyond soliciting feedback from the learners, and should focus on the outcomes of learning, changes in behaviors, and ultimately improvement in patient outcomes.

The aforementioned educational development model must be considered within the context of the local systems, resources, and available expertise. National curricula developed by professional organizations based on consensus among experts can play a significant role in supporting the efforts of surgical educators. Such curricula could be used as developed or modified based on the unique needs of the individual residency programs and the available resources.

Educational Theories and Constructs

Learning may be defined as the process of acquiring new knowledge that results in the desired change. Learning theories, which are the underpinnings of all medical education, rely on research in education and help educators to better comprehend how learners learn. Learning theories stem from the social sciences rather than the natural sciences; consequently, they provide a set of organized principles rather than descriptions of natural laws that are universally applicable.

In addition, it is important to recognize that instead of one foundation, learning theories form many small foundations that can be interconnected to create a composite of thought and meaning. In general, these learning theories differ from each other in their view of how learning occurs and which factors influence learning along with knowledge retention and transfer.[10] A construct to better conceptualize these foundations is provided below, but there are many other equally valid and reliable ways to connect the learning theories. Surgical educators should use these theoretical constructs in designing education and training programs that effectively address learners' needs.

Cognitive Learning Theories

Cognitive learning theories, which posit that learning is an active process, focus on how learners discover and use new knowledge effectively. Instead of focusing on learner behaviors, cognitive learning theories focus on how the brain absorbs, processes, and stores information, and then retrieves it when needed at a future time. Central to these learning theories is the belief, as outlined by Jean Piaget, PhD, that the brain grows and develops in discrete stages. A variety of contemporary learning principles relating to desired difficulty, the testing effect, and forced retrieval, originate from cognitive learning theories.

Educators using cognitive learning theories typically view learning as a discrete change in the overall state of knowledge. Therefore, the instructional sessions may focus on pretest to posttest changes, repetition of units of work, and demonstrations or rehearsals. Also, major focus is placed on methods to support memory through advanced organizers, mnemonics, analogies, and decisional algorithms. Feedback, which is important to ensure that the correct memory linkages are formed, may be as simple as right or wrong. Knowledge transfer is enhanced by optimally processing or chunking large amounts of learned information.

For example, suppose that Dr. C. McBurney is teaching a review session on acute appendicitis to entering surgery residents. Using a cognitive approach, she may start the session with a quick pretest to see how much the residents remember about appendicitis from their medical student years. Based on these results, Dr. McBurney may use the rest of the didactic time to discuss elements of the patient history, physical examination, and laboratory findings that are classic for appendicitis, as well as the atypical presentation and treatment of nonperforated and perforated appendicitis. Dr. McBurney may then use a posttest to see how much new knowledge the residents have acquired from the review session.

Behaviorist Learning Theories

Behaviorist learning theories posit that all learners are essentially sponges waiting to absorb knowledge through external passive mechanisms. The original behaviorist theory, developed by B.F. Skinner, PhD, argues that all learning occurs in response to either rewards or punishments.[11] Behaviorist learning theories are often used to better comprehend why learners exhibit behaviors that are either consistent with or seemingly opposed to effective learning strategies.

Educators using behaviorist learning theories typically view learning as a probable outcome that can be influenced by structuring the correct instructional sessions or stimuli. These sessions usually focus on measurable behavioral outcomes compared to a baseline, with an emphasis on learning basic concepts before moving to more advanced levels. Educators who use this approach also focus on methods to reinforce positive learning through feedback and tangible rewards. Feedback should be constructive to encourage behavioral changes, and knowledge transfer should be enhanced through the creation of positive learning environments.

Returning to the example above, suppose that Dr. McBurney would like to add in some behaviorist aspects to the review session on acute appendicitis. In this situation, Dr. McBurney may ask the residents to take turns and demonstrate how they may change their standard history-taking and focus on assessing atypical pain in the patient with appendicitis. Next, she may ask the residents to demonstrate how they perform an appropriate physical examination on a mannequin within the context of atypical presentation of appendicitis. Effective feedback from Dr. McBurney would be important in improving the performance of the residents. Finally, Dr. McBurney may ask each learner to write down the orders needed to admit the patient from the emergency department and then the postoperative orders after the appendectomy.

Constructivist Learning Theories

Constructivist learning theories differ from cognitive and behaviorist schools of thought in that knowledge is seen as a relative, instead of an absolute, concept. At their philosophical core, cognitive behaviorists believe that the educator's role is to reproduce in the learner an accurate reflection of the body of knowledge; whereas, constructivists believe that each learner may construct a different meaning from the same sets of facts or knowledge based on their past experiences.

The two primary types of constructivist theories are cognitive constructivism and social constructivism. Cognitive constructivism focuses on the individual learner and grew from Dr. Piaget's work.[12] Modern interpretations of social constructivism are developed from the research of Lev Vygotsky, PhD, which emphasizes that community and cultural connections mediate the process of knowledge acquisition and retention.[13]

One example of a constructivist-based learning theory is experiential learning theory developed through the work of David Kolb, PhD.[14] Dr. Kolb posited that learning occurs through a four-stage cycle of concrete experience, reflective observation, abstract conceptualization, and active experimentation (Figure 1). New knowledge and behaviors are reinforced each time the learner progresses through all four stages. Acquisition of correct knowledge and skills requires feedback to the learner throughout the cycle.[15]

Another example of a constructivist-based learning theory is social cognitive theory (formerly known as social learning theory) pioneered by Albert Bandura, PhD.[16] Dr. Bandura believed that learning is a continuous and dynamic interplay between a learner's personal factors (values, goals, previous knowledge and experience, and motivations); the learning activities; and the learning environment (both in-person and virtual).

Figure 1. Kolb's experiential learning cycle

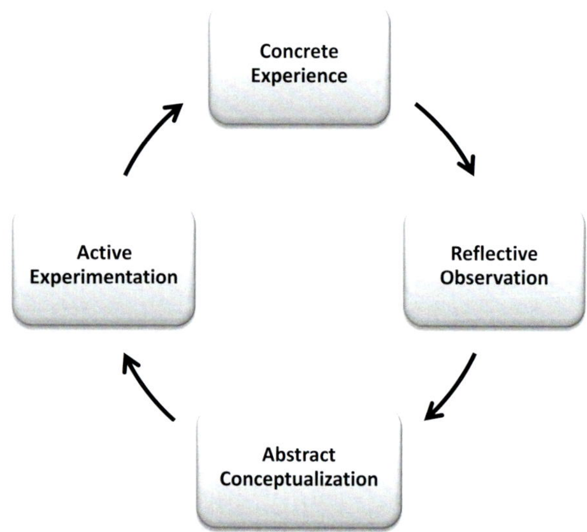

Figure 2. Maslow's hierarchy of needs

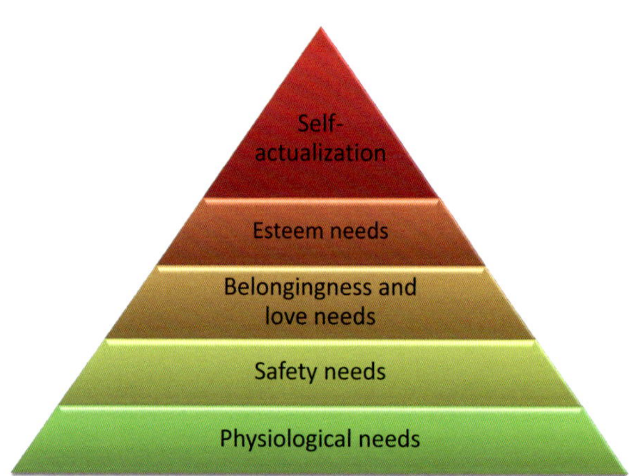

Central to social cognitive learning theory is helping learners discover and modulate their self-regulation and self-efficacy. Self-regulated learning stems from the self-directed learning theory which emphasizes personal autonomy, self-management in learning, independent learning, and learner control of instruction that catalyzes lifelong learning.[17] Constructive feedback is again needed for accurate self-efficacy and appropriate goal setting and attainment. Effective learner remediation strategies typically rely on aspects of self-regulated learning theory.[18,19]

Another example of constructivist learning theory is adult learning theory, which is more commonly referred to as adult learning principles, pioneered by Malcolm Knowles, PhD.[20] Dr. Knowles believed that learning occurred along a developmental continuum that evolved from pedagogical (how children learn) principles to andragogical (how adults learn) principles. This continuum does not necessarily correlate with the chronologic age of the learner, and may instead be more influenced by the learner's motivation and readiness to learn.

Abraham Maslow, PhD, developed the "hierarchy of needs," which argues that all humans have basic needs (physiological and safety); psychological needs (self-esteem, belonging, and love); and self-fulfillment needs (self-actualization) (Figure 2).[21]

Constructivist learning theory would argue that all learners strive for self-actualization and just require the right tools, coaching, and resources to set their own goals, objectives, and pathways. Therefore, to fully incorporate adult learning principles into teaching sessions, a surgical educator should take the following steps:

1. Establish a safe learning environment
2. Involve learners in determining their learning needs and planning their curriculum
3. Encourage learners to identify learning resources and pursue individualized learning plans
4. Teach learners approaches to self-assess their knowledge and skills

Educators who use constructivist learning theories view learning as situationally dependent; thus, to enhance learners' intrinsic motivation to learn, it is important to construct educational experiences that occur in realistic environments and feature authentic tasks that are within each individual's realm of experience. For example, educators could enhance a learner's memory by using multiple iterations of scenarios with learning goals and objectives that emphasize both the similarities and differences; this approach demonstrates to the learner the need for flexibility. Specific methods using this approach include apprenticeships, debates, and simulation. Importantly, successful constructivist learning sessions require the learner to have already mastered the basic cognitive and behavioral approaches.

In the example with Dr. McBurney, she may use constructivist learning theories to structure the didactic session at the simulation center to focus on a variety of patient cases that involve different presentations of acute appendicitis. This instructional method is best suited for residents who already know how to take a history, perform a physical examination, and interpret diagnostic tests. Instead, it focuses on the real-life nuances of distinguishing between the many possible sources of right lower quadrant abdominal pain. At the conclusion of the session, Dr. McBurney asks the residents to reflect on what they learned and how they would apply those lessons to the next patient they see with acute abdominal pain.

Mythological Learning Theory Concepts
No description of learning theories would be complete without also discussing approaches to learning that do not appear to be supported by evidence.

The first concept is the idea that effective teaching is both easy and natural in medical education. Effective teaching is a complex interaction between the teacher and the learner. Constructive teaching typically requires the same behaviors in the teachers as is expected of the learners, including a lifelong commitment to improving and adapting, and the use of role-modeling to effectively demonstrate discipline and self-regulation.

Another learning theory myth relates to the concept of learning styles, which argues that each individual learns differently and should be matched to a specific instructional modality. Numerous learning style inventories exist, including the Kolb Learning Style Inventory, VAK (visual, auditory, kinesthetic), and VARK (VAK + representational). Unfortunately, many of the constructs that underpin the learning styles assessment through these instruments are contradictory. Furthermore, the empirical evidence supporting the grouping of learners by learning styles is weak. Generally, the learning style of an individual appears to be situational at best and likely fluctuates depending on the learning tasks involved and the person's overall intrinsic and extrinsic motivation to learn.

Lastly, the idea that the learners just need an effective learning environment in which to teach themselves is unconfirmed in the medical education literature. On the contrary, learners tend to be inaccurate in their self-assessments of their knowledge gaps and often do not effectively manage their learning opportunities.[22] This mismatch is not the learners' fault, but rather a lack of mechanisms to assess their own learning or lack of experience to know what they do not know. Instead, given the expanding repertoire of medical and surgical knowledge and skills, now more than ever learners need effective educators to support their learning through well-planned and executed learning sessions.

Assessment and Evaluation

In addition to a solid comprehension of learning theories and constructs, surgical educators also must have appropriate command of current methods to assess learners and to evaluate educational programs. Although the terms assessment and evaluation are often used interchangeably, the two terms are different and must be used correctly.

Assessment focuses on the learners, whereas evaluation involves the measurement of the effectiveness of a curriculum or a learning plan. Assessment is a "systematic method of obtaining information used to draw inferences about characteristics of people," according to the *Standards for Educational and Psychological Testing,* created by the American Educational Research Association, American Psychological Association, and the National Council on Measurement in Education.[23] Because professionals make various assessments every day, assessments may seem simple and straightforward; however, meaningful assessments of health professions learners can be complex. Comprehending the educational underpinnings that create this complexity will help the surgical educator to conduct meaningful assessments.

Reasons for Complexity in Assessments
Is assessment difficult? Most individuals can identify an exceptional actor, athlete, or dancer, even if the assessor has no training in that specific domain, which would suggest that assessment is easy. Yet rigorous, evidence-based assessments needed to make important decisions are more complex. This complexity occurs in any of the assessment frameworks commonly used in medical education, including ABMS/ACGME Core Competencies, ACGME/American Board of Surgery (ABS) Milestones, or Entrustable Professional Activities. Comprehending the underpinnings of this complexity will help the educator use established assessment frameworks and build new ones.

The first domain of complexity relates to *the level of performance being assessed*, for which Miller's pyramid is a useful taxonomy.[24] The four levels of Miller's pyramid can assess whether the learner: *Knows* (can recall facts); *Knows How* (can apply the knowledge and understand high level concepts); *Shows How* (can display the trait of interest in an artificial environment); and *Does* (can perform in the real environment) (Figure 3).

Figure 3. Miller's pyramid

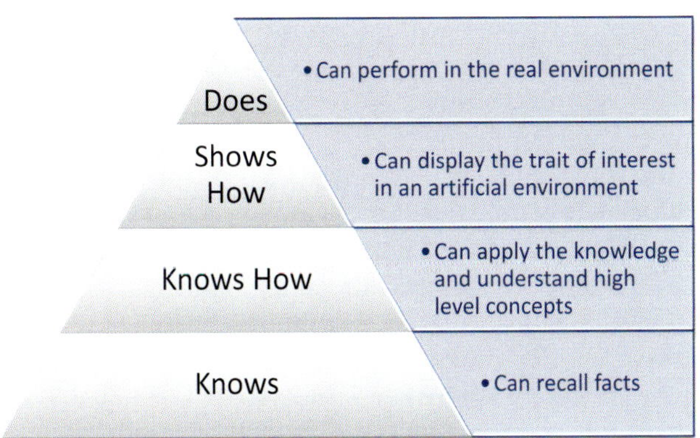

Using the core competencies as a framework, the assessment of medical knowledge can be relatively easy, as written tests can readily provide information about the learner's knowledge. Assessment of the other core competencies involves greater complexity. Assessment of patient care and technical skills should be conducted in workplace settings and in the simulation environment. A variety of structured assessment methods including Objective Structured Clinical Examinations (OSCE) and Objective Structured Assessment of Technical Skills (OSATS) can be very useful in this regard.

Assessments of interpersonal and communication skills and professionalism should be conducted in workplace settings and through simulation-based methods such as an OSCE. Assessment methods for these competencies must take into consideration certain nuances. For example, most learners know what appropriate professional conduct is, so it is of little value to establish at the *know* or *knows how* level. Even at the *shows how* level, most learners will conduct themselves appropriately in an artificial environment. Yet we know problems with professionalism exist in workplace environments, where assessments can yield valuable information to allow appropriate inferences to be drawn. In the workplace, certain questions need to be answered, such as: How will the assessment be conducted? What assessment methods are needed? Who will perform the assessment? and What is considered the appropriate level of skill? Just as multiple variables create complexity in a scientific experiment, the variables associated with assessments in workplace environments create complexity and must be controlled as much as possible for the assessments to be meaningful.

The second domain of complexity results from *variability in the data.* Despite well-established definitions, assessments sometimes are conducted with insufficient rigor, which creates variability in the data. In the aforementioned example relating to the assessment of professional behaviors in the workplace, variability results from the different levels of rigor needed for evidence of validity, how the assessment is performed, who performs the assessment, and the planned use of the assessment. Some common terms used with respect to the planned use of the assessment are formative and summative, which focus on the goal of the assessment, and low- and high-stakes, which focus on the consequences of the assessment. Formative assessment is helpful in providing feedback to the learners on how they are progressing toward the achievement of preestablished outcomes or objectives. Such assessment occurs during the course of learning and can provide information to the learner about what has been learned and what needs additional study. The principal goal of summative assessment is to serve as a final measure of how well learners have achieved the goals and objectives. A summative assessment typically occurs at the end of a course of study. Effective feedback is essential to improve knowledge and skills following formative assessment. Feedback may also be coupled with summative assessment; however, its role in this context is more limited. The "This Week in SCORE" quizzes and ABSITE are examples of formative assessments, whereas the ABS Qualifying and Certifying Examinations are summative assessments.

The planned use of the results of assessment may be in *low-stakes* or *high-stakes settings,* yet another domain of complexity. If the consequences of an unsatisfactory assessment result are less severe, it would be considered a low-stakes assessment. Many formative assessments are low stakes, as are assessments that may be performed repetitively with intervening education until a satisfactory result is achieved. High-stakes assessments have a major impact on the learner if the result is unsatisfactory. Surgical educators are familiar with such assessments as they are common throughout medical education – for example, the Medical College Admission Test (MCAT), United States Medical Licensing Examination (USMLE) Steps 1 and 2, and ABS Qualifying and Certifying Examinations. Poor performance may negatively impact the learner's career.

No matter what the planned use, the assessment needs to yield *valid and reliable results* if appropriate inferences are to be made about the learner's knowledge and skills. In the realm of assessment, validity refers to the accuracy of the assessment results, and reliability refers to the reproducibility of the results. Of note, validity and reliability relate to the results of the assessment and not the validity and reliability of the assessment method or tool. Assessment tools or tests are never summarily valid or invalid; rather, assessment results are evaluated for evidence of validity and this evidence needs to be based on the intended use of the results.[23, 25, 26] For example, assessment tools such as checklists, global ratings, and simulators are not valid by themselves. The results of the assessments must be evaluated and demonstrate evidence of validity, which is developed from multiple sources, as outlined below.

- *Evidence based on test content:* The assessment must evaluate the content of the domain of interest, which must be defined using an appropriate methodology. Examples of such evidence include the development of the blueprint of a written assessment by content experts or the determination of tasks relating to a procedure that will be assessed in a simulated environment.
- *Evidence based on response process:* This evidence focuses on the process of assessing the learner and may relate to the test itself, the instructions given, or even the method of scoring or development of composite scores. Any possible sources of error in the process must be minimized. Examples of such evidence include review of the assessment and scoring methods, and of strategies for implementation of the assessment.

- *Evidence based on internal structure:* This evidence focuses on the reproducibility or reliability of the assessment. With the currently accepted unitary theory of validity, reliability is not an entity unto itself but is a part of the validity evidence. Considering that any assessment results that lack evidence of reliability are considered invalid, folding reliability into the evidence for validity is appropriate. Evidence of validity requires sufficient reliability for it to be meaningful. If an assessment produces different results each time it is used, the results cannot be considered valid. An example of such evidence includes data from psychometric analysis of the reliability of the assessment method.
- *Evidence based on relationship to other variables:* This evidence is the most familiar to surgical educators. For example, a commonly used construct argues that individuals with greater experience perform better than those with lesser experience. Although this would be considered convergent evidence, discriminant evidence is equally important. Discriminant evidence would be provided by lack of correlation between an assessment result and some construct known to be distinct from the construct of interest. Examples of such evidence include comparison of the assessments of learners at two levels within the construct of interest, and comparing the results of the performance of a learner using the construct of interest with the results of the learner's performance using another assessment construct.
- *Evidence based on the consequences of testing:* This evidence most closely relates to the intended use of the assessment results, which should match the use and lead to more benefit than harm. For example, if the assessment of surgeons to become board certified was so difficult that very few became board certified, the individual learners and the general population would be harmed; however, if it were too easy, the general population could also be harmed. An example of such evidence includes data from appropriate standard setting used to make pass/fail decisions.

The level of evidence needed is directly related to the use of the results. For a low-stakes formative assessment, limited validity evidence may be needed other than to ensure the content is appropriate, the task is performed correctly, and no bad habits are learned. A much higher standard is necessary for summative and high-stakes assessments. High-stakes settings require stronger evidence from multiple sources. Content is still important, but so are reliability and evidence based on other variables. In addition, the process should be rigorous. To claim evidence based on a difference noted between experts and novices is a weak construct. For example, how much faith should you place in an assessment that can discriminate between a PhD mathematician and a second grader learning multiplication tables? Plenty if that is your goal, but none if the goal is to determine the mathematics class placement for two high school students of varying abilities.

The underpinnings of evidence of validity in assessment are important, including how the assessment is performed and who performs the assessment. How an assessment is performed can rely on objective, subjective, or "subjectively-objective" data. Each method is associated with evidence for, as well as threats to, validity.

Few surgical assessments are truly objective. For example, measurement of defined factors, such as number of procedures, time required to perform the procedures, and similar variables, have limitations. Case logs allow learners to record the number and type of cases being performed. Perceived competence and expected outcomes of practicing physicians often are based on how many cases they have performed. For example, becoming a Center of Excellence for bariatric surgery requires that the individual surgeons at the center must have performed at least 50 bariatric procedures. Many studies in cardiac, vascular, and pancreatic surgery suggest that high-volume centers have better outcomes, thereby equating volume with competence. However, limited evidence of validity exists for use of numbers in assessing the competence of individual surgeons, as some may require more procedures to acquire competence than others. Also, the critical number of procedures to demonstrate competence may be different for each learner based on the types of cases. A learner facile with laparoscopic surgery may need few cases for competence in laparoscopy when compared with the peers but may require more vascular surgery cases than the peers to achieve the same level of competence in vascular surgery. Therefore, case logs show that the learner has had adequate opportunities to develop competence but are not a reliable method of assessing individual competence.

Subjective assessments also are common. Often a single question is asked on an end-of-rotation questionnaire that requires the rater to assess the learner's overall operative ability. Similarly, for recredentialing of practicing surgeons, a single question may be the only item used in the assessment. Many issues such as bias are present when such broad-based assessments are used, many of them resulting from the raters. The issues include ratings based on general impressions and not on assessments of specific competencies, failure to recall details, and inflation of assessments through reporting of the good results more frequently than the bad.[27] Again, these inconsistencies result in threats to evidence of validity.

A variety of tools have been developed to minimize the threat to validity and to add some objectivity to subjective assessments. For example, specific criteria may be added to assessments of performance through direct observations.

Such assessments may be considered subjectively-objective. These assessments can be broadly divided into global ratings or procedure-specific ratings tools, such as checklists. Each method has its own evidence for and threats to validity. To study global ratings across a range of cases, Doyle and colleagues used a global rating scale based on the OSATS and the Global Operative Assessment of Laparoscopic Skills (GOALS) to assess residents at multiple levels on 15 different general surgical procedures. Scores improved with increasing resident years, demonstrating evidence of validity, and when the results of a resident's performance were assessed over time, the scores were similar, also yielding evidence of reliability.[28]

The other option is to use a procedure-specific checklist during the assessment. The evidence of validity for checklist-based assessments varies. Regehr and colleagues reported that in the simulated environment of an OSCE, global rating scales were superior to checklists especially when completed by experts.[29] Vassilou and colleagues demonstrated similar results within the context of laparoscopic cholecystectomy, comparing a global rating scale (GOALS) to a procedure-specific checklist; the checklist had an inferior interrater reliability and the checklist scores were not significantly different between novice and expert surgeons.[30] Other researchers have demonstrated much better validity and reliability evidence for procedure-specific checklists. Beard and colleagues compared a 30-point task-specific checklist to a generic global rating scale used to assess operative competence during carotid endarterectomy, and noted that both the checklist and the global rating scale differentiated between two groups (trainees and practicing surgeons), which provided some evidence that both methods yield valid results.[31]

The final area of complexity in assessment relates to determining performance at the satisfactory level based on defined standards. Specific standard-setting methods are beyond the scope of this chapter, but the overarching concept of normative-referenced and criterion-referenced standards is an educational underpinning that significantly affects assessment. Normative-referenced passing standards are based on comparing an individual's assessment results with those of the rest of the cohort being assessed, whereas criterion-referenced standards are based on a predetermined level that remains unchanged based on the performance of the group assessed. Either method creates challenges and complexities. Using the ACGME/ABMS core competencies as an example, standards could be established with either method. Again, medical and surgical knowledge can be reasonably assessed either way. A test blueprint can be developed requiring that all information should be known, using a criterion-referenced standard; however, it is difficult to apply this model and cover a large breadth of topics. A normative-referenced approach is most often used in these situations.

In assessments of other core competencies, using either approach can become more complex. For example, one would expect all learners to behave professionally at a set level, so to fail a certain percentage as required in a normative-referenced method seems arbitrary; yet, establishing the criteria for this competency could also appear arbitrary, as it raises the question of what criteria should be used. Must the learner act professionally 70 percent or 100 percent of the time? One may be too lenient and the other too challenging, though an admirable goal.

With the desire to move toward competency-based education, criterion-referenced assessment appears to be advantageous, but this approach still creates challenges. For example, criterion-referenced assessment and entrustable professional activities would appear an ideal match in that the learner is entrusted once the individual has met the preestablished criteria. But again, this approach creates complexity by requiring a determination of the entrustable activities that could encompass the entire domain of surgery, designing the criteria for each activity, and determining if all or a percentage of the chosen activities must be performed at the entrustment level.

Program evaluations also need to be conducted with sufficient rigor to provide meaningful data that are actionable. Information from such evaluations is critical to determining the effectiveness of the educational program and in making requisite changes based on this information. The Kirkpatrick Model is used widely for the purpose of program evaluation and includes four levels (Figure 4).[32] Level 1 focuses on the reaction of the learners and includes subjective feedback about the program and its relevance to the learners' needs. Level 2 focuses on learning and objectively addresses whether the learners have acquired the requisite levels of knowledge, skills, or other competencies. Level 3 focuses on behavioral changes, and addresses the application of the knowledge or skills learned to the real environments. This requires objective measurements of carefully selected variables to assure the accuracy of the evaluation. Level 4 focuses on results and addresses the outcomes of the educational program in real settings.

Figure 4. Kirkpatrick model

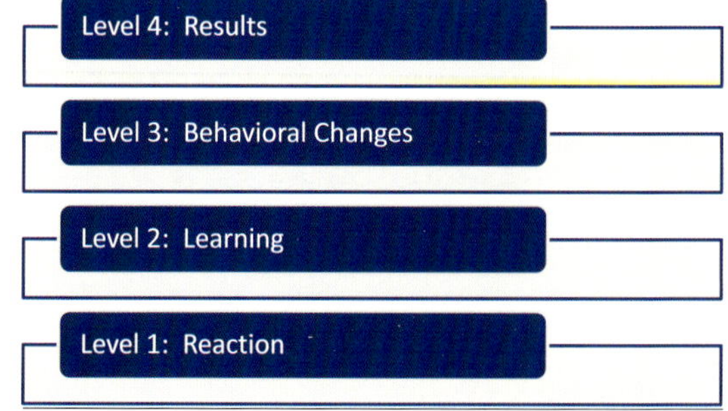

Numerous confounding variables in various environments of surgical care make it difficult to infer causality and to link patient care outcomes to an educational program, especially when participation in the educational program and the assessment of performance and outcomes in real environments are widely separated in time.

The educational theories and constructs, and the principles of assessment and evaluation articulated above should form the basis for effective education and training programs. The ACS Division of Education has used these underpinnings to create innovative programs that are establishing new benchmarks.

Innovative ACS Division of Education Programs that Address Surgery Resident Education

Since the ACS Division of Education was established in 2001, a spectrum of innovative education and training programs have been developed and launched, founded on educational underpinnings, including theories, constructs, and principles articulated previously in this chapter. Many of these programs are based on the use of simulation. Simulation-based education programs include the use of sound educational underpinnings to address various competencies and incorporate deliberate practice and mastery learning in competency-based models.[33] Simulation-based education can address the competencies of cognitive skills, patient care skills, procedural skills, interpersonal and communication skills, and professionalism. The innovative programs of the Division of Education encompass the continuum of surgical careers from the early years of training through the duration of surgical practice and focus specifically on the transitions from one level to the next during this progression.

Innovative Curricula

The ACS Division of Education has addressed the important transition from medical school to surgery residency through the following innovative programs that are based on sound educational underpinnings:

- A modular curriculum, developed in collaboration with the Association of Program Directors in Surgery (APDS) and the Association for Surgical Education (ASE), is aimed at preparing fourth-year medical students for surgery residency training. This ACS/APDS/ASE Resident Prep Curriculum ("Boot Camp") includes 45 peer-reviewed modules that focus on clinical, procedural, and non-technical skills, and 23 of these modules have been designated as essential by the experts involved with the development of the curriculum.
- The ACS Fundamentals of Surgery Curriculum® (ACS FSC) addresses the cognitive and decision-making skills of entering surgery residents through novel case-based simulations. The program has established a new standard in cognitive simulation-based surgical education. ACS FSC addresses 14 domains through 108 peer-reviewed case scenarios. Low-stakes, formative assessments are built into the program and allow the faculty to share valuable feedback with the residents about their strengths and gaps in cognitive skills. Advanced cases that involve the use of a similar simulation-based education model are currently being developed for the more senior residents. ACS FSC is designed to anticipate clinical scenarios that entering surgery residents will encounter in clinical settings and prepare them to anticipate these situations, think through them critically, and approach them with a degree of confidence and safety that is essential for delivery of optimal patient care.
- The ACS Surgery Resident Objective Structured Clinical Examination (ACS OSCE) includes 10 OSCE stations that are aimed at promoting patient safety and involve the use of standardized patients. The program, which includes a robust assessment model with excellent evidence of validity, is designed to assess the clinical skills of entering surgery residents and provides the opportunity to share constructive feedback to improve resident performance.[34]
- The ACS Entering Resident Readiness Assessment (ACS ERRA) program is a rigorous assessment program that uses a key features approach to focus on the cognitive, decision-making, and patient management skills of entering surgery residents.[35] The key features approach used in this innovative program yields high reliability with relatively short testing times. Results from ACS ERRA are shared with the respective program directors and their residents, with the goal of developing individualized learning plans to address the gaps identified. ACS ERRA includes 140 critical decisions in 40 cases within 20 topics across 10 clinical domains. Advanced modules that involve the key features approach are currently being developed for senior-level residents.
- The ACS/APDS Surgery Resident Skills Curriculum addresses the technical skills of surgery residents and is composed of three sets of modules: The 16 Phase I Modules address basic tasks and skills and are aimed at entering surgery residents; the 15 Phase II Modules focus on complete procedures and may be used to assess the technical skills of residents during various years of surgery training; and the 10 Phase III Modules focus on teamwork skills. The ACS/APDS Surgery Resident Skills Curriculum is designed to yield formative assessment data that may be used to address performance gaps. These three sets of modules may be integrated into a residency program to create a foundational curriculum and can help program directors organize the designated training time.
- ACS Objective Assessment of Skills in Surgery (ACS OASIS) is a novel program that involves rigorous assessments of technical skills of surgery residents at two levels, using a multi-station format. The modules for the second-year residents are currently being pilot-tested and development of the modules for the fourth-year surgery residents has commenced.

In addition, the ACS Division of Education has created novel e-learning programs to address the other competencies, including interpersonal and communication skills, professionalism, and patient safety.

Innovative Network of Simulation Centers

In 2005, the ACS Division of Education launched the program for accreditation of simulation centers based on specific standards and criteria.[36] These accredited simulation centers are called ACS-accredited Education Institutes (ACS-AEIs). The ACS-AEIs are accredited at two levels – Comprehensive and Focused.

- The Comprehensive ACS-AEIs are multidisciplinary and are engaged in advancing the field of simulation-based education through innovation and cutting-edge scholarship. They serve as valuable organizational resources to promote patient safety and as sites for training future leaders in the domain of simulation-based surgical education. The requirements for space, facilities, and personnel are more stringent for the Comprehensive ACS-AEIs as compared to the Focused ACS-AEIs.
- The Focused ACS-AEIs generally serve a single group of learners and are more limited in their scope of activities.

The ACS-AEIs offer unique education and training opportunities to residents. In 2020, the total number of ACS-AEIs was 98. A Consortium of these ACS-AEIs has been created to pursue cutting-edge activities, share valuable information, cross-fertilize ideas across the Consortium, and collaboratively advance the field of simulation-based surgical education.

Innovative Faculty Development Programs

Faculty development is essential in designing standard-setting education programs that result in a major positive impact on residency training. Faculty development remains a major focus of the ACS Division of Education and includes several innovative programs that are establishing new national and international benchmarks. The faculty development efforts are aimed at surgeon educators as well as non-surgeon surgical educators. The specific programs of the division in the domain of faculty development are described below.

- The ACS Surgeons as Educators Course, now in its 28th year, is the flagship of all faculty development programs aimed at surgeon educators. The course is comprehensive and covers the breadth of surgical education through effective and interactive modules. Immersive methods are used throughout the course and are founded on the educational underpinnings articulated in this chapter. The ACS Surgeons as Educators Course has had a profound positive impact on the careers of many surgeon educators who have, in turn, served as mentors for other surgeon educators and have made major contributions to advance surgical education.
- The novel ACS Certificate Program in Applied Surgical Education Leadership (CASEL) is for surgeon educators who want to pursue an advanced program after they have successfully completed specific faculty development courses, such as the ACS Surgeons as Educators Course, and possess sufficient surgical education experience. The modules of CASEL are delivered over a period of time and address important topics aimed at developing future leaders in surgical education. A key component of CASEL is a requirement to design and implement a novel surgical education project at their home institutions under the guidance of mentors who are selected from a pool of nationally renowned surgical educators. The mentors guide the progress of the CASEL participants during the year-long program and monitor their progress along with the CASEL faculty and ACS senior staff. The participants are supported in their professional work throughout the year and the effort culminates in the presentation of a final report on the project the following year. Satisfactory completion of the project and presentation of the final report are requirements for award of the Certificate of Completion for CASEL.

The ACS Academy of Master Surgeon Educators™

The ACS Academy of Master Surgeon Educators is an innovative program that was created by the ACS Division of Education in 2017 to recognize and engage master surgeon educators from across the surgical specialties and create a vibrant academy to innovate and elevate surgical education to the next level. The activities include identifying far-reaching surgical education opportunities, significantly advancing surgical education through cutting-edge scholarship, and providing mentorship to the junior surgeon educators. Individuals apply for membership in one of three categories: Member, Associate Member, and Affiliate Member. The Members must meet stringent admission criteria through demonstration of career-long landmark contributions to surgical education and must meet the high standards and criteria for admission. Associate Members must have made noteworthy contributions to surgical education and demonstrated their commitment to advancing this field. They must meet the standards and criteria for this category of membership. Both Members and Associate Members must be Fellows of ACS. Affiliate Members are non-surgeons who support the goals of the Academy. Individuals are selected for membership in all three categories through a process of stringent peer review and are inducted into the Academy annually. In 2020, the total membership of the Academy was 223 and growing.

During the early stages of the Coronavirus Disease 2019 (COVID-19) pandemic, the Academy embarked on an ambitious project to address the pandemic-related challenges and opportunities, and to transform surgery residency training for the future. This monumental effort has resulted in collection of data on the pandemic's impact on surgery residency training, development of novel educational methods, and dissemination of valuable information nationally and internationally. Transformational changes in surgery residency programs resulting from these endeavors will continue to be a foundation for innovation long after the pandemic. The Academy is also creating a disaster plan for surgery residency training to address national, regional, or local crises that may affect surgery residency training in the future. The Academy's programs and projects are founded on the sound educational underpinnings articulated in this chapter.

Tables 1 and 2 highlight the innovative programs of the ACS Division of Education and provide information on the target audience and the principal goals of each program.

There are many other programs developed by the ACS Division of Education and other entities that may be used to complement the teaching programs for residents. These can be found at *facs.org/education/division-of-education.*

Table 1. Critical ACS Division of Education programs for residents based on sound educational underpinnings

Title of ACS Program or Product	Target Audience	Principal Goals of the Program
ACS/APDS/ASE Resident Prep Curriculum ("Boot Camp")	Fourth-year Medical Students preparing for surgery residency	To prepare medical students for entry into surgery residency training through a modular curriculum with essential and optional modules; heavy emphasis on the use of simulation.
ACS Fundamentals of Surgery Curriculum® (ACS FSC)	Entering Surgery Residents	To support the learning needs of residents in the domain of cognitive skills through standard-setting, innovative simulation-based cases.
ACS Surgery Resident Objective Structured Clinical Examination (ACS OSCE)	Entering Surgery Residents	To objectively assess with high reliability the clinical skills of residents to promote patient safety, and provide opportunities to share constructive feedback.
ACS Entering Resident Readiness Assessment (ACS ERRA)	Entering Surgery Residents	To rigorously assess cognitive, decision-making and patient management skills of residents with high reliability, using the innovative 'key features' approach. Allows benchmarking data to be shared with residency programs to create individual learning plans and address educational gaps.
ACS/APDS Surgery Resident Skills Curriculum	Surgery Residents	To teach and formatively assess technical skills of residents through three sets of modules that focus on: 1) basic skills, 2) complete procedures, 3) teamwork skills.
ACS Objective Assessment of Skills in Surgery (ACS OASIS)	PGY2 and PGY4 Surgery Residents	To rigorously assess essential technical skills of second- and fourth-year residents along with the opportunity to share feedback.
ACS-Accredited Education Institutes (Simulation Centers)	Practicing Surgeons, Surgery Residents, and Surgical Teams	To accredit and create a national network of simulation centers that offer state-of-the-art simulation-based training to various learners using standardized modules, objectively assess performance, and advance the field of simulation-based surgical education.

Table 2. ACS Division of Education programs based on sound educational underpinnings to support and recognize surgery faculty

Title of ACS Program	Target Audience	Principal Goal of the Program
ACS Surgeons as Educators Course	Surgeon Educators	To provide surgeon educators essential knowledge and skills in the theory and practice of state-of-the-art surgical education through interactive modules.
ACS Certificate Program in Applied Surgical Education Leadership (CASEL)	Advanced Surgeon Educators	To provide surgeon educators advanced educational content and to offer individualized, practical leadership experiences, that include completion of projects at the home institutions, leading to award of a certificate.
ACS Academy of Master Surgeon Educators™	Preeminent and Nationally and Internationally Renowned Surgeon Educators	To recognize preeminent surgeon educators based on rigorous standards and criteria, and engage them in pursuing innovative surgical education programs and advancing surgical education.

Conclusion

Residency training in surgery continues to evolve dramatically because of unprecedented changes in health care and monumental advances in surgical education. Novel educational approaches in residency training must address the core competencies through innovative programs that are founded on sound educational underpinnings, including well-established theories, constructs, and principles. This solid foundation is necessary to create and implement effective programs that continually improve residency training, patient care provided by residents, and patient outcomes. The ACS Division of Education remains steadfast in its commitment to developing new and innovative training programs that positively impact both surgery resident training and the care of surgery patients.

Acknowledgment

The authors would like to acknowledge the outstanding support of Linda K. Lupi, MBA, in the preparation of this book chapter.

References

1. Sachdeva AK, Blair PG, Lupi LK. Education and training to address specific needs during the career progression of surgeons. *Surg Clin N Am*. 2016;96(1):115-128.
2. Sachdeva AK, Loiacono LA, Amiel GE, Blair PG, Friedman M, Roslyn JJ. Variability in the clinical skills of residents entering training programs in surgery. *Surgery*. 1995;118(2):300-309.
3. Napolitano LM, Savarise M, Paramo JC, et al. Are general surgery residents ready to practice? A survey of the American College of Surgeons Board of Governors and Young Fellows Association. *J Am Coll Surg*. 2014;218(5):1063-1072.
4. Mattar SG, Alseidi AA, Jones DB, et al. General surgery residency inadequately prepares trainees for fellowship: results of a survey of fellowship program directors. *Ann Surg*. 2013;258(3):440-449.
5. Sachdeva AK, Flynn TC, Brigham TP, et al. Interventions to address challenges associated with the transition from residency training to independent surgical practice. *Surgery*. 2014;155(5):867-882.
6. Thomas PA, Kern DE, Hughes MT, Chen BY, eds. *Curriculum development for medical education: A six step approach*. Baltimore, MD: Johns Hopkins University Press, 2016.
7. American Board of Medical Specialties. Standards for the ABMS Program for Maintenance of Certification (MOC). January 15, 2014. https://www.abms.org/wp-content/uploads/2020/11/standards-for-the-abms-program-for-moc-final.pdf. Accessed February 4, 2021.
8. Eno C, Correa R, Stewart NH, et al. *ACGME milestones guidebook for residents and fellows*. 2020. https://www.acgme.org/Portals/0/PDFs/Milestones/MilestonesGuidebookforResidentsFellows.pdf. Accessed February 4, 2021.

9. Steinert Y, Mann K, Centeno A, Dolmans D, Spencer J, Gelula M, Prideaux D. A systematic review of faculty development initiatives designed to improve teaching effectiveness in medical education: BEME guide no. 8. *Med Teach.* 2006;28(6):497-526.
10. Schunk DH. *Learning theories: An educational perspective.* New York, NY: Macmillan, 1991.
11. Skinner BF. *About behaviorism.* New York, NY: Vintage Books, 1976.
12. Piaget J. The role of action in the development of thinking. In: Overton WF, Gallagher JM, eds. *Knowledge and development.* Boston, MA: Springer, 1977.
13. Vygotsky LS. *Mind in society: The development of higher psychological processes.* Cambridge, MA: Harvard University Press, 1978.
14. Kolb, DA. *Experiential learning: Experience as the source of learning and development.* Englewood Cliffs, NJ: Prentice-Hall, 1984.
15. Yardley S, Teunissen PW, Dornan T. Experiential learning: AMEE guide no. 63. *Med Teach.* 2012;34(2):e102-115.
16. Bandura A, Walters RH. *Social learning theory.* Oxford, England: Prentice-Hall, 1977.
17. Candy PC. *Self-direction in lifelong learning.* San Francisco, CA: Jossey-Bass, 1991.
18. Sandars J, Cleary TJ. Self-regulation theory: applications to medical education: AMEE guide no. 58. *Med Teach.* 2011;33(11):875-886.
19. Andrews MA, Kelly WF, DeZee KJ. Why does this learner perform poorly on tests? Using self-regulated learning theory to diagnose the problem and implement solutions. *Acad Med.* 2018;93(4):612-615.
20. Knowles MS, Holton RA III, Swanson RA. *The adult learner, 7th ed.* Burlington, MA: Elsevier, 2011.
21. Maslow AH. A theory of human motivation. *Psych Rev.* 1943;50(4):370-396.
22. Kirschner PA, Sweller J, Clark RE. Why minimal guidance during instruction does not work: an analysis of the failure of constructivist, discovery, problem-based, experiential, and inquiry-based teaching. *Ed Psych.* 2006;41(2):75-86.
23. American Educational Research Association, American Psychological Association, National Council on Measurement in Education, and Joint Committee on Standards for Educational and Psychological Testing. *Standards for educational and psychological testing.* Washington, DC: American Educational Research Association, 2014.
24. Miller GE. The assessment of clinical skills/competence/performance. *Acad Med.* 1990;65(9Suppl):S63-S67.
25. Messick S. Validity. In: Linn RL, ed. *Educational measurement, 3rd ed.* New York: American Council on Education/Macmillan, 1989:13-103.
26. Kane MT. Validation. In: Brennan RL, ed. *Educational measurement, 4th ed.* New York, NY: American Council on Education/Praeger Series on Higher Education, 2006:17-64.
27. Williams RG, Klamen DA, McGaghie WC. Cognitive, social and environmental sources of bias in clinical performance ratings. *Teach Learn Med.* 2003;15(4):270-292.
28. Doyle JD, Webber EM, Sidhu RS. A universal global rating scale for the evaluation of technical skills in the operating room. *Am J Surg.* 2007;193(5):551-555.
29. Regehr G, MacRae H, Reznick RK, Szalay D. Comparing the psychometric properties of checklists and global rating scales for assessing performance on an OSCE-format examination. *Acad Med.* 1998;73(9):993–997.
30. Vassilou MC, Feldman LS, Andrew CG, et al. A global assessment tool for the evaluation of intraoperative laparoscopic skills. *Am J Surg.* 2005;190(1):107-113.
31. Beard JD, Choksy S, Kahn S, Vascular Society of Great Britain and Ireland. Assessment of operative competence during carotid endarterectomy. *Br J Surg.* 2007;94(6):726-730.
32. Kirkpatrick DL, Kirkpatrick JD. *Evaluating training programs: The four levels, 3rd ed.* San Francisco, CA: Berrett-Koehler Publishers Inc., 2006.
33. Chauvin SW. Applying educational theory to simulation-based training and assessment in surgery. *Surg Clin N Am.* 2015;95:695-715.
34. Sudan R, Lynch TG, Risucci DA, Blair PG, Sachdeva AK. American College of Surgeons Resident Objective Structured Clinical Examination (ACS OSCE): a national program to assess clinical readiness of entering PGY-1 surgery residents. *Ann Surg.* 2014;260(1):65-71.
35. Sullivan ME, Park YS, Liscum K, Sachdeva AK, Blair PG, Gesbeck M, Bordage G. The American College of Surgeons Entering Resident Readiness Assessment program: development and national pilot testing results. *Ann Surg.* 2020;272:194-198.
36. Sachdeva AK, Pellegrini CA, Johnson KA. Support for simulation-based surgical education through American College of Surgeons-Accredited Education Institutes. *World J Surg.* 2008;32(2):196-207.

AMERICAN C
SURGEONS A
OF SURGEON
COLLEGE OF
AMERICAN C
SURGEONS A
OF SURGEON
COLLEGE OF
AMERICAN C
SURGEONS A

CHAPTER 3

On Optimal Oversight, Governance, and Management of Graduate Medical Education Programs in Surgery

Lead Author
E. Christopher Ellison, MD, FACS, MAMSE

Co-Authors
L.D. Britt, MD, MPH, DSc(Hon), FACS, FCCM, MAMSE, FRCSEng(Hon), FRCSEd(Hon), FWACS(Hon), FRCSI(Hon), FCS(SA)(Hon), FRCS(Glasg)(Hon)
Julie A. Freischlag, MD, FACS, FRCSEd(Hon), DFSVS, MAMSE
Amy N. Hildreth, MD, FACS
Benjamin T. Jarman, MD, FACS
Jeffrey B. Matthews, MD, FACS, MAMSE
John R. Potts III, MD, FACS, MAMSE
Linda R. Archer, PhD
Molly Brittain, MEd
Katherine L. Files, MBA
Mitchell C. Sokolosky, MD

CHAPTER 3

On Optimal Oversight, Governance, and Management of Graduate Medical Education Programs in Surgery

Common acronyms and their meanings

Acronym	Meaning
AAES	American Association of Endocrine Surgeons
AAMC	Association of American Medical Colleges
ABMS	American Board of Medical Specialties
ABS	American Board of Surgery
ACGME	Accreditation Council for Graduate Medical Education
ACS	American College of Surgeons
AEI	Accredited Education Institutes
AMSE	Academy of Master Surgeon Educators™
AOA	American Osteopathic Association
APDS	Association of Program Directors in Surgery
ASE	Association for Surgical Education
CCC	Clinical Competency Committee
CEO	Chief Executive Officer
CLER	Clinical Learning Environment Review
CMS	Centers for Medicare and Medicaid Services
COVID-19	Coronavirus Disease 2019
CPR	Common Program Requirements
DEI	Diversity, Equity, and Inclusion
DGME	Direct GME Payment
DIO	Designated Institutional Official
EPAs	Entrustable Professional Activities
ERAS	Electronic Residency Application Service
GME	Graduate Medical Education
GMEC	Graduate Medical Education Committee
HR	Human Resources
IME	Medicare Indirect Medical Education Payments
IR	Institutional Requirements
M&M	Morbidity and Mortality
NRMP	National Resident Matching Program
NSQIP	National Surgical Quality Improvement Program
OR	Operating Room
PD	Program Director
PEC	Program Evaluation Committee
PPE	Personal Protective Equipment
QA	Quality Assurance
QI	Quality Improvement
RC	Review Committee
SI	Sponsoring Institution
VA	Department of Veteran's Affairs

Executive Summary

This chapter reviews essential elements for successful management of a residency program in surgery, including the optimal oversight and governance of graduate medical education (GME) programs. Although the focus is on general surgery, common themes apply to all surgical residency programs. Through strong collaboration, the education leadership team of training programs will be better able to achieve the goal of training safe and competent surgeons who are prepared for independent practice.

This chapter answers the following questions:

1. What key components are necessary for the optimal management, oversight, and governance of a successful GME program in surgery?
2. What are the key elements of the Institutional Requirements (IR) and Common Program Requirements (CPR) established by the Accreditation Council for Graduate Medical Education (ACGME)?
3. What are the roles of the program director (PD), designated institutional official (DIO), department chair, and chief executive officer (CEO)?
4. How can programs best align and comply with external educational regulatory organizations?
5. What key institutional resources are needed and how can programs assure optimal support for residents and faculty?
6. What are the most effective strategies for leadership to develop resident autonomy while maintaining high-quality care and patient safety?

Key Elements for Optimal Oversight, Governance, and Management

Six elements are essential for the optimal management, oversight, and governance of the successful administration of GME surgery programs. These fundamentals are as follows:

- Understanding of and compliance with ACGME requirements
- A supportive and collaborative leadership team
- Adequate resource allocation
- Continuous program evaluation and prospective quality improvement (QI)
- Opportunities for assessment and feedback for trainees, faculty, and institutional leaders
- A culture that is conducive to education and training while also focused on QI and patient safety

Details regarding each of these components are discussed throughout this chapter.

The ACGME Institutional Requirements and Common Program Requirements

Surgical training is a complex system, which the ACGME regulates. Each ACGME-accredited local surgical program must function under the authority and oversight of an ACGME-accredited sponsoring institution (SI).[1]

The ACGME has both IR and CPR that each SI must meet to ensure that financial, educational, and clinical resources are available.[1, 2] The ACGME requirements specify the necessary resources, curriculum, and environment of an accreditable program, as well as the duties of the PD and faculty members. The ACGME also has specialty Review Committees (RC); for general surgery, it is the RC for Surgery. The RCs assess programs' compliance with ACGME IR and CPR.

Institutional Requirements

The ACGME looks at institutional commitment and governance for residency training programs. According to the ACGME requirements, each SI must have a written statement of the teaching hospital's commitment to GME, which must be submitted to the ACGME every five years.

This document must be signed by the DIO, the institution's senior management, and a representative of the SI's governing body. The DIO and GME Committee (GMEC) must have authority and responsibility for the oversight and administration of the SI's programs and responsibility for assuring compliance with ACGME CPR, specialty/subspecialty-specific program requirements, and IR (see Table 1 for role of DIO). The inclusion of a signatory from the SI's faculty governing body or medical staff administrative committee helps ensure that faculty are aware of and committed to the support of the GME programs. While the SI is responsible for providing appropriate resources, the institution's GMEC is responsible for oversight and compliance with the IR and provides oversight of resident/fellow stipends and fringe benefits.

Table 1. The role of the Designated Institutional Official

- Review of ACGME Program Information forms
- Participate in funding and position negotiations with affiliated hospitals
- Conduct educational workshops for programs
- Conduct mock site visits for programs
- Establish GME institutional policies
- Work with the GME Office on program and resident matters
- Meet as needed with PDs
- Meet with Residents/Fellows regarding GME concerns
- Attend Resident Council, House Staff, and Faculty Governance meetings

The ACGME IR also sets expectations for the optimal resources to support program administration, including protected time for the PD and program administrator, professional development for the PD and core faculty members, and other resources.[2]

Common Program Requirements

The ACGME considers its general requirements, which are found in its CPR, fundamental to GME. The CPR require that SIs ensure adequate resources for resident education and specify the resources that must be provided. Documentation of these resources is necessary to maintain accreditation and to support efforts to expand the complement of residents.

Among the CPR are six core competencies that residents are expected to develop before they enter surgical practice. These core competency areas are closely tied to the American Board of Surgery's (ABS) Continuous Certification program mandates and are as follows:

- Patient care
- Interpersonal and communication skills
- Medical knowledge
- Professionalism
- Practice-based learning
- Systems-based practice

ACGME Review Committees

The ACGME RCs assess the residency program and determine whether the program complies with ACGME requirements. The RCs develop and assess the requirements specific to individual specialties, which the ACGME publishes and updates.[3]

The RCs establish the maximum number of trainees for each ACGME-accredited program.[1,3] This approved complement is based on the program's capacity to meet the training requirements for each specialty. General surgery programs may admit no more residents/fellows than the approved complement without prior approval from the RC for Surgery. A decision to increase the number of trainees in a residency program is determined on the basis of available clinical resources, case numbers, and fellowships that may compete for these resources.

The RC assesses how well the program complies with the mandates by reviewing information supplied by the PD, residents, and faculty and submitted to the ACGME through annual reports and surveys administered to the residents and faculty members. The RC conducts periodic site visits (every 10 years), which consist of personal interviews and reviews of documents. All new program requirements and significantly altered existing program requirements that the ACGME or the RC propose are open to public comment.

The RCs also determine whether training programs have adequate resources to expand its complement of trainees. Determining whether a program has the necessary resources requires a detailed discussion in the residency program's education committee. The PD is responsible for leading this discussion. If resources are sufficient, the committee should prepare, approve, and submit a request to the SI's GMEC. If the GMEC approves and guarantees a funding source for resident salaries and benefits, the increase request should be submitted to the ACGME specialty RC through the Accreditation Data System available at *www.acgme.org/globalassets/pfassets/programresources/440_requests_for_changes_in_resident_complement.pdf*. Program expansion proposals occur at regularly scheduled meetings of the RC, which are listed under the "Meetings and Educational Activities" tab on the ACGME website at *www.acgme.org*. The PD and GMEC should provide a document describing the educational rationale for the requested increase, details on resources available, and evidence that the increase will not adversely affect the educational program.

The Institutional Leadership Team: Roles and Responsibilities

Leadership of a thriving surgical training program requires a team approach with dedicated leadership at several levels, including the PD, the DIO, and administrative leaders, such as the CEO.

The Program Director

The PD is critical to team success for many reasons—not the least of which is serving as the nexus between the residents and other members of the leadership team. The PD must work both within the framework of the requirements specified by the ACGME, as well as in harmony with the governing regulations of the SI and the clinical site(s) where the residents work.

The PD must be consistently visible and involved with faculty and leadership at the primary clinical site and affiliated sites that provide resident education and clinical experience. The PD should influence decisions that affect residency training at the primary and affiliated sites. This responsibility is accomplished through the PD and the core teaching faculty serving on hospital and medical staff committees, such as the credentials committee, operating room (OR) committee, QI committee, and medical records committee. The PD's role in decision-making should be codified in the written residency affiliation agreements of the primary and affiliated clinical teaching sites.

The DIO recommends appointment of the PD, which requires approval from the SI's GMEC. In addition, the PD must have the full support of the department chair(s) or chief(s) of surgery at the program's primary clinical site and affiliated sites. The PD acts with the support of the DIO and must comply with the policies of the SI.

To create and maintain a program that rises to the highest standards requires that the PD receive consistent and effective guidance from academic and SI leaders. The PD is responsible for ensuring that the daily administration and supervision of the residency program meets or exceeds ACGME standards. Academic and institutional leaders must provide learners with appropriate resources and support for an optimal educational experience. For an example of an organizational chart for surgical residency program oversight, see Figure 1.

The GMEC must approve a new PD, and the program's policies and procedures must adhere to the SI's policies. By participating in the GMEC, the PD enables the program to stay abreast of GME-related activities within the SI, the primary clinical site, and any affiliates. In addition, the PD can inform and influence GMEC actions. If the GMEC does not have a surgeon PD or a surgical resident member, the PD should monitor the committee's actions by attending meetings or reviewing the meeting minutes.

The Designated Institutional Official

Designated by the SI, the DIO is responsible for overseeing each of the SI's ACGME-accredited programs. In collaboration with the GMEC and the PD, the DIO ensures compliance with ACGME requirements. Together, the DIO and PD serve as program advocates to ensure the SI provides appropriate resources to ensure an optimal professional and learning environment.

Each SI must have a DIO with the authority to oversee and administer each of the SI's ACGME-accredited programs and a GMEC composed of the DIO, PD, at least two residents, and a QI or patient safety officer.[2] The DIO must review and approve information submitted by the program to the ACGME and the program's annual evaluation, action plan, and 10-year self-study.

The DIO facilitates collaborative relationships among the PD and the SI's CEO and the CEOs of affiliated clinical sites and ensures CEO(s) participate in leadership team activities as needed. As SI administrative leaders increasingly participate in graduate education, the DIO and PD must help CEOs understand residency program needs and align their guiding principles with the residency program's educational goals and the requirements of national governing bodies such as the ACGME.

Figure 1. Organizational chart for surgical residency program oversight (example)

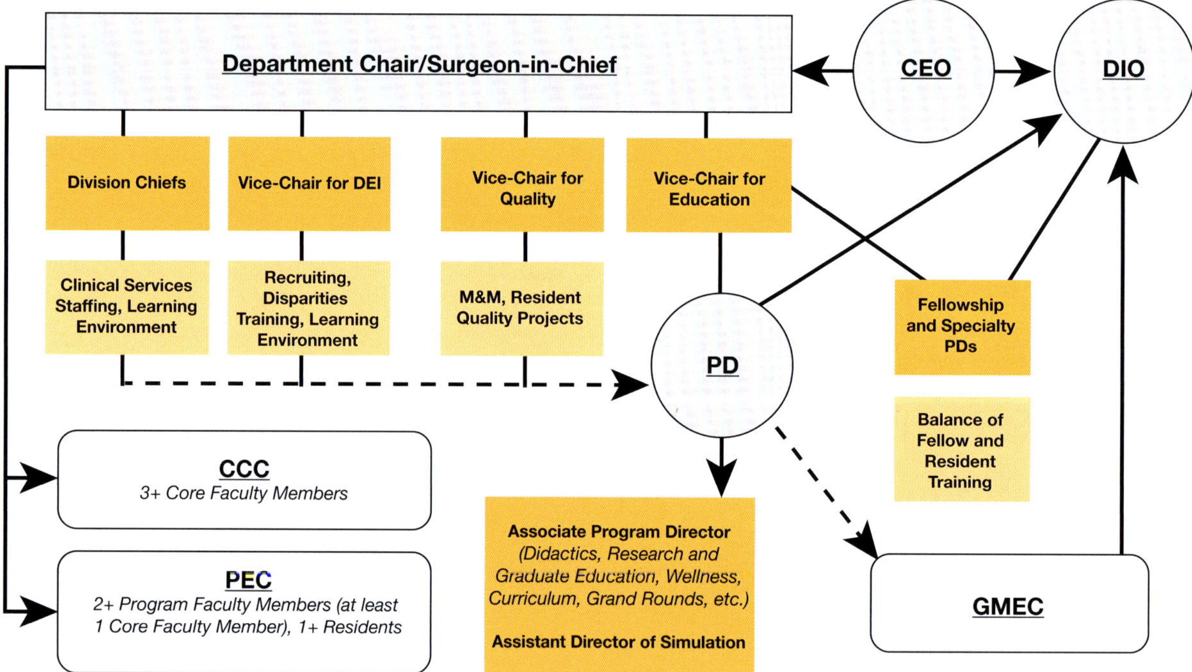

The DIO also helps the PD manage underperforming residents and disciplinary issues. In contrast to the PD, who may be closer to the resident, the DIO can provide an objective assessment and recommend learning opportunities to address challenges. The DIO also is involved in resident grievance and due process activities.

The DIO should know the institution's human resources (HR) policies and procedures and advise the PD dealing with professionalism and misconduct issues. The DIO educates SI personnel about a resident's simultaneous roles as employee and learner. If remediation is needed, the DIO may advocate for a remediation plan. For instance, the DIO can help determine if a professionalism issue is because of an academic deficiency that can be remediated or a misconduct issue that could result in dismissal. The DIO should work closely with the institution's legal team, especially if dismissal is under consideration.

The successful DIO plays a key role by responding quickly to resident concerns and improving the quality and timeliness of communication between residents and the administration, which raises morale, decreases anxiety, and allows residents to focus on education and patient care.

General Surgery Residency Program Designations

History. General surgery residency programs are categorized by a variety of labels by different organizations. There have been a multitude of changes and expectations in graduate medical education over the past 20 years which have rendered current program designations obsolete and consistency is needed. Residency programs are based in a variety of health care environments with variable amounts of undergraduate medical education, bench or clinical research, academic support, and clinical volume. Common to all programs are ACGME requirements for scholarly activity.

What is the big deal? Programs are commonly referred to as "academic" and "non-academic." Within the realm of surgery residency where all programs have accreditation standards to meet for scholarly activity – there are not "non-academic" programs and the term is offensive. "Community" is also utilized to describe programs – but there are substantial differences between a "community" hospital without structured education/research when compared to well established and resourced "community" hospitals that provide medical and surgical education.

Need for consistent designations. The consistent designation of programs serves to better understand program resources and learning environments. Program types are frequently utilized in surgery literature but they are not consistent and it is unclear how the terms used are generated and assigned to individual programs.

Current program designations

Association of Program Directors in Surgery

1. Independent
2. Military
3. University

American Board of Surgery (for research purposes only)

1. Independent
2. Military
3. University

Review Committee for Surgery

No specific distinction made

Association of American Medical Colleges - FREIDA

1. University-based
2. Community-based
3. Military-based
4. Community-based/University-based
5. Other
6. Osteopathic recognition/focus

"Independent" residency programs are located in medical centers that are independent of a medical school, or geographically distinct from an affiliated medical school. Faculty and residents in these programs pursue academic work and provide the most current, cutting edge surgical care. Education affiliation between independent programs and medical schools are common-place and depend on the nature of that affiliation – the term "hybrid" is sometimes used to describe them. Independent programs are characterized by a tendency to be smaller (average 3-5 residents per year), high operative volumes, research opportunities, and few, if any coexistent fellowship programs. Residents who graduate from independent programs successfully pursue general surgery practice or additional fellowship training.

"Military" programs are those programs affiliated with branches of the U.S. Armed Forces. Applicants are selected through prior military obligations such as the Reserved Officer Training Corps (ROTC) or Health Professions Scholarship Program (HPSP). These programs provide unique opportunities to serve military beneficiaries throughout the world. Residents who graduate from military programs successfully pursue general surgery practice or additional fellowship training.

"University" programs are academic centers where the primary hospital is also the primary clinical teaching site for an affiliated medical school. University hospitals are characterized by a tendency to be larger (average 5-7 residents per year), the presence of additional learners in surgical subspecialties and fellowships, high operative volumes, and support to pursue bench research or dedicated research time. Residents who graduate from university programs successfully pursue general surgery practice or additional fellowship training.

The Association of American Medical Colleges (AAMC) utilizes "community-based" instead of "independent" owing to the broad scope of medical students represented with highly variable accreditation requirements among different specialties of medicine. General surgery residency programs do not exist where there is not a higher level of academia to meet ACGME standards and the presence of focused and continuous education. There are "community" hospitals with limited structure for scholarly activity and without medical school affiliations, and general surgery residencies do not belong in this category.

PD Interaction with the Department Chair, DIO, and CEO
The surgery PD often asks the department chair or chief of surgery how to manage the teaching faculty. The DIO and the CEO also can provide essential support to the PD.

The DIO helps the program maintain accreditation and compliance with ACGME requirements and helps the PD establish policies related to resident performance issues. Up to one-third of surgery residents require remediation at some point.[4] A well-defined pathway is essential to effective remediation and contributes to the success of these residents.

In addition, the PD must have resources to draw upon when a resident is unresponsive to remediation. Establishing shared and consistent definitions of remediation processes is important to enable training programs to achieve ACGME goals, hold the medical profession accountable, and engender the public trust. The remediation process varies across training programs due, in part, to the lack of standardized definitions for terms such as *good standing, remediation, probation,* and *termination.*[5] Hence, the DIO should work with the PDs and GMEC to establish uniform definitions and processes. Clear guidance for handling interventions through coaching, remediation, and dismissal should be established across the institution, including when the PD should involve the DIO and other leaders.

CEO support is also critical to the success of GME programs. Although not specifically outlined in ACGME requirements, the CEO must ensure the SI's culture prioritizes and supports education and training across all GME programs. For example, a teaching hospital's CEO should provide resources to address safety and personnel issues in the residency program.

The PD must ensure that the residency program fits the educational culture the CEO has established. The CEO also must provide resources and financial support to retain resilient and engaged faculty and learners and to maintain adequate case volumes for residents. The CEO's support is essential if residency programs are to have adequate funding. Meeting many new ACGME requirements will require increased investment from the SI.

In addition to space, facilities, and equipment, optimal GME requires financial support and staff resources. Establishing and increasing this support, as necessary, requires open and honest discussions within the SI that include the DIO, PD, the department chair or chief of surgery, hospital representatives, and occasionally the CEO.

The DIO and PD must have clearly identified funding sources for salary, benefits, and support for academic growth for the PD and associate and assistant PDs. This funding should be allocated in proportion to the "percent effort" required to administer the residency and specified by the specialty's ACGME RC. In addition, the SI's education budget for the offices of the DIO, PD, and other necessary staff must be clearly identified and include the full spectrum of necessary resources, including faculty time, staffing, equipment, space, and other items specified in the ACGME IR.

Leadership in Crisis
The Coronavirus Disease 2019 (COVID-19) pandemic has highlighted the importance of effective clinical and educational leadership during a crisis. Both the DIO and CEO should play leadership roles during a crisis, providing essential support to the PDs. CEOs should:

- Provide adequate personal protective equipment (PPE)
- Work with the PDs to quickly establish a safe learning environment and support the transition to distance learning and telehealth
- Proactively develop policies about patient care, PPE, and visitation to protect the safety of residents, patients, faculty, students, staff, visitors, and the institution
- Coordinate a response between other regional hospitals as well as public health officials

External Verification, Regulatory, and Educational Bodies

Successful surgical residency programs must interact and comply with the rules promulgated by multiple external entities. Among these bodies are certifying and accrediting groups, government agencies, and professional education and development organizations at the local, state, and national levels.

Certifying and Accrediting Bodies
Certifying and accrediting bodies, include not only the ACGME, but also the ABS and the American Osteopathic Association (AOA) certifying boards, which certify program graduates under the auspices of the American Board of Medical Specialties (ABMS).

The ACGME accredits fellowship programs that provide additional training after completion of a general surgery residency, including, pediatric, vascular, and cardiothoracic surgery. Some fellowship programs may be accredited by organizations such as the Fellowship Council,[6] The Transplant Accreditation & Certification Council (TACC),[7] and the American Association of Endocrine Surgeons (AAES).[8]

Educational activities that are designed to improve surgical knowledge and skills (for example, simulation-based education) also may be accredited. For example, the American College of Surgeons (ACS) awards accreditation to teaching facilities when they fulfill the requirements to become an ACS-accredited Educational Institute (ACS-AEI).[9]

Government Regulatory and Licensing Entities

Residency programs need to confirm that residents and faculty are licensed to practice medicine and surgery in their state. State licensing boards frequently require that residency programs report disciplinary actions involving residents.

The U.S. government, as a major funder of GME, also has some regulatory control over surgical training. The Congressional Research Service estimates the average annual cost per trainee across specialties to be $112,000 to $129,000.[10] In 2015, federal investment in GME was estimated to be $16 billion, including support through Medicare, the Children's Hospitals Graduate Medical Education Program, the Teaching Health Center Graduate Medical Education Program, and the Department of Veterans' Affairs (VA).[11]

Funding sources may vary by SI and may include multiple sources of funding within each SI. However, the largest source of financial support for GME is Medicare, which, in 2016, paid teaching hospitals an estimated $3.79 billion in direct GME payments (DGME) and $7.4 billion in indirect GME payments (IME).[12] Medicare only funds its share of the costs of a hospital's approved residency/fellowship costs; in many states, Medicaid provides support as well. Any remaining costs must be paid by SI funding sources.

Medicare funding for GME training programs cover the additional costs associated with a teaching hospital and is provided through DGME and IME. DGME covers resident/fellow stipends and benefits, faculty salaries, GME office expenses, accreditation fees, educational space, and recruitment costs. IME covers the increased costs associated with the more complex patients teaching hospitals often treat. The DGME and IME payments, which are derived from separate formula-based payments set by federal statute, are made directly to the teaching hospital, regardless of its ACGME SI designation.[11]

In 1997, the Balanced Budget Amendment capped the number of residency positions that may receive Medicare funding. Teaching hospitals may train more residents and fellows than their cap but will not receive funding for those additional positions. Some teaching hospitals may raise the training cap by adding rural training tracks or receiving cap redistribution because of hospital closures.

Because the government provides most of the funding for GME, residency programs will be required to provide accurate, timely reports of the identities of residents on duty at each government-funded clinical site. Reports usually are submitted to the administration of the individual teaching site and then forwarded to the relevant federal agency.

Professional Organizations for Residents, Faculty, and Educators

Two national organizations provide valuable services to most residency programs and their applicants. The Electronic Residency Application Service (ERAS), a function of the AAMC, provides uniform information on applicants to a program. The National Resident Matching Program (NRMP) provides a mechanism for residency programs to identify and matriculate applicants.

For surgeons and other educational professionals associated with surgical residency programs, membership in two organizations provides valuable opportunities for knowledge acquisition, professional development, and influence in GME. The Association for Surgical Education (ASE) is open to all surgical educators. For PDs, membership and participation in the Association of Program Directors in Surgery (APDS) provides access to new research, interaction with colleagues, and informative discussions that will improve the understanding of requirements and actions of the ACGME, the RC, and the certifying boards.

The ACS Academy of Master Surgeon Educators (AMSE) is a new organization that recognizes surgeons who have demonstrated excellence in surgical education. The Academy provides a forum for the presentation and discussion of topics of importance to surgical educators. Through a dedicated, members-only listserv, the organization offers a useful resource to surgical educators.

Ensuring Success of Programs and Residents

To ensure optimal success of a residency program, the program must be evaluated continuously for areas of improvement. Likewise, residents and faculty must be regularly assessed.

Continuous Program Evaluation and Improvement
The PD and core faculty should regularly evaluate the program to identify opportunities to improve the curriculum and resident experience, including case logs and the resident and faculty evaluations of each assignment. The resident education curriculum must include appropriate experiences in both real and simulated settings.

In addition, adequate activities supporting scholarship, such as clinical and basic research and scientific writing, should be made available and have the support of all participating faculty.

Regular, documented assessments of individual resident performance are required to effectively affirm resident progress. Resident evaluation of the faculty should focus on the quality of faculty teaching and availability. Faculty assessment of residents and resident evaluation of faculty may be conducted using both formal and informal processes.

The PD, with assistance from a program evaluation committee (PEC), should regularly assess the overall curriculum and expected skill acquisition components as established by the ACGME. This process includes establishing benchmarks and recording achievement of the ACGME-mandated milestones to be tailored to the individual resident through the clinical competency committee (CCC).

Opportunities for Evaluation and Feedback
GME is a two-way process. Residents must be able to both receive and give feedback and constructive criticism without fear of retaliation. The CCC is the forum where meetings with the residents occur biannually. Evaluations should be clearly communicated to the trainee along with plans for remediation as needed and a written discussion summary should be provided to the trainee and included in the resident's file. The summary should document milestones and satisfaction of other ACGME mandates. In addition, the CCC needs to be involved with biannual assessments of the residents, which the PD or assigned mentor should share with the resident.

If program deficiencies are discovered that negatively affect resident performance, it is imperative to address these issues at all levels and through the PEC. If the underlying problem is systemic or institutional, then the DIO should be consulted before effecting change.

Likewise, the residents should be offered opportunities to give feedback to the PD regarding faculty performance, the learning environment, and so on. This summation should include written reports and can be facilitated by regularly scheduled meetings of the residents, the PD, and other faculty as needed. Resident feedback should be shared with the faculty and become part of their portfolio.

The Resident/Fellow Forum
Every program should have a resident/fellow forum which allows communication regarding their working environment.[1] Any resident or fellow must have the opportunity to directly raise concerns to the forum and the forum must have the option to convene without faculty members, administrators, or the DIO. The option to present concerns that arise from this forum directly to the DIO and GMEC should be in place.

Establishing a Culture Conducive to Optimal Learning
The program's success depends on the development and preservation of a culture of inquiry and learning. When faculty are committed to treating trainees as colleagues, this relationship helps create a positive learning environment. Treating a trainee as a colleague in learning implies mutual respect, consideration of each other's opinions, and a conjoined philosophy to find solutions that lead to better patient care. Objective evaluation of the teaching culture can be accomplished through the annual resident survey, ACGME Clinical Learning Environment Review (CLER), and a formal objective culture evaluation tool administered by the department and institution.

Other cultural requirements include a clear focus on diversity, equity, and inclusion (DEI), resiliency training, and resident well-being.

Achieving and Documenting Resident Clinical Proficiency
The ACGME's move to standardize resident education and require demonstrated objective clinical proficiency has created a need for more accurate documentation of resident competencies. For example, hospitals now require certification of competency before allowing a provider to independently perform bedside procedures. The CEO and chief medical officer, along with the DIO and PDs, must provide educational programs and certification for bedside procedures. Steps in the process include: knowledge acquisition, skills acquisition, and practice; performance of procedures under direct supervision; and certification by the PD or someone equally qualified.

The ACS and the APDS have established a three-phase skills curriculum for all surgery residents (see Chapter 2). Phase 1 focuses on basic surgical skills using instructional modules followed by a verification of proficiency assessment. Phase 2 includes 15 modules that address specific advanced skills and procedures. Phase 3 includes 10 modules that adress team-based skills.[13]

Knowledge acquisition may require assigned readings and/or tutorial videos explaining the indications, contraindications, and steps required to successfully complete the procedure. Typically, residents are expected to complete and log a critical number of successfully performed procedures with graduated responsibility before the PD considers advancing them from direct to indirect supervision. The list of resident names and certified procedures can then be uploaded to an online procedure certification database that supervisors, nurses, and other teammates can access as needed to verify credentials.

Faculty Support

GME support for faculty is divided into compensation and faculty development. Compensation is unique for each institution and varies according to whether the faculty is volunteer or full-time. For institutions with full-time faculty, support may depend on developing a compensation system that recognizes educational effort. Although the SI should provide educational support to its programs and faculty, individualized programs and departments could also design a curriculum to support faculty development.

All surgeons can improve their teaching skills through learning and practice. Effective educators also need to be able to effectively assess and provide feedback to residents. Curricula to develop PDs and faculty members are available in many SIs. An individual residency program also may design and implement its own curriculum for its teaching faculty members, and numerous resources are available to help develop faculty. For example, the APDS *Program Director's Handbook* is an excellent resource for both the PD and all members of the teaching faculty. The *Journal of Surgical Education* (*www.journals.elsevier.com/journal-of-surgical-education*) and *The Journal of Graduate Medical Education* (*www.jgme.org/*), address a range of topics pertinent to the development of teaching faculty members in surgery. A variety of excellent resources in faculty development, such as the Surgeons as Educators Course, are available through the ACS. For details, go to *www.facs.org/education/roles/educators.*

Quality Resources and the Quality Improvement Process

Quality assurance (QA) for resident-run services and procedures should include mechanisms in addition to the traditional weekly morbidity and mortality (M&M) conference, such as:

- The College's National Surgical Quality Improvement Program (ACS NSQIP®) Risk Calculator (*https://riskcalculator.facs.org/RiskCalculator/*) to document preoperative risk assessment
- Real-time data tracking of outcomes supplemented with comparisons to appropriate risk-adjusted national benchmark data
- A readily available technical skills assessment tool (smartphone based) to document progression to independence[14]
- A clearly defined protocol for escalation of attending involvement, including clearly defined mandatory triggers for greater attending participation
- Rules should be in place for consultation and/or transfer to another service when appropriate

An excellent resource that provides information on quality benchmarks and methods for achieving a culture of high-reliability is the ACS *Optimal Resources for Surgical Quality and Safety*, the "Red Book."

Achieving Resident Autonomy, Patient Safety, and High-Quality Care

Many factors, including work-hour limitations, pressure to enhance OR efficiency, medicolegal responsibility considerations, and billing and compliance concerns challenge the development of resident autonomy within surgical training programs. The anxiety about successful management of complications that emerge when a resident provides surgical care is real. However, residents must engage in independent decision-making and performance of operative procedures (including the management of postoperative complications) to achieve self-confidence and progress to independent practice. Collaboration among PDs, department chairs, medical staff leaders, and patient care team members can create oversight and supervision mechanisms to foster progressive resident autonomy and ensure patient safety and high-quality outcomes. Whether the pilot or the co-pilot lands a 787 is unknown to most passengers as long as the procedure is done appropriately and adequately supervised to assure equivalent quality and safety.

Supervision of Residents

The ACGME defines different forms of resident supervision within the CPR.[1] Direct supervision is defined by the physical presence of the supervising physician. Indirect supervision refers to the situation in which the supervising physician is either immediately available in the hospital or available by telephone or another electronic modality.

At the conclusion of residency, the PD must attest to the ability of the surgical graduate to practice autonomously. It is essential that the PD have adequate opportunity to assess a resident practicing with minimal supervision. In aviation, pilots in training fly initially with expert instructors observing and able to intervene if necessary. This allows them to assess objectively the trainee's decision-making but intervene in the event of a safety issue.

The CPR do not distinguish the OR environment from other sites of care. The ACGME stipulates that each patient have an identifiable, appropriately credentialed, and privileged attending physician who is responsible and accountable for the care of the patient and that this information be provided to the patient and the entire surgical care team. Health care institutions, through their medical staff structure, implement policies regarding physician rounding and documentation. Each residency program must specify roles and responsibilities for residents and fellows at each level of training on each assignment and in circumstances that require escalation and communication to attending physicians.

Regulations Regarding Resident Autonomy in the OR

The Centers for Medicare & Medicaid Services (CMS) established rules for billing in teaching settings in 1997 and 2002 that require direct attending involvement and participation in key portions of procedures. Third-party payors may not recognize billing modifiers and will not reimburse services performed by residents without direct attending participation. Direct supervision of residents during the critical portion of the procedure is necessary to satisfy billing requirements. Thus, the surgeon must be physically present in the OR with the resident and patient during the critical portion of an operation; the decision to scrub in is left to the individual surgeon based on case complexity, patient acuity, and the level of training and ability of the respective resident. Other noncritical portions of a procedure can be accomplished with indirect supervision.[11]

Progressive Transfer of Responsibility

Transfer of autonomy to a resident with the goal of conditional independence should occur in a graduated fashion based on the achievement of specific milestones. A resident should receive specific approval from the PD to move to the next level of autonomy based on inputs, including review of prior assessments, formal intraoperative assessments, appropriate skills training, case log experience, and ACGME milestone progression. Typical procedures appropriate for conditional independence at each level should be specified by the program director in consultation with the CCC.

To inform the assessment process, the ACGME RC for Surgery introduced Milestones 2.0 in July 2020.[15] These milestones specify five levels of progressive achievement in ACGME-defined core competencies. For details, go to *www.acgme.org/Portals/0/PDFs/Milestones/SurgeryMilestones.pdf?ver=2020-09-01-152718-110*.

The RC also recently increased the requirement for teaching assistant cases to further develop autonomy. To allow a trainee to be entrusted to complete the core activities of a general surgeon without supervision, the ABS, in collaboration with the RC and the APDS, is testing the feasibility of Entrustable Professional Activities (EPAs) as an assessment framework.[16] The ABS is conducting five EPAs-based pilot projects: the evaluation and management of inguinal hernia, right lower quadrant pain and appendicitis, gallbladder disease, and blunt or penetrating trauma, as well as the provision of general surgical consultation to other health care providers.

Acute care general surgery services are an increasingly popular vehicle for general surgery residency programs to foster progressive resident autonomy in and out of the OR.[17] Essential features include specification of types of cases appropriate for a resident-run service and criteria for transfer to subspecialty services.

Preoperative informed consent discussion with the patient should disclose and specify the roles of the resident and attending surgeon, including for the critical portion of the procedure.[18] Patient education and buy-in are critical to ensure public trust and transparency in residency training.

Review Process for Resident Performance

Residents must be exposed to the peer-review process to emphasize QI and to establish career-long habits of focused review of individual practice patterns and outcomes. This necessity pertains not only to learning clinical knowledge and technical skills, but also to understanding QI and fostering professionalism. Residents progress toward independence from demonstration, to step-by-step instruction, to coaching.[19,20] Evaluation of progress toward autonomy should consider operative planning, including positioning, equipment, entry, and exposure; effectiveness of communication with anesthesiologists, OR staff, patients, and family; knowledge of technical steps, including pitfalls; and the recognition of personal limitations, including the need to ask for help.

Residents can demonstrate the development of confidence and responsibility in a number of ways, such as the ability to guide junior residents through essential operations. Residents develop surgical judgment through evaluation and management consultations, review of perioperative management decisions, and communication with consultants and attending surgeons. A weekly QI conference with program or team leadership can provide additional oversight by reviewing management decisions and the identifying system-based quality issues. The Quality In-Training Initiative: An ACS NSQIP Collaborative (*https://qiti.acsnsqip.org/ACS_NSQIP_2017_QITI_Curriculum.pdf*) is an excellent resource for instituting a QI process in a surgical residency.

Conclusion

The optimal oversight, management, and governance of GME in surgery requires a committed, collaborative leadership team. Institutional leadership must create a culture conducive to education that enables residents to develop autonomy, while maintaining high-quality care and protecting patient safety.

Suggested Readings

Accreditation Council for Graduate Medical Education. Learn at ACGME. Available at: https://dl.acgme.org/. Accessed September 29, 2020.

American Board of Surgery. The American Board of Surgery Booklet of Information 2020-2021. Available at: https://www.absurgery.org/xfer/BookletofInfo-Surgery.pdf. Accessed October 16, 2021.

American College of Surgeons. ACS NSQIP Surgical Risk Calculator. Available at: https://riskcalculator.facs.org/RiskCalculator/. Accessed September 29, 2020.

American College of Surgeons. ACS Resources for Educators. Available at: https://www.facs.org/education/roles/educators. Accessed September 29, 2020.

American College of Surgeons. The Quality In-Training Initiative: An ACS NSQIP Collaborative. Available at: https://qiti.acsnsqip.org/ACS_NSQIP_2017_QITI_Curriculum.pdf. Accessed September 29, 2020.

Association of Program Directors in Surgery. The Association of Program Directors in Surgery PD Handbook. Available at: https://apds.org/program-directors/pd-handbook. Accessed September 29, 2020.

Ellison EC, Spanknebel K, Stain SC, et al. Impact of the COVID-19 pandemic on surgical training and learner well-being: report of a survey of general surgery and other surgical specialty educators. *JACS* in press. Available at: https://www.journalacs.org/action/showPdf?pii=S1072-7515%2820%2932308-5.

Hoyt DB, Ko CY. *Optimal Resources for Surgical Quality and Safety*. Chicago, IL: American College of Surgeons; 2017.

Journal of Surgical Education. Available at: https://www.journals.elsevier.com/journal-of-surgical-education. Accessed September 29, 2020.

Ma OJ, Hedges JR, Jerris R, Newgard CD. The academic RVU: ten years developing a metric for and financially incenting academic productivity at Oregon Health & Science University. *Acad Med.* 2017:92;1138-1144.

Manthey DE and Fitch M. Stages of competency for medical procedures. *Clin Teach.* 2012;9(5):317-319.

The Journal of Graduate Medical Education. Available at: https://www.jgme.org/. Accessed September 29, 2020.

United States Government Accountability Office. Physician Workforce: HHS needs better information to comprehensively evaluate graduate medical education funding; GAO-18-240; March 2018. Available at: https://www.gao.gov/products/gao-18-240. Accessed November 5, 2021.

References

1. Accreditation Council for Graduate Medical Education. ACGME Program Requirements for Graduate Medical Education in General Surgery Accessed July 1, 2020. Available at: https://acgme.org/Portals/0/PFAssets/ProgramRequirements/440_GeneralSurgery_2020.pdf?ver=2020-06-22-085958-260
2. Accreditation Council for Graduate Medical Education. ACGME Institutional Requirements. Available at: https://www.acgme.org/globalassets/PFAssets/ProgramRequirements/800_InstitutionalRequirements_2021.pdf?ver=2021-02-19-090632-820&ver=2021-02-19-090632-820. Accessed October 16, 2021.
3. Accreditation Council for Graduate Medical Education. ACGME Specialty Requirements. Available at: https://www.acgme.org/Specialties. Accessed August 17, 2020.
4. Yaghoubian A, Galante J, Kaji A, et al. General surgery resident remediation and attrition: a multi-institutional study. *Arch Surg.* 2012;147(9):829–833.
5. Smith JL, Lypson L, Silverberg M, et al. Defining uniform processes for remediation, probation, and termination in residency. *West J. Emerg Med.* 2017;18:110-113.
6. Fellowship Council. Directory of Fellowships. Available at: https://fellowshipcouncil.org/directory-of-fellowships/. Accessed July 31, 2020.

7. American Society of Transplant Surgeons. Abdominal Transplant Surgery Fellowship. Available at: https://asts.org/training/transplant-accreditation-certification-council. Accessed July 31, 2020.
8. American Association of Endocrine Surgeons. Endocrine Surgery Fellowships. Available at: https://www.endocrinesurgery.org/fellowships. Accessed August 17, 2020.
9. American College of Surgeons. American College of Surgeons Accredited Education Institutes. Available at: https://www.facs.org/education/accreditation/aei. Accessed August 17, 2020.
10. Congressional Research Service. Federal support for graduate medical education: an overview. Updated December 2018. Available at: https://crsreports.congress.gov/product/pdf/R/R44376. Accessed October 16, 2021.
11. Congressional Research Service. In focus. Medicare graduate medical education payments: an overview. Updated February 2019. https://crsreports.congress.gov/product/pdf/IF/IF10960.
12. Association of American Medical Colleges. Medicare payments for graduate medical education: what every medical student, resident, advisor needs to know. April 2019. https://aamc-black.global.ssl.fastly.net/production/media/filer_public/64/77/6477adae-c4c6-4e0e-8c6f-adcdabf2bdec/dgme_-_medicare_gme_payments_what_you_need_to_know_-_20190430.pdf.
13. American College of Surgeons, Association of Program Directors in Surgery. ACS/APDS Surgery Resident Curriculum. Available at: https://www.facs.org/education/program/resident-skills.
14. George BC, Bohnen JD, Schuller MC, Fryer JP. Using smartphones for trainee performance assessment: a SIMPL case study. *Surgery*. 2020;167(6):903-906.
15. Edgar L, Roberts S, Holmboe E. Milestones 2.0: a step forward. *J Grad Med Educ*. 2018;10(3):367-369.
16. Brasel KJ, Klingensmith ME, Englander R, et al. Entrustable professional activities in general surgery: development and implementation. *J Surg Educ*. 2019;76(5):1174-1186.
17. Kantor O, Schneider AB, Rojnica M, et al. Implementing a resident acute care surgery service: improving resident education and patient care. *Surgery*. 2017;161(3):876-883.
18. Bryan AF, Bryan DS, Matthews JB, Roggin KK. Toward autonomy and conditional independence: a standardized script improves patient acceptance of surgical trainee roles. *J Surg Educ*. 2020;77(3):534-539.
19. Mellinger JD, Williams RG, Sanfey H, et al. Teaching and assessing operative skills: from theory to practice. *Curr Probl Surg*. 2017;54(2):44-81.
20. Sakran JV, Ko C, Hoffman RL. The ACS NSQIP quality in-training initiative: educating residents to ensure the future of optimal surgical care. American College of Surgeons Bulletin. Available at: https://bulletin.facs.org/2013/11/the-acs-nsqip-quality-in-training-initiative-educating-residents-to-ensure-the-future-of-optimal-surgical-care/. Published November 1, 2013. Accessed September 29, 2020.

AMERICAN
SURGEONS
OF SURGEO
COLLEGE O
AMERICAN
SURGEONS
OF SURGEO
COLLEGE O
AMERICAN
SURGEONS

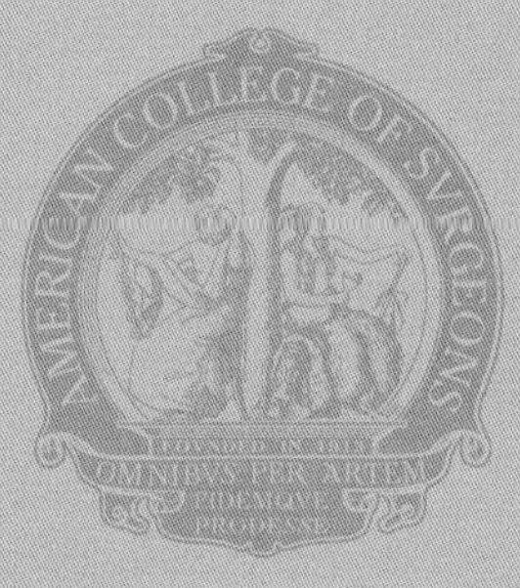

CHAPTER 4
Core Knowledge for Residency Training

Lead Author

John A. Weigelt, MD, DVM, MMA, FACS, MAMSE

Co-Authors

Daniel L. Dent, MD, FACS

James C. Hebert, MD, FACS

CHAPTER 4

Core Knowledge for Residency Training

Executive Summary

Modern surgical training and its supporting curriculum are founded on core knowledge. It is essential to define and frame a curriculum to manage the program and expectations of learners. The core knowledge curriculum becomes the road map for modern surgical training and skills development. Training in assessment, professionalism, and implementation of successful practice are based on this foundation.

Introduction

Surgery training programs must ensure that surgeons know and practice safe and effective patient care when they enter the surgical workforce. Achieving this goal requires a systematic curriculum to provide trainees with skills and knowledge not only in preoperative, intraoperative, and postoperative care, but also in the nonoperative competencies needed to manage patients. Although textbooks serve as a guide to general surgery topics, they are not intended to serve as a curriculum for general surgery training programs.

The first part of this chapter identifies curriculum topics a general surgeon should master during training. All general surgery training programs should address these curriculum priorities, which align with the description of core knowledge for a general surgeon promulgated by the American Board of Surgery (ABS) (these descriptions are available on the ABS website at *www.absurgery.org).*

This chapter also identifies curricular topics that are relevant but not critical components of a general surgeon's core knowledge base. While they take lower priority and less time in a properly constructed curriculum, they are important in the development of an optimal understanding of general surgery and the ability to perform general surgery procedures. By establishing a hierarchal curriculum, faculty and trainees can better allocate their time and energy while they acquire the knowledge and skills necessary for successful clinical practice.

The second part of this chapter offers a variety of methods in the implementation of an effective general surgery curriculum. We offer methods intended to help general surgery training programs provide this curriculum. As medical education continues to evolve and adapt based on the needs of trainees and the ongoing changes in technology, our approach acknowledges these changes while offering methods to empower faculty and enable trainees to acquire the knowledge appropriate for a general surgeon. Surgical education occurs along a continuum that requires a commitment to lifelong learning; our emphasis in this chapter is on one important aspect of that education and our intent is to bring clarity and increase access to an ever-growing body of knowledge. However, trainees must remember that the residency program is only one step in their education; as they enter practice and care for patients, they must embrace lifelong learning.

Defining Core Knowledge for Residency Training

General surgeons need to master the knowledge and techniques necessary to successfully manage the preoperative, operative, and postoperative care of patients with a broad spectrum of diseases that can present for emergent or elective surgical care. Some disease categories are more common than others and require more depth and breadth of knowledge. For less common conditions, surgeons must recognize when they need additional knowledge and have a system to obtain it.

Necessary skills for a general surgeon include diagnostic acumen and technical ability to perform surgical interventions. The ABS developed an accepted definition of the scope of practice of a general surgeon, which is available at *www.absurgery.org*.

The ABS definition identifies seven major categories:

- Alimentary tract
- Abdomen and its contents
- Breast, skin, and soft tissue
- Endocrine system
- Surgical critical care
- Surgical oncology
- Trauma

A training program must plan how trainees will gain the knowledge sufficient to manage patients presenting with diseases in these seven categories. Clinical rotations, which focus on many of these categories, enable trainees to learn while caring for actual patients. Conferences and other educational experiences supplement the clinical rotation experience. These activities vary from program to program based on the structure of the clinical rotations segment of the curriculum. Variations in resource availability and the commitment and teaching talent of the faculty mean that some program experiences will be more robust than others. Programs need to recognize shortcomings in resources or faculty and address them by providing supplementary educational content.

The program director (PD) conducts an educational needs assessment and develops a strategic plan tailored to improve their individual program and its unique strengths and weaknesses. An analysis of the education quality of each ABS-defined topic area will help PDs devise this improvement plan. This process could compare the program's experience with a surgical textbook or a more detailed disease-based taxonomy. A program's ABS In-Training Examination (ABSITE) scores offer another way to identify areas that need improvement. To judge the curriculum quality, a set of specific and measurable knowledge, skills, and abilities for each resident will be necessary for all seven ABS categories. The ABS has identified eight specific clinical care domains where these knowledge, skills, and abilities can be defined and monitored:

- Coagulation abnormalities
- Endoscopy—colonoscopy, endoscopy, laparoscopy
- Fluid and electrolyte management
- Imaging use to facilitate patient management
- Infectious disease and antibiotic management
- Metabolism and nutrition
- Pain management
- Shock and resuscitation

How a training program addresses each skill set will depend upon its educational resources. Some of these clinical categories may be taught or learned through self-study and supplemented through clinical experience. Additionally, some categories require defined educational programs, whereas others do not. Regardless, all categories require educational activities to provide the necessary content.

Basic educational programs that can enable trainees to attain expertise in the core knowledge areas of general surgery include:

- Advanced Cardiac Life Support (ACLS)
- Advanced Trauma Life Support® (ATLS®)
- Fundamentals of Laparoscopic Surgery (FLS)
- The ABS Flexible Endoscopy Curriculum (ABS-FEC)

The ABS has identified five surgical specialty areas of clinical care that are important for training but not necessarily critical to a general surgeon's core knowledge base. Although comprehensive knowledge in these areas requires training beyond general surgery, a trained general surgeon should understand common problems in these areas. The curriculum should anticipate that a general surgeon may need to manage clinical problems in these five categories:

- Burns
- Pediatric surgery
- Thoracic surgery
- Transplantation
- Vascular surgery

Each training program must determine how best to provide these additional educational opportunities for trainees to learn key content in these specialties. Each program also will need to assess a trainee's knowledge of conditions and diseases within these categories that includes a record of clinical exposure to these categories, didactic time spent on associated topics, and self-study assignments. These specialty topics, however, should not drive the program's curriculum.

Applying Core Knowledge

Training programs provide residents with multiple opportunities to develop and enhance their core knowledge, including clinical rotations and operating experience.

Clinical Rotations

Clinical rotations should foster learning in the seven primary areas a general surgeon needs to master. A set of written objectives for each clinical rotation should ensure that all trainees have the opportunity to acquire the clinical knowledge and skills associated with each primary area.

Teaching sessions should be formally structured to supplement clinical rotations so that residents can gain knowledge in each of the following areas:

- Coagulation abnormalities
- Endoscopy—colonoscopy, endoscopy, laparoscopy
  - FLS
  - ABS-FEC
- Fluid and electrolyte management
- Imaging use to facilitate patient management
- Infectious disease and antibiotic management
- Metabolism and nutrition
- Pain management
- Shock and resuscitation
- ACLS
- ATLS

These clinical rotations may include a variety of teaching methods, such as:

- Orientation sessions
- Boot camps that provide concentrated, intense knowledge delivery and skills training
- Conferences
- Teaching conferences
  - Grand rounds
  - Journal clubs
  - Specialty conferences

Written objectives for each teaching activity should be prepared and described in terms of SMART objectives. Here is what "SMART" stands for, with parenthetical examples of each objective related to teaching how to tie sutures:

Specific (tie under tension)
Measurable (demonstrate on skills apparatus and closing midline incision)
Attainable (easily attained through structured learning and practice)
Relevant (critical to every surgical procedure)
Time-based (straightforward approximation under tension during years 1-2; tying deep and tying blind under tension during years 3-4)

Three additional examples of clinical service objectives are provided in Appendix A, which could be adopted into the SMART model.

Milestones developed by the Accreditation Council for Graduate Medical Education (ACGME) can serve as a template to assess trainee performance and document how well they have attained the knowledge, skills, attitudes, and other attributes in each of the six ACGME competency areas. Documented in a semi-annual resident performance review reported to the ACGME, these milestones can help track trainee growth and development. They do not represent objectives for learning activities nor do they relate to a specific postgraduate year of education; milestones may be achieved earlier or later according to expectations for individual trainees and/or the peer group. The milestone achievements of individual trainees may determine if they advance or graduate.

Using SMART goals to implement core content complements the milestones and Entrustable Professional Activities (EPAs) that help ensure the resident curriculum has clear training objectives.

Operative Case Experience

A surgical training program also must include operative experience. Each residency program must assess in writing how a trainee's operative experience aligns with ABS expectations of core and advanced essential general surgery procedures. Although breadth and volume of experience are important, assessments should emphasize assessment of critical steps, complexity, and outcomes, and not just quantity of cases (Appendix B).

Each procedural experience must provide an opportunity for the resident to grow in knowledge and skill. As such, the surgical faculty should create an environment to optimize growth opportunities, which should include routine preprocedural assessment of the resident's preparation and knowledge and an intraoperative assessment of the resident's technical and decision-making skills.

To evaluate a program's breadth of operative experience, start by comparing it to the ABS Surgical Council on Resident Education (SCORE) list of operative procedures (see Appendix C). Next, programs should design rotations to ensure that each resident has adequate exposure to these procedures. The SMART format of goals and objectives for operative procedures will help the resident identify the salient points for each of these operations.

Another excellent resource to view experienced surgeons demonstrating these core operations is accessible in the American College of Surgeons (ACS) Online Video Library (see Appendix D) and the ACS Multimedia Atlas of Surgery Volumes (see Appendix E). These two resources provide in-depth, highly detailed educational content for a variety of procedure types across many body systems.

Teaching Methods for Effective Knowledge Delivery

Sources of information for a general surgery curriculum are varied, and include textbooks, the ABS SCORE curriculum, review of current literature, and so on.

Textbooks

Textbooks form the backbone of a general surgery program. They usually present the material by broad topics, an organ system, or specific diseases, such as gastric adenocarcinoma. They also may include chapters about fundamental aspects of surgical patient care, such as shock, fluid and electrolytes, and wound healing. Although textbooks provide information key to a general surgeon's foundation of learning, traditionally they do not always contain the most current information because they are updated only every four to five years. Electronic textbooks are updated more frequently, however, and have become the new standard.

A curriculum may use textbooks in many ways. A textbook may be incorporated into postgraduate education as a study guide for residents, becoming a self-study tool to complement other parts of the curriculum, including patient experience, or a resident may use specific reading assignments to review an entire textbook each year. Still another way would be to review a textbook every five years along with material presented throughout the training period. Many textbooks include tests that can be incorporated into these assignments or used in self-study.

The ABS SCORE Curriculum

The ABS SCORE was developed in 2006 as a not-for-profit consortium of principal organizations in U.S. surgical education; in 2019, it merged with ABS. The organizations participating in the collaborative effort that led to SCORE include the ABS, ACS, American Surgical Association (ASA), Association of Program Directors in Surgery (APDS), Association for Surgical Education (ASE), Review Committee (RC) for Surgery of the ACGME, and Society of American Gastrointestinal and Endoscopic Surgeons (SAGES). The main objective of SCORE is to develop resources to support a national curriculum for general surgery training.

The topics in SCORE are organized according to the six ACGME competencies and presented as didactic modules that reflect the learning objectives of those competencies. For most U.S. residency programs, SCORE is one of the main sources of curricular content, featured in a programmatic way, or used as a self-study activity. The ABS uses SCORE to drive its content for assessment and examinations. Programs must subscribe to SCORE to use the material.

SCORE, the goals of which are largely clinical rotation objectives, can be employed to meet the specific objectives of a program. Ideally, for programs to develop the appropriate assessment tools, these objectives could be written as modular objectives to be administered in the rotations. SCORE organizes topics in a way that supports this modular concept. Adult learners learn best when they can easily recognize a need-to-know topic while taking care of their patients. In other words, assigned readings should coincide with what a specific resident needs to know on the current rotation.

Current and Critical Literature Review

There are many ways to become familiar with current and critical literature. These include subscribing to specific journals, receiving e-mails promoting monthly journal content, reviewing listings of journal contents and electronic e-mail journal watches, using Internet resources (for example, PubMed, Google Scholar, and others), perusing formal, published systematic reviews, and studying evidence-based consensus statements published by consortia (for example, the Cochrane Collaboration Database and the Agency for Healthcare Research and Quality's Systematic Review Data Repository). Residents should become familiar with each of these types of resources to determine which are best suited to their professional growth.

Residents also may join journal clubs to read primary literature, learn how to critically evaluate a study, defend or critique a study's findings, and even how to write effectively for publication in the scientific literature. To create an additional forum for residents and faculty to become colleagues in learning, journal clubs should select relevant articles for discussion, include faculty guidance, and expedite resident participation. Journal clubs should have a clear structure and process objectives to make the activity valuable for all learners. This activity should be introduced early in residency training so that junior residents develop the habit, discipline, and confidence to read and assess active literature and defend their understanding in an open forum. Journal clubs should be composed of residents who are of a similar age or stage of development as a surgeon.

Residents may be motivated to review the scientific literature either by interesting clinical cases that may stimulate a search for relevant scientific articles or by a topical approach to supplement didactic sessions in the curriculum that require the use of primary literature.

One approach that engages both residents and practicing surgeons in the scientific literature is *Selected Readings in General Surgery*—a publication of the ACS (available in the Publications section of the ACS website at *www.facs.org*). This publication was started as a resident education program by Robert McClelland, MD, FACS, at the University of Texas Southwestern School of Medicine, Dallas, in the late 1960s; it was offered as a limited subscription service beginning in 1973 and became available nationally in the mid-1970s. In 2005, Dr. McClelland retired and gave the publication to the ACS, where Lewis M. Flint, MD, FACS, MAMSE, has shepherded it to become a go-to electronic resource and standalone curriculum for general surgery. The program, which is available by subscription, uses past and current articles to highlight information across the breadth of general surgery to help residents and practicing surgeons expand their scope of knowledge.

Simulation-Based Education

Simulation-based education is an essential tool for training surgical residents. Simulation reproduces real-life scenarios and builds resident competency by tailoring education to appropriate levels of complexity and cultivating specific clinical and technical skills. Optimal delivery of this education occurs through activities ranging from practicing incisions and suturing on an orange, to more complex technical skills labs simulating high-fidelity scenarios, such as robotics exercises and virtual reality. This training can improve and reinforce residents' confidence in their surgical techniques through practice, provide a bridge for learning prior to the operating room, and improve performance of procedures requiring multidisciplinary collaboration and teamwork. Ultimately, this targeted skills training benefits surgeons and the health care systems by significantly reducing patient risk and increasing quality of care.

Simulation also may be used to train residents as teachers. For example, simulation in the residents as teachers (RaT) programs allow residents to practice their teaching skills in a controlled learning environment, which enhances the quality of their teaching and feedback.

In 2005, the ACS launched the ACS-accredited Education Institutes (ACS-AEI) program to verify and recognize a national network of simulation centers that offer state-of-the-art simulation-based training to various learners using standardized modules and objective assessments of performance. This comprehensive accreditation program promotes patient safety, develops new education and technologies, identifies best practices, and encourages research and collaboration. It also offers virtual grand rounds and seminars to reinforce the highest standards in simulation-based education (*www.facs.org/education/accreditation/aei)*. Integrating simulation-based education into surgical residency programs enables surgeons to address future challenges in medicine with precision, skill, and confidence. Additional resident education resources available from the ACS are discussed in Chapter 6.

Anatomic Study

Another important resource for surgical education is the renewed study of anatomy, which for many surgical residents was last studied in their first year of medical school. An anatomy lab, as part of an ACS-AEI offering, or part of the anatomy department in a medical school is a wonderful resource for residents to have access to review anatomy, learn exposure, and explore in-depth concepts briefly discussed as a medical student. Another wonderful resource built into a surgical residency program stems from the development of relationships with anatomic pathologists within the institution or the medical examiner if in close proximity to the residency training facilities. This is often an opportunity for residents to see anatomy unlike their previous exposure to cadavers or inanimate or computerized anatomic simulation.

Attaining and Applying Medical Knowledge

Just as objectives and metrics must be applied to patient care and other competencies, so they must be applied to medical knowledge. For instance, objectives regarding patient care can be identified by rotations based on residents' exposure to patients; similar expectations should be applied to medical knowledge. Unfortunately, the sheer volume of medical knowledge can overwhelm and intimidate the trainee.

To improve how we address the acquisition of appropriate medical knowledge as residents progress through a training program, start by providing guidance on how to use reference material, including textbooks and current literature. Learning objectives for medical knowledge must recognize individual learning styles as well as programmatic expectations. Start by listing expectations that emphasize a resident's progressive responsibility to meet training program objectives and achieve timely personal development. Table 1 offers trainees a model to attain and apply medical knowledge over the five years they spend in a program. Like milestones, these levels are not specific to postgraduate year, but rather to the progress of each resident.

Table 1. Model to attain and apply medical knowledge (MK) during and after a training program

Five distinct levels of attaining and applying medical knowledge (MK)	Level of Training	Methods to approach MK within a training program with expected interventions
Access to medical knowledge	Level 1	a. Identify basic surgical textbook (often chosen by program). b. Establish a personal reading program aimed at acquiring MK pertinent to level of training. c. Program may have reading program with specific objectives/assignments.
Correlate MK with clinical exposure	Level 2	a. Focused reading from basic surgical textbook based on clinical experiences.
Broaden MK in relationship to clinical experience	Level 3	a. Variations and nuances of MK related to a specific topic attained by broadening source of information. b. This will require new sources of information such as current literature or textbooks on specific topics. c. An example: A case of cholelithiasis will offer opportunity to access MK about other disease states involving the gallbladder.
Organize/collate information into retrievable information	Level 4	a. Focus recall of MK useful in clinical practice. b. Integrate MK with other competencies fostering a practice pattern and recognizable professional activity.
Scope of MK allows information to flow into patient care activity	Level 5	a. Point of care MK complete. b. References used for review and new developments consistent with lifelong learning.

Professional Behavior Core Knowledge

Surgical education has long emphasized ability and availability as key components of surgeon behavior, and all programs are structured to help residents attain these traits. Affability also is recognized and included as a key component of a surgeon's behavior; in fact, the success of a surgical practice may depend on the affability of its surgeons.
In order to become affable, residents should first understand what it means. An affable person is easy to talk to, friendly, and approachable; it is a trait common to those who are outgoing, benevolent, sociable, and courteous. For general surgeons, affability is strongly associated with effective communication skills. Most residency programs have an idea of their residents' relative communication skills, but it is difficult to find metrics to assess affability. Nevertheless, the program's challenge is to assess, improve, and document these communication skills. An effective surgeon approaches all situations with empathy and a positive attitude. This defines an aspect of interpersonal relationships most recently referred to as emotional intelligence. Emotional intelligence can be learned, measured, and targeted for improvement. Emphasis on developing and promoting emotional intelligence should be a specific goal of training.

The ACGME recognized the need for appropriate communication skills in 2008 when it designated "interpersonal and communication skills" as one of the six core competencies (Figure 1). More specific to surgery, the ACS describes professionalism, including interpersonal and communication skills, as it applies to surgeons in its Statements on Principles at *www.facs.org/about-acs/statements/stonprin*.

Residents must demonstrate interpersonal and communication skills that result in the effective exchange of information and collaboration with patients, their families, and health professionals.

Expectations include:

- Communicate effectively with patients, families, and the public, as appropriate, across a broad range of socioeconomic and cultural backgrounds.
- Communicate effectively with physicians, other health professionals, and health-related agencies.
- Work effectively as a member or leader of a health care team or other professional group.
- Act in a consultative role to other physicians and health professionals; and maintain comprehensive, timely, and legible medical records, if applicable.

Figure 1. ACGME Competencies for Interpersonal and Communication Skills

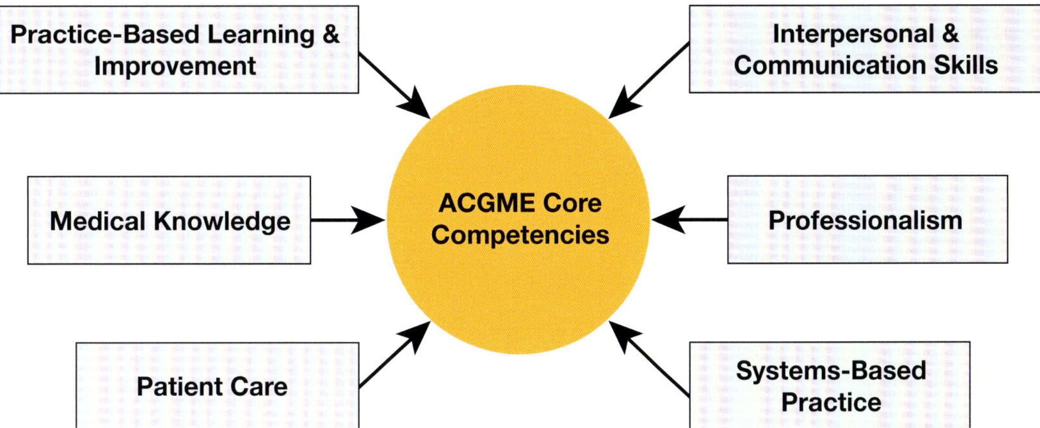

Affable surgeons are good communicators. Unfortunately, tools to assess communication skills are inexact and varied. Most tools measure performance of the team, not the individual. The ABS recognizes the importance of communication in daily surgical practice and emphasizes it as a core EPA, which the ABS is currently evaluating for inclusion in residency training.

Essential Elements for Teaching Effective Communication Skills

Effective communication should be a common goal of faculty and trainees. The variability of communication skills among surgeons, whether they are trainees or faculty, shows why a training curriculum must enhance communication. One effective way to teach these skills is through faculty modeling. There are other ways to develop communications skills, such as through role playing grounded in real-life examples.

Faculty Modeling

Faculty modeling is the most effective way to establish the expectations and culture necessary for residents to develop their communication skills. Residents should observe faculty-patient relations, with an emphasis on patient communication techniques. Resident-patient communication should be observed by faculty, and constructive feedback from faculty should help surgical residents adjust and develop their communication and emotional intelligence skills. Sometimes, a program is structured so that faculty-patient communication occurs without the resident present to observe, or resident-patient communication occurs in isolation. Similar isolation may occur during a formal consultation. Thoughtful attempts should be made to enhance transparency. Some faculty may, in fact, not be suited for modeling patient communication.

Developing Communications Skills

Basic communication skills can be developed through activities that model and teach listening skills, respectful vocabulary, the power of pausing, introspection, and practice through role playing.

Specific communications activities for a surgical curriculum should include setting care goals; obtaining informed consent (the indications, the contraindications, alternative forms of therapy, the anticipated results, and the risks or complications); using shared decision-making; explaining surrogate decision-making; delivering bad news; explaining a complication or adverse outcome honestly; and facilitating an end-of life discussion (including the five phases of death and dying). Residents also need to learn how to interact with nurses, administrative staff, non-surgeon medical colleagues, and peers. For example, residents might collaboratively practice respectful consideration of peers' clinical judgments or obtaining information from a patient or family member. Another collaborative activity might involve the simulation of a surgical consultation by nurses or other specialists. Role playing between internal medicine and general surgery residents with faculty facilitation can be especially useful.

These activities should focus on authentic problems in which the resident must keep the patient needs in the center and seek to do the right thing for the individual patient. Residents must learn how to discuss alternatives, listen to patient concerns, and practice shared decision-making. Some urgent health care conditions, such as traumatic injury or other urgent conditions, may limit effective communication, but in all other clinical situations the surgeon should take the time to listen and communicate.

Conclusion

In this chapter, we described how a program curriculum should encompass the core knowledge a general surgeon must obtain, as well as related topics with which they should be familiar. We showed how to implement a curriculum through hands-on experiences, such as those gained on clinical rotations and through operative experience, as well as through other teaching methods, such as textbooks, the ABS SCORE curriculum, literature review, simulation-based education, and anatomic study. Finally, we defined the professional behavior to which all general surgeons must aspire, including how residents can become affable, adept communicators expressing inspired emotional intelligence.

Two themes run throughout this chapter. The first is the importance of setting milestones for residents and measuring their accomplishments against those objectives. Before they leave the residency program, each resident should have the knowledge and skills necessary to practice safely and effectively, as well as a lifelong commitment to learning.

Appendix A

Examples of Clinical Service Objectives

1. Surgical Critical Care (SCC): Ventilator Management
2. Alimentary Tract—GERD
3. Trauma

Surgical Critical Care (SCC): Ventilator Management

Postgraduate Year (PGY) Level	Objectives for Ventilator Management	Measurement
PGY1	1. List three (3) different ventilator modes. 2. Identify a common use for each mode.	1. Pre- and post-test for these knowledge objectives
PGY2	1. List indications for ventilator support. 2. Describe the assessment for possible weaning from mechanical ventilation.	1. Pre- and post-test 2. Clinical rounds based on rotation evaluations
PGY3	1. Demonstrate a set of ventilator settings for a 70 kg patient who was just intubated for hypoxemia. 2. Choose two (2) methods to increase oxygenation in a ventilated patient. 3. Describe effect of PEEP during mechanical ventilation.	1. Posttests/quizzes 2. Clinical rounds based on rotation evaluations 3. Case conference participation including presentation which should be kept in personal folio
PGY4	1. Illustrate steps to manage progressive hypoxemia while on mechanical ventilation. 2. Describe rescue methods of ventilation for an ARDS patient.	1. Clinical rounds based on rotation evaluations 2. Case conference participation including presentation which should be kept in personal folio 3. Number and quality of presentations if an ICU rotation part of curriculum
PGY5	1. Describe barotrauma and volutrauma as related to mechanical ventilation. 2. Explain the difference between a pressure and volume mode of ventilation.	1. Clinical rounds based on rotation evaluations 2. Case conference participation including presentations which should be kept in personal folio

Alimentary Tract—GERD

PGY Level	Objectives	Measurement
PGY1	1. Describe and can identify normal anatomy of the esophagus, GE junction, stomach, and vagus nerves during common operations. 2. Demonstrate knowledge of normal esophageal and gastric physiology and the pathophysiology of typical GERD. 3. Demonstrate knowledge of usual symptoms in patients with typical GERD. 4. Describe common tests used in the diagnosis of typical GERD – (pH monitoring, manometry, EGD, UGI). 5. Demonstrate knowledge to use information to develop a differential diagnosis for patients with symptoms of GERD. 6. Demonstrate basic knowledge of surgical and non-surgical treatments of patients with GERD. 7. Describe the routine postoperative course including nutritional modification. 8. Describe the steps to identify and manage simple postoperative problems (pain, fever, bleeding, hypotension, oliguria, gas-bloat, dysphagia, and so on) occurring after fundoplication.	1. Pre- and post-test for these knowledge objectives 2. Case conference presentation and clinical rounds assessment by rotation evaluations 3. Clinical performance assessed by rotation evaluations 4. Lab allowing anatomic dissections – hands-on or virtual
PGY2	1. Describe common variations in anatomy (for example, replaced left hepatic artery, accessory left hepatic artery, variations in the vagus nerves) during fundoplication. 2. Demonstrate knowledge of pathophysiology of patients with atypical GERD (for example, bile reflux). 3. Interpret common tests used in the diagnosis of GERD – (pH monitoring, manometry, EGD, UGI). 4. Describe the significance of metaplasia and dysplasia on esophageal biopsies. 5. Demonstrate ability to position a patient and identify sites for port placement during laparoscopic fundoplication. 6. Describe indications and contraindications for fundoplication. 7. Articulate the steps of a typical 360° fundoplication. 8. Describe the evaluation of complex postoperative problems (such as, esophageal perforation).	1. Pre- and post-test 2. Case conference presentation and clinical rounds assessment by rotation evaluations 3. Clinical performance assessed by rotation evaluations 4. Lab allowing anatomic dissections – hands-on or virtual 5. Simulation lab for endoscopic skills
PGY3	1. Identify normal anatomy and variations during fundoplication. 2. Demonstrate knowledge of the impact of patient factors on pathophysiology and the treatment of patients with GERD. 3. Describe the indications and technique for esophageal biopsy. 4. Describe the management of patients with metaplasia (Barrett esophagus) and dysplasia found on esophageal biopsy. 5. Describe the management of esophageal stricture. 6. Describe the management of complex postoperative complications (such as sepsis, esophageal perforation).	1. Pre- and post-test 2. Case conference participation including presentations which should be kept in personal folio 3. Clinical performance assessed by rotation evaluations 4. Lab allowing anatomic dissections – hands-on or virtual 5. Simulation lab for endoscopic skills

PGY Level	Objectives	Measurement
PGY4	1. Identify normal anatomy and variations during complex anti-reflux procedures such as revisions. 2. Describe the work-up and management of a patient with recurrent GERD symptoms after anti-reflux surgery. 3. Describe the management of patients with severe underlying medical conditions and GERD. 4. Articulate the indications for partial fundoplication. 5. Describe the techniques of diaphragmatic closure and the indications and techniques for mesh placement.	1. Pre- and post-test 2. Case conference participation including presentations which should be kept in personal folio 3. Clinical performance assessed by rotation evaluations 4. Simulation lab for endoscopic skills 5. Operative experience including procedural numbers and competency assessment
PGY5	1. Articulate the implications of varying anatomy on the steps of initial and redo anti-reflux procedures. 2. Demonstrate comprehensive knowledge of the varying patterns of disease presentation and alternative and adjuvant treatments of patients with GERD. 3. Describe in detail the steps of anti-reflux procedures and diaphragm closure including redo surgery. 4. Describe indications and techniques for esophageal lengthening. 5. Describe in detail surgery to treat esophageal perforations.	1. Pre- and post-test 2. Case conference participation including presentations which should be kept in personal folio 3. Clinical performance assessed by rotation evaluations 4. Operative experience including procedural numbers and competency assessment

Trauma

PGY Level	Objectives for Assessment of the Trauma Patient	Measurement
PGY1-2	1. Recognition of Trauma Activation Criteria – Intubation – Tube thoracostomy – IV fluid/blood resuscitation 2. Achieve sonographic skills set for FAST 3. Have basic videos of interventional procedures 4. Recognition of need for specialty consultation (for example, orthopaedics for femur fracture)	1. ATLS completion 2. Simulation lab performance 3. Achievement of skill competency in simulation lap for surgical procedures 4. Complete ultrasound course for FAST exam 5. Clinical performance assessed by rotation evaluations 6. View basic videos of procedures
PGY3-4	Recognition of need for operative intervention – Laparotomy – Thoracotomy – Vascular exploration	1. Clinical performance on rotation assessed by rotation evaluations 2. Competency assessment in simulation lab 3. Consider Advanced Trauma Operative Management (ATOM®) for assessment 4. Case conference participation including presentations which should be kept in personal folio
PGY4-5	Meet comprehensive needs of the trauma patient – Performance of operative procedures (abdomen, thorax, soft tissue) – Coordinates comprehensive care with consultants – Provides care for special populations (for example, pediatric, elderly, pregnant, anticoagulated)	1. Clinical performance on rotation 2. Case conference participation including presentations which should be kept in personal folio 3. Evaluation of procedural number 4. Achievement of competency in basic operative exposures 5. Communication skills with other health care providers

Appendix B

Examples of key knowledge/learning for surgical procedures

1. Cholecystectomy for cholelithiasis
2. Sigmoid colectomy for diverticulitis
3. Herniorrhaphy for inguinal hernia

Cholecystectomy for Cholelithiasis

Normal Anatomy	• Gallbladder has four anatomic areas: fundus, body, infundibulum, and neck. • Serosa present except where it is adherent to liver. • No muscularis mucosa or submucosa. • Cystic artery (CA), usually a branch of the RHA, supplies blood supply and divides into anterior and posterior branches at the gallbladder neck. • Cystic duct (CD) drains the gallbladder into the common bile duct (CBD). It has valves (spiral valves of Heister) that are not functional but may make cannulation difficult. • Anatomic variations of the CA in relationship to the CD exist. • Anatomic variations of the CD entering the CBD exist. • The CD and the extrahepatic biliary system include the right and left bile duct system draining into the CBD. • The CBD terminates at the Sphincter of Oddi in the 2nd portion of the duodenum.
Physiology/Pathophysiology	• The liver produces 500-1000 mL of bile daily in response to neurogenic, humoral, and chemical stimuli. • The gallbladder stores bile and delivers it to the duodenum after a meal or other stimuli. Cholecystokinin (CCK) is the main stimulus to gallbladder emptying. • Stones form when the bile is supersaturated especially with cholesterol. • Cholesterol stones (80 percent) are most common in Western countries. They are radiolucent, soft, and multi-faceted. • Pigment stones (20 percent) can also form and are composed of calcium bilirubinate. They are small, brittle, and spiculated. They often occur in patients with hemolytic disorders.
Causes, risk factors, epidemiology	• Gallbladder disease is most associated with gallstones. • Obstruction by a stone in the cystic duct is the usual cause. • Uncontrollable risk factors include age, race, gender, and family history. • Controllable risk factors include diet, obesity, and medications. • Native Americans and Mexican Americans have a very high risk of cholelithiasis.
Describe/elicit presenting signs/symptoms and development a differential diagnosis list	• The most consistent symptoms are right upper quadrant (RUQ) pain. • Nausea and vomiting also may be present, and all symptoms can be elicited by a fatty meal. • Fever is present with acute cholecystitis. • Because upper abdominal pain is common, a differential diagnosis must include inflammatory changes in the stomach, liver, and pancreas. • Some pain profiles will also mimic myocardial conditions and even pneumonia.
Identify/ describe physical exam findings	• Pain is usually in the RUQ, but can also be epigastric and radiating to the back. • A Murphy sign may also be present. • Jaundice is rarely apparent with a diagnosis of biliary colic or cholecystitis.
Describe pertinent laboratory tests needed	• Biliary colic from chronic cholelithiasis is associated with normal labs. • Acute cholecystitis is associated with a leukocytosis, bilirubin elevation (usually < 4 mg/mL), and mild elevation in alkaline phosphatase and transaminases.
Describe indications/ contraindications for imaging studies	• Ultrasound examination of the gallbladder is the imaging study of choice. • In certain cases biliary radionuclide scanning (HIDA) may help in unusual cases. • CT scanning is not helpful.

Describe operative treatment options; essential steps	• Cholecystectomy is indicated for biliary colic and acute cholecystitis; laparoscopic procedure is preferred. • Perioperative antibiotics given for acute cholecystitis, but not necessary for biliary colic diagnosis. • Tube cholecystostomy may be necessary in severe cases or in critically ill patients. Essential steps: • Identifying the critical view of safety before dividing the CA and CD. • Dissecting in the plane between the serosa of the GB and the GB wall. This should be done avoiding injury to the GB and bile spillage. • A cholangiogram may be done if there are risk factors for CBD stones or anatomy is confusing.
Describe nonoperative treatment options	• No appropriate nonoperative options exist.
Common complications	• Infection: Intra-abdominal abscess and surgical site infection (SSI) not common; gallbladder injury during dissection and stone soilage possibly increases risk. • Bleeding. Injury to liver bed, CA ligation fails. • Thermal injury to adjacent organs: From electronic dissection. • CBD injury: Mistaken identification of CBD with injury that can vary from minor laceration to total transection.
Pitfalls	• Misdiagnosis especially if a diagnosis of biliary dyskinesia is considered. • Indications for IOC. • Anatomic variations of CA and CD.
Assist with surgery/patient management	• Perioperative care – PGY1-5. • Surgical assistant – PGY2-3.
Perform surgery or management independently	• PGY3-5.

Sigmoid Colectomy for Diverticulitis

Normal anatomy	• Sigmoid colon is 'S'-shaped portion of the distal colon beginning at the pelvic brim and terminating at the rectum at about the S3 level. The luminal diameter is narrower than the proximal portions of colon. • Morphology and histology: The mucosa is simple columnar epithelium with goblet cells and crypts of Lieberkuhn extending to the muscularis mucosa. Deeper are the submucosa and the muscularis propria consisting of circular inner layer and longitudinal layer divided into 3 distinct bands, teniae coli – one located on the mesenteric portion and two on the anti-mesenteric portion. Fatty appendages, epiploic appendix, are found on the mesenteric side of the anti-mesenteric teniae. Most of the sigmoid and mesentery are enveloped by a thin layer of visceral peritoneum. • Blood supply: Sigmoid branches of the inferior mesenteric artery are contained within the mesentery. Marginal branches course around the colon circumference and penetrate the colon wall at the mesenteric sides of the taenia. • Relationship to other structures: Bladder, ureters, iliac vessels, uterus, tubes and ovaries, vagina, small bowel, psoas muscle, and abdominal wall.
Physiology/ Pathophysiology	• The sigmoid contracts to propel stool to the rectum. It has no absorptive function of consequence. • Contraction leads to high pressures over time that can lead to hypertrophy of muscularis which in turn can lead to the narrowing of the lumen and higher pressures that cause herniation of the mucosa and submucosa (false diverticulum) through defects at the sites of the penetrating vessels along the teniae. • True versus false diverticula. Ninety-five percent (95%) of false diverticula are in the sigmoid colon and account for most cases of diverticulitis. • Microscopic perforations usually enclosed by epiploic appendix or sigmoid mesentery which can lead to pericolonic inflammation, phlegmon, abscess formation, free perforation with generalized peritonitis, and/or fecal peritonitis. • Hinchey classification of severity. • Fistulae – colovesical, colovaginal, and colocutaneous. • Obstruction – large or small bowel, ureteral.
Causes, risk factors, epidemiology	• Incidence increases with age. • Low-fiber diet high in animal fat. • Obesity. • Smoking. • Medications – steroids, opioids, and NSAIDS. • Routine vigorous exercise may decrease risk.
Describe/elicit presenting signs/ symptoms and development a differential diagnosis list	• Persistent lower abdominal or left lower quadrant pain, may be associated with nausea or vomiting. • Fever. • History of constipation and occasionally mild diarrhea (paradoxical). • More severe cases with general abdominal pain and occasional distention. • Differential – ureteral stone, urinary tract infection (UTI), ischemic colitis, inflammatory bowel disease, irritable bowel disease, appendicitis, ovarian pathology, PID, and colon cancer.
Identify/ describe physical exam findings	• Simple disease with normal temperature or mild fever. • Left lower quadrant tenderness, local.
Describe pertinent laboratory tests needed	• CBC and differential. • Urinary analysis (UA). • Other tests may be needed depending on patient's comorbidities.
Describe indications-contraindications for imaging studies	• CT scan with IV contrast should be done in most cases.

Describe operative treatment options; essential steps	• Resection with primary anastomosis with or without diverting ileostomy for recurrent diverticulitis that is quiescent, chronic colovesical or colovaginal fistula, and for patients with more severe disease but without significant patient risk factors or vascular instability. • Hartmann procedure for severe disease. • Drainage with diverting colostomy for severe cases where resection is deemed unsafe. • Laparoscopic versus open. Essential steps: • Preoperative marking for stoma. • Positioning on the table. • Foley catheter. • Skin prep including vaginal prep when needed. • Mobilization of sigmoid. • Identifying sigmoid rectum junction. • Identifying optimal proximal resection line. • Protecting ureters and other structures such as use of ureteral stents, intraoperative identification of ureters. • Mobilization of left colon for tension-free anastomosis or colostomy including freeing the splenic flexure. • Steps in stapled and hand-sewn anastomosis. • Steps in performing end-descending colostomy. • Steps in performing diverting ileostomy.
Describe nonoperative treatment options	• Milder cases can be treated with rest, diet modification, and antibiotics. • Some abscess can be treated with percutaneous drainage in addition to rest, diet modification, and antibiotics.
Common complications	• SSI. • Deep space abscess. • Anastomotic leak if primary anastomosis performed. • Ureteral injury. • Bladder injury. • Bleeding from iliac and mesenteric vessels, spleen capsule. • Enterostomy.
Pitfalls	• Extensive inflammation making dissection difficult with risk to injuring adjacent structures. • Failure to adequately identify and preserve ureters. • Failure to resect to rectum and to normal proximal colon to remove all high-pressure zone. • Failure to mobilize proximal colon sufficiently for tension-free anastomosis or stoma. • Potential for splenic injury when mobilizing flexure.
Assist with surgery/ patient management	• Perioperative care – PGY1-5. • Surgical first assistant – PGY2-3.
Perform surgery or manage independently	• Resident has demonstrated sufficient knowledge, clinical skills, and operative technical skill under supervision.

Herniorrhaphy for Inguinal Hernia

Normal anatomy	• Inguinal canal is defined by a posterior floor that is formed by the transversalis fascia, anteriorly by the external oblique aponeurosis, inferiorly by the inguinal and lacunar ligaments, and superiorly by the internal oblique and transversalis abdominus muscles and aponeuroses. • In men, the inguinal canal contains the spermatic cord which consists of the vas deferens, the testicular artery, the cremasteric artery, the ilioinguinal nerve, the genital branch of the genitofemoral nerve, the pampiniform plexus of veins, and the cremaster muscle. • In women, the inguinal canal contains the round ligament of the uterus. • The external iliac vessels lie posterior to the inguinal floor.
Physiology/ Pathophysiology	• An inguinal hernia protrudes through the inguinal floor. A direct hernia protrudes through floor medial to the inferior epigastric vessels. An indirect hernia represents embryonic failure of closure of the processus vaginalis and is found lateral to the inferior epigastric vessels. The sigmoid contracts to propel stool to the rectum. It has no absorptive function of consequence. • Contraction leads to high pressures over time that can lead to hypertrophy of muscularis, which in turn can lead to narrowing of the lumen and higher pressures that cause herniation of the mucosa and submucosa (false diverticulum) through defects at the sites of the penetrating vessels along the teniae. • True versus false diverticula. Ninety-five percent (95%) of false diverticula are in the sigmoid colon and account for most cases of diverticulitis. • Microscopic perforations usually enclosed by epiploic appendix or sigmoid mesentery which can lead to pericolonic inflammation, phlegmon, abscess formation, free perforation with generalized peritonitis, and/or fecal peritonitis. • Hinchey classification of severity. • Fistulae – colovesical, colovaginal, and colocutaneous. • Obstruction – large or small bowel, ureteral.
Causes, risk factors, epidemiology	• More common in males. • Connective tissue disorders. • Increased intra-abdominal pressure: chronic cough, ascites, and peritoneal dialysis. • Obesity. • Smoking.
Describe/elicit presenting signs/ symptoms and development a differential diagnosis list	• Groin bulge. • Often associated with lifting or straining. • May be intermittent and reduce spontaneously or with active effort. • Differential – abscess, lymph node, and muscle strain.
Identify/ describe physical exam findings	• Inspection of groin for bulge, may change in size with cough or Valsalva. • Palpable bulge on palpation of the inguinal canal. May be elicited by cough or Valsalva.
Describe pertinent laboratory tests needed	• Diagnosis can usually be made by physical exam.
Describe indications-contraindications for imaging studies	• CT may help exclude the diagnosis in a patient with an unconvincing exam. Imaging rarely necessary in patient with hernia on exam.

Describe operative treatment options; essential steps	• Inguinal herniorrhaphy may be performed open (anterior approach) or laparoscopically or robotically (via extraperitonal or transabdominal preperitoneal approach). Essential steps: • Positioning on the table. • Foley catheter. • Skin prep including scrotal prep when needed. • Dissection through external oblique aponeurosis into inguinal canal. • Identify and protect or divide ilioinguinal nerve. • Identify hernia sack, typically anteromedial to the spermatic cord. • Safely reduce sack and its contents. • Repair inguinal floor, with or without mesh. • Close inguinal canal (anterior approach).
Describe nonoperative treatment options	• Minimally symptomatic cases can be treated nonoperatively with patient instructed about potential need to seek care urgently in the case of hernia incarceration. • Patients who are poor operative risks or have chronically elevated intra-abdominal pressure may be considered for nonoperative management.
Common complications	• Ilioinguinal nerve injury. • Groin/scrotum hematoma. • Testicular artery injury necessitating orchiectomy. • Recurrence. • Inguinodynia. • SSI.
Pitfalls	• Injury to hernia sack contents. • Failure to identify ilioinguinal nerve with ligation causing inguinodynia. • Complex hernias – sliding hernia, pantaloon hernia, and recurrent hernia. • Failure to place mesh tacks correctly (laparoscopic or robotic approach) resulting in chronic pain. • Failure to obtain hemostasis resulting in postoperative hematoma.
Assist with surgery/ patient management	• Perioperative care – PGY1-5. • Surgical first assistant – PGY1-3.
Perform surgery or management independently	• Resident has demonstrated sufficient knowledge, clinical skills, and operative technical skill under supervision.

Appendix C

Core Operative Procedures as Listed in ABS SCORE Curriculum
Including Resident Expectations
Accessed July 2020

Category #	Patient Care Category	Type	Level	Patient Care Topic	Describe operative treatment options	Assist with surgery/ Patient management	Perform surgery/ Manage independently
1	Abdomen - General	Operation/ Procedure	Core	Abdominal Exploration	X	X	X
1	Abdomen - General	Operation/ Procedure	Core	Peritoneal Dialysis Catheter Insertion	X	X	X
2	Abdomen - Hernia	Operation/ Procedure	Core	Diaphragmatic Hernia - Repair	X	X	X
2	Abdomen - Hernia	Operation/ Procedure	Core	Inguinal and Femoral Hernia - Repair	X	X	X
2	Abdomen - Hernia	Operation/ Procedure	Core	Miscellaneous Hernias - Repair	X	X	X
2	Abdomen - Hernia	Operation/ Procedure	Core	Ventral Hernia - Repair	X	X	X
3	Abdomen - Biliary	Operation/ Procedure	Core	Cholecystectomy with or without Cholangiography	X	X	X
3	Abdomen - Biliary	Operation/ Procedure	Core	Cholecystostomy	X	X	X
3	Abdomen - Biliary	Operation/ Procedure	Core	Choledochoenteric Anastomosis	X	X	X
3	Abdomen - Biliary	Operation/ Procedure	Core	Common Bile Duct Exploration and Choledochoscopy	X	X	X
4	Abdomen - Liver	Operation/ Procedure	Core	Hepatic Abscess - Drainage	X	X	X
4	Abdomen - Liver	Operation/ Procedure	Core	Hepatic Biopsy	X	X	X
5	Abdomen - Pancreas	Operation/ Procedure	Core	Pancreatectomy - Distal	X	X	X
5	Abdomen - Pancreas	Operation/ Procedure	Core	Pancreatic Debridement	X	X	X
5	Abdomen - Pancreas	Operation/ Procedure	Core	Pancreatic Pseudocyst - Drainage	X	X	X
6	Abdomen - Spleen	Operation/ Procedure	Core	Splenectomy	X	X	X
7	Alimentary Tract - Esophagus	Operation/ Procedure	Core	Anti-reflux Procedures	X	X	X

Category #	Patient Care Category	Type	Level	Patient Care Topic	Describe operative treatment options	Assist with surgery/ Patient management	Perform surgery/ Manage independently
8	Alimentary Tract - Stomach	Operation/ Procedure	Core	Gastrectomy - Partial/total	X	X	X
8	Alimentary Tract - Stomach	Operation/ Procedure	Core	Gastroduodenal Perforation - Repair	X	X	X
8	Alimentary Tract - Stomach	Operation/ Procedure	Core	Gastrostomy	X	X	X
8	Alimentary Tract - Stomach	Operation/ Procedure	Core	Vagotomy and Drainage	X	X	X
9	Alimentary Tract - Small Intestine	Operation/ Procedure	Core	Adhesiolysis	X	X	X
9	Alimentary Tract - Small Intestine	Operation/ Procedure	Core	Ileostomy and ileostomy Closure	X	X	X
9	Alimentary Tract - Small Intestine	Operation/ Procedure	Core	Small Intestinal Resection	X	X	X
10	Alimentary Tract - Large Intestine	Operation/ Procedure	Core	Appendectomy	X	X	X
10	Alimentary Tract - Large Intestine	Operation/ Procedure	Core	Colectomy - Partial	X	X	X
10	Alimentary Tract - Large Intestine	Operation/ Procedure	Core	Colectomy - Total and Subtotal	X	X	X
10	Alimentary Tract - Large Intestine	Operation/ Procedure	Core	Colostomy and Colostomy Closure	X	X	X
11	Alimentary Tract - Anorectal	Operation/ Procedure	Core	Anal Sphincterotomy	X	X	X
11	Alimentary Tract - Anorectal	Operation/ Procedure	Core	Anorectal Abscess - Drainage	X	X	X
11	Alimentary Tract - Anorectal	Operation/ Procedure	Core	Anorectal Fistula - Repair	X	X	X
11	Alimentary Tract - Anorectal	Operation/ Procedure	Core	Hemorrhoids - Management	X	X	X
11	Alimentary Tract - Anorectal	Operation/ Procedure	Core	Perianal Condylomas - Excision	X	X	X
12	Endoscopy	Operation/ Procedure	Core	Bronchoscopy and Bronchoalveolar Lavage	X	X	X

Category #	Patient Care Category	Type	Level	Patient Care Topic	Describe operative treatment options	Assist with surgery/ Patient management	Perform surgery/ Manage independently
12	Endoscopy	Operation/ Procedure	Core	Esophagogastroduodenoscopy	X	X	X
12	Endoscopy	Operation/ Procedure	Core	Lower GI Endoscopy	X	X	X
13	Breast	Operation/ Procedure	Core	Axillary Sentinel Lymph Node Biopsy and Lymphadenectomy	X	X	X
13	Breast	Operation/ Procedure	Core	Duct Excision	X	X	X
13	Breast	Operation/ Procedure	Core	Excisional Breast Biopsy and Partial Mastectomy	X	X	X
13	Breast	Operation/ Procedure	Core	Mastectomy - Simple, Modified Radical, and Radical	X	X	X
13	Breast	Operation/ Procedure	Core	Percutaneous Breast Biopsy and Cyst Aspiration	X	X	X
15	Skin and Soft Tissue	Operation/ Procedure	Core	Melanoma - Wide Excision	X	X	X
15	Skin and Soft Tissue	Operation/ Procedure	Core	Pilonidal Cystectomy	X	X	X
15	Skin and Soft Tissue	Operation/ Procedure	Core	Sentinel Lymph Node Biopsy for Melanoma	X	X	X
15	Skin and Soft Tissue	Operation/ Procedure	Core	Skin/Soft Tissue Lesions - Excisional and Incisional Biopsy	X	X	X
15	Skin and Soft Tissue	Operation/ Procedure	Core	Soft Tissue Infections - Incision, Drainage, Debridement	X	X	X
16	Surgical Critical Care	Operation/ Procedure	Core	Intubation and Difficult Airway	X	X	X
16	Surgical Critical Care	Operation/ Procedure	Core	Nutritional Support	X	X	X
16	Surgical Critical Care	Operation/ Procedure	Core	Ultrasound Use for Intravascular Access	X	X	X
16	Surgical Critical Care	Operation/ Procedure	Core	Vascular Access	X	X	X
17	Trauma	Operation/ Procedure	Core	Abdominal Exploration for Trauma	X	X	X
17	Trauma	Operation/ Procedure	Core	Cardiac Injury - Repair	X	X	X
17	Trauma	Operation/ Procedure	Core	Duodenal and Pancreatic Injury - Operations	X	X	X
17	Trauma	Operation/ Procedure	Core	Esophageal Injury - Repair	X	X	X

Category #	Patient Care Category	Type	Level	Patient Care Topic	Describe operative treatment options	Assist with surgery/ Patient management	Perform surgery/ Manage independently
17	Trauma	Operation/ Procedure	Core	Fasciotomy	X	X	X
17	Trauma	Operation/ Procedure	Core	Focused Assessment with Sonography for Trauma (FAST)	X	X	X
17	Trauma	Operation/ Procedure	Core	Gastrointestinal Tract Injury - Repair	X	X	X
17	Trauma	Operation/ Procedure	Core	Hepatic Injury - Packing and Repair/Resection	X	X	X
17	Trauma	Operation/ Procedure	Core	Neck Injuries - Management	X	X	X
17	Trauma	Operation/ Procedure	Core	Splenectomy/ Splenorrhaphy	X	X	X
17	Trauma	Operation/ Procedure	Core	Urinary Tract Injuries - Operations	X	X	X
17	Trauma	Operation/ Procedure	Core	Vascular Injuries - Operations	X	X	X
17	Trauma	Operation/ Procedure	Core	Wounds, Major - Debride/ Suture	X	X	X
18	Vascular - Arterial Disease	Operation/ Procedure	Core	Amputations - Lower Extremity	X	X	X
18	Vascular - Arterial Disease	Operation/ Procedure	Core	Embolectomy/ Thrombectomy - Arterial	X	X	X
18	Vascular - Arterial Disease	Operation/ Procedure	Core	Lower Extremity Bypass	X	X	X
19	Vascular - Venous	Operation/ Procedure	Core	Vena Cava Filter Insertion	X	X	X
19	Vascular - Venous	Operation/ Procedure	Core	Venous Insufficiency/Varicose Veins - Operation	X	X	X
20	Vascular - Access	Operation/ Procedure	Core	Arteriovenous Graft/Fistula	X	X	X
20	Vascular - Access	Operation/ Procedure	Core	Vascular Exposure - Principles	X	X	X
20	Vascular - Access	Operation/ Procedure	Core	Venous Access Devices - Insertion	X	X	X
22	Thoracic Surgery	Operation/ Procedure	Core	Exploratory Thoracotomy - Open and Thoracoscopic	X	X	X
22	Thoracic Surgery	Operation/ Procedure	Core	Partial Pulmonary Resections - Open and Thoracoscopic	X	X	X
22	Thoracic Surgery	Operation/ Procedure	Core	Tube Thoracostomy and Thoracentesis	X	X	X

Category #	Patient Care Category	Type	Level	Patient Care Topic	Describe operative treatment options	Assist with surgery/ Patient management	Perform surgery/ Manage independently
23	Pediatric Surgery	Operation/ Procedure	Core	Inguinal Hernia - Repair	X	X	X
23	Pediatric Surgery	Operation/ Procedure	Core	Intussusception - Operation	X	X	X
23	Pediatric Surgery	Operation/ Procedure	Core	Malrotation - Operation	X	X	X
23	Pediatric Surgery	Operation/ Procedure	Core	Meckel's Diverticulum - Excision	X	X	X
23	Pediatric Surgery	Operation/ Procedure	Core	Pyloromyotomy	X	X	X
23	Pediatric Surgery	Operation/ Procedure	Core	Umbilical Hernia - Repair	X	X	X
24	Plastic Surgery	Operation/ Procedure	Core	Complex Wound Closure	X	X	X
24	Plastic Surgery	Operation/ Procedure	Core	Skin Grafting	X	X	X
25	Genitourinary	Operation/ Procedure	Core	Cystostomy	X	X	X
25	Genitourinary	Operation/ Procedure	Core	Nephrectomy	X	X	X
26	Gynecology and Obstetrics	Operation/ Procedure	Core	Hysterectomy and Salpingo-Oophorectomy	X	X	X
26	Gynecology and Obstetrics	Operation/ Procedure	Core	Surgical Considerations of the Pregnant Patient	X	X	X
27	Head and Neck	Operation/ Procedure	Core	Lymph Node Biopsy	X	X	X
27	Head and Neck	Operation/ Procedure	Core	Tracheostomy	X	X	X

Advanced Operative Procedures as Listed in ABS SCORE Curriculum Including Resident Expectations Accessed July 2020

Category #	Patient Care Category	Type	Level	Patient Care Topic	Describe operative treatment options	Assist with surgery/ Patient management	Perform surgery/ Manage independently
3	Abdomen - Biliary	Operation/ Procedure	Advanced	Bile Duct Cancer - Operation	X	X	
3	Abdomen - Biliary	Operation/ Procedure	Advanced	Bile Duct Injury, Iatrogenic - Acute Repair	X	X	
3	Abdomen - Biliary	Operation/ Procedure	Advanced	Bile Duct Neoplasms - Operation	X	X	
3	Abdomen - Biliary	Operation/ Procedure	Advanced	Gallbladder Cancer - Operation	X	X	
3	Abdomen - Biliary	Operation/ Procedure	Advanced	Ultrasound of the Biliary Tree	X	X	
4	Abdomen - Liver	Operation/ Procedure	Advanced	Hepatic Ultrasound - Intraoperative	X	X	
4	Abdomen - Liver	Operation/ Procedure	Advanced	Segmentectomy/Lobectomy	X	X	
5	Abdomen - Pancreas	Operation/ Procedure	Advanced	Ampullary Resection for Tumor	X	X	
5	Abdomen - Pancreas	Operation/ Procedure	Advanced	Pancreatectomy - Total	X	X	
5	Abdomen - Pancreas	Operation/ Procedure	Advanced	Pancreatic Ultrasound - Intraoperative	X	X	
5	Abdomen - Pancreas	Operation/ Procedure	Advanced	Pancreaticoduodenectomy	X	X	
5	Abdomen - Pancreas	Operation/ Procedure	Advanced	Pancreatitis, Chronic - Operative Management	X	X	
7	Alimentary Tract - Esophagus	Operation/ Procedure	Advanced	Cricopharyngeal Myotomy with Zenker Diverticulum - Excision	X	X	
7	Alimentary Tract - Esophagus	Operation/ Procedure	Advanced	Esophageal Perforation - Repair/Resection	X	X	
7	Alimentary Tract - Esophagus	Operation/ Procedure	Advanced	Esophagectomy/ Esophagogastrectomy	X	X	
7	Alimentary Tract - Esophagus	Operation/ Procedure	Advanced	Esophagomyotomy (Heller)	X	X	

Category #	Patient Care Category	Type	Level	Patient Care Topic	Describe operative treatment options	Assist with surgery/ Patient management	Perform surgery/ Manage independently
7	Alimentary Tract - Esophagus	Operation/ Procedure	Advanced	Paraesophageal Hernia - Repair	X	X	
8	Alimentary Tract - Stomach	Operation/ Procedure	Advanced	Morbid Obesity - Operation	X	X	
8	Alimentary Tract - Stomach	Operation/ Procedure	Advanced	Postgastrectomy Syndromes - Revisional Procedures	X	X	
11	Alimentary Tract - Anorectal	Operation/ Procedure	Advanced	Anal Cancer - Excision	X	X	
11	Alimentary Tract - Anorectal	Operation/ Procedure	Advanced	Rectal Cancer - Abdominoperineal Resection and Pelvic Exenteration	X	X	
11	Alimentary Tract - Anorectal	Operation/ Procedure	Advanced	Rectal Cancer - Transanal Resection	X	X	
11	Alimentary Tract - Anorectal	Operation/ Procedure	Advanced	Rectal Prolapse - Repair	X	X	
14	Endocrine	Operation/ Procedure	Advanced	Adrenalectomy	X	X	
14	Endocrine	Operation/ Procedure	Advanced	Ultrasound of the Thyroid	X	X	
15	Skin and Soft Tissue	Operation/ Procedure	Advanced	Ilioinguinal-Femoral Lymphadenectomy	X	X	
15	Skin and Soft Tissue	Operation/ Procedure	Advanced	Soft Tissue Sarcoma - Resection	X	X	
16	Surgical Critical Care	Operation/ Procedure	Advanced	Noninvasive and Invasive Cardiac Pacing	X	X	
17	Trauma	Operation/ Procedure	Advanced	Hand Tendon Repairs	X	X	
17	Trauma	Operation/ Procedure	Advanced	Thermal Injuries - Operations	X	X	
18	Vascular - Arterial Disease	Operation/ Procedure	Advanced	Abdominal and Aortoiliac Aneurysm - Repair	X	X	
18	Vascular - Arterial Disease	Operation/ Procedure	Advanced	Aortoiliac Reconstruction for Occlusive Disease	X	X	
18	Vascular - Arterial Disease	Operation/ Procedure	Advanced	Carotid Endarterectomy	X	X	

Category #	Patient Care Category	Type	Level	Patient Care Topic	Describe operative treatment options	Assist with surgery/ Patient management	Perform surgery/ Manage independently
18	Vascular - Arterial Disease	Operation/ Procedure	Advanced	Endovascular Intervention Principles	X	X	
18	Vascular - Arterial Disease	Operation/ Procedure	Advanced	Extra-Anatomic Bypass	X	X	
18	Vascular - Arterial Disease	Operation/ Procedure	Advanced	Graft-Enteric Fistula - Management	X	X	
18	Vascular - Arterial Disease	Operation/ Procedure	Advanced	Mesenteric Occlusive Disease - Operation	X	X	
18	Vascular - Arterial Disease	Operation/ Procedure	Advanced	Peripheral Aneurysms - Repair	X	X	
18	Vascular - Arterial Disease	Operation/ Procedure	Advanced	Superior Mesenteric Artery Embolectomy/ Thrombectomy	X	X	
18	Vascular - Arterial Disease	Operation/ Procedure	Advanced	Ultrasound in the Diagnosis and Management of Vascular Diseases	X	X	
21	Transplantation	Operation/ Procedure	Advanced	En Bloc Abdominal Organ Retrieval	X	X	
21	Transplantation	Operation/ Procedure	Advanced	Live Donor Hepatectomy	X	X	
21	Transplantation	Operation/ Procedure	Advanced	Live Donor Nephrectomy	X	X	
21	Transplantation	Operation/ Procedure	Advanced	Liver Transplantation	X	X	
21	Transplantation	Operation/ Procedure	Advanced	Pancreas Transplantation	X	X	
21	Transplantation	Operation/ Procedure	Advanced	Renal Transplantation	X	X	
23	Pediatric Surgery	Operation/ Procedure	Advanced	Branchial Cleft Anomaly - Excision	X	X	
23	Pediatric Surgery	Operation/ Procedure	Advanced	Chest Wall Deformity - Repair	X	X	
23	Pediatric Surgery	Operation/ Procedure	Advanced	Diaphragmatic Hernia - Repair	X	X	
23	Pediatric Surgery	Operation/ Procedure	Advanced	Esophageal Atresia/ Tracheoesophageal Fistula - Repair	X	X	
23	Pediatric Surgery	Operation/ Procedure	Advanced	Gastroschisis/ Omphalocele - Repair	X	X	
23	Pediatric Surgery	Operation/ Procedure	Advanced	Hirschsprung's Disease - Operation	X	X	

Category #	Patient Care Category	Type	Level	Patient Care Topic	Describe operative treatment options	Assist with surgery/ Patient management	Perform surgery/ Manage independently
23	Pediatric Surgery	Operation/ Procedure	Advanced	Imperforate Anus - Operation	X	X	
23	Pediatric Surgery	Operation/ Procedure	Advanced	Intestinal Atresia/Stenosis - Repair	X	X	
23	Pediatric Surgery	Operation/ Procedure	Advanced	Meconium Ileus - Operation	X	X	
23	Pediatric Surgery	Operation/ Procedure	Advanced	Necrotizing Enterocolitis - Operation	X	X	
23	Pediatric Surgery	Operation/ Procedure	Advanced	Orchiopexy	X	X	
23	Pediatric Surgery	Operation/ Procedure	Advanced	Thyroglossal Duct Cyst - Excision	X	X	
26	Gynecology and Obstetrics	Operation/ Procedure	Advanced	Cesarean Section	X	X	
27	Head and Neck	Operation/ Procedure	Advanced	Modified Neck Dissection	X	X	
27	Head and Neck	Operation/ Procedure	Advanced	Parotidectomy	X	X	

Appendix D

American College of Surgeons Online Videos

More than 2,000 videos are available in a wide selection of body system and procedure type, and new videos are added each year.

The library contains the following categories of videos:

- Bariatric Surgery
- Cardiothoracic Surgery
- Challenging and Unusual Problems in Surgery
- Colon and Rectal Surgery
- Endocrine Surgery
- General Surgery
- Hepatobiliary Surgery
- Hernia Surgery
- Highlights from International Meetings
- Neurological Surgery
- Obstetrics and Gynecology
- Orthopaedic Surgery
- Otolaryngology–Head and Neck Surgery
- Pancreas Surgery
- Pediatric Surgery
- Surgical History
- Trauma Surgery
- Urologic Surgery
- Vascular Surgery

Appendix E

ACS Multimedia Atlas of Surgery Volumes
Expert surgeons provide detailed, step-by-step instruction using a combination of video, illustration, and intraoperative photos to clarify specific points of each procedure.

Bariatric Surgery Volume

- A comprehensive, atlas-style text, this volume includes 48 chapters presenting open and laparoscopic surgical techniques for treating bariatric disorders.

Liver Surgery Volume

- A comprehensive, atlas-style text, this volume includes 41 chapters presenting hepatobiliary repair techniques using open and laparoscopic methods.

Pancreas Surgery Volume

- A comprehensive, atlas-style text, this volume includes 36 chapters presenting both open and laparoscopic surgical techniques for treating pancreatic disease states.

Hernia Surgery Volume

- A comprehensive, atlas-style text, this volume includes 28 chapters presenting hernia repair techniques using open and laparoscopic methods.

Colorectal Surgery Volume

- A comprehensive, atlas-style text, this volume includes 26 chapters presenting open and laparoscopic surgical techniques for treating colorectal disorders.

Suggested Readings

Accreditation Council for Graduate Medical Education. Surgery Milestones. Available at: www.acgme.org/Portals/0/PDFs/Milestones/SurgeryMilestones.pdf. 2019.

American College of Surgeons. Task Force on Professionalism. Code of Professional Conduct. *J Am Coll Surg*. 2004;199(5):734-735.

Aryal KR, Pereira J. E learning in surgery. *Indian J Surg*. 2014;76(6):487-493.

Barry L, Blair PG, Cosgrove EM, et al. One year, and counting, after publication of our ACS "Code of Professional Conduct". *J Am Coll Surg*. 2004;199(5):736-740.

Cate OT. A primer on entrustable professional activities. *Korean J Med Educ*. 2018;30(1):1-10.

Cate OT. Nuts and bolts of entrustable professional activities. *J Grad Med Educ*. 2013;5(1):157-158.

Emanuel EJ. The inevitable reimagining of medical education. *JAMA*. 2020;323(12):1127-1128.

Kapadia MR, Kieran K. Being affable, available, and able is not enough: prioritizing surgeon-patient communication. *JAMA Surg*. 2020;155(4):277-278.

Lindeman B, Sarosi GA. Competency-based resident education: the United States perspective. *Surgery*. 2020;167(5):777-781.

Miloslavsky EM, Sargsyan Z, Heath JK, Kohn R, Alba GA, Gordon JA, Currier PF. Simulation Resident-as-Teacher Program. *J Hosp Med*. 2015;12;767-772.

Monday LM, Gaynier A, Berschback M, et al. Outcomes of an online virtual boot camp to prepare fourth-year medical students for a successful transition to internship. *Cureus*. 2020;12(6):e8558. Published 2020 Jun 11.

Ogbeiwi O. Why written objectives need to be really SMART. Br J Health Care Manag. 2017;23:324-336.

Redlich P, Webb T, Weigelt J. (2018). Role of protected block curriculum in surgical education. 10.5772/intechopen.72120.

Surgical Council on Resident Education. SCORE Curriculum. Available at: https://www.surgicalcore.org/.

Webb TP, Weigelt JA, Redlich PN, Anderson RC, Brasel KJ, Simpson D. Protected block curriculum enhances learning during general surgery residency training. *Arch Surg*. 2009;144(2):160-166.

AMERICAN
SURGEONS
OF SURGEONS
COLLEGE OF
AMERICAN
SURGEONS
OF SURGEONS
COLLEGE OF
AMERICAN
SURGEONS

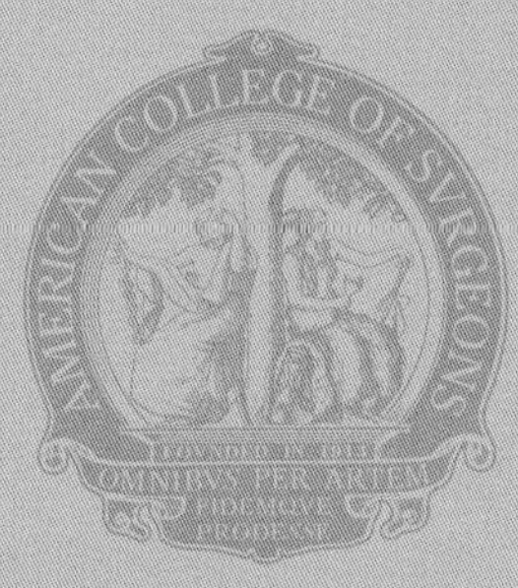

CHAPTER 5

Curriculum: Core Professional and Doctoring Skills

Lead Author

Anna M. Ledgerwood, MD, FACS

Co-Authors

Charles E. Lucas, MD, FACS

J. Wayne Meredith, MD, FACS, MCCM, MAMSE

CHAPTER 5

Curriculum: Core Professional and Doctoring Skills

Executive Summary

Foundational to surgical care is the trust a surgeon earns from the patients they serve. Gaining the trust of a patient is the premise upon which healing and surgical skills can be delivered. To be a surgeon is to be a doctor first.

What It Means to Be a Doctor

What Is a "Doctor?"
Although the term "doctor" derives from Latin and means teacher, many new definitions have evolved. A scholarly person who completes a graduate degree program and who has extensive knowledge in a specific area may be awarded the doctor of philosophy degree (PhD). The term "doctor" may be used as a verb meaning to "doctor somebody" or "treat somebody." A medical connotation of "doctor" refers to a skilled, learned professional who uses knowledge and skill to treat a patient and to teach self-care to the patient. Regardless of which definition is used in daily medical practice, the patient expects the doctor to look and behave in a professional manner and to convey concern for the patient.

Medical Doctor
The ingrained behavior required to become a professional medical doctor begins in early childhood when parents, relatives, neighbors, and teachers help to form a sense of social integration with family, neighbors, and schoolmates; it continues throughout the high school and college years. Medical schools and surgical residency programs should assess candidates for the presence of these behaviors. The surgical residency should hone these qualities as the learner adapts to the challenges of providing extraordinarily complex care to patients from many different backgrounds. The surgical faculty should lead by example and consistently display the qualities of an excellent surgeon, such as scientific knowledge, technical skill, team leadership, and emotional intelligence.

The maturation of a physician falls into three broad areas of how we learn: the affective domain, the cognitive domain, and the psychomotor domain.[1]

The Affective (Feeling) Domain

The affective domain involves feelings, emotions, and attitudes. It encompasses the physician qualities that lead to a positive relationship between physician and patient. Many aspects of the affective domain contribute to how mature surgeons should comport themselves around patients and colleagues.

First Impressions: Meeting the Patient
Physician Attire
Attire can create a lasting first impression. Societal changes over the years have changed what a physician wears while seeing patients. After World War II, male physicians would almost always wear a coat and tie and female physicians a conservative dress in the office or during hospital rounds. After weekend church services, some physicians even wore formal attire when seeing patients. Physician dress customs during patient encounters have become considerably relaxed since then. For example, some surgeons, after operating in the morning, will see their office patients in the afternoon in their surgical greens (or blues or oranges) and a white coat.

These dress code changes raise the question: What does a patient expect when being examined by a physician in the outpatient setting? The authors' experience, supported by peer-reviewed research, suggests that patients expect professional attire. A multicenter study in Japan found that physician attire influenced patient satisfaction with the care provided to them, with older patients preferring a shirt and tie with a white coat and younger patients satisfied with casual attire with a white coat.[2] A multicenter study in the U.S. found that physician attire affects patients' perception of good care and confidence in their physicians. Most patients preferred a shirt and a tie along with a white coat to surgical scrubs with a white coat.[3]

Additionally, these studies found that the patients preferred their physicians to be properly attired during hospital visits on weekends. Older patients, in particular, downgraded the wearing of surgical scrubs at any time. Patients followed in an orthopaedic clinic wanted to see their physicians properly attired and expressed that if a house officer wore surgical scrubs they should also wear a clean white coat.[4] The orthopaedic fellows in adult reconstructive surgery at the Newton Wellesley Hospital in Massachusetts are informed that: "Adult Reconstruction Fellows at NWH are expected to make rounds on patients in professional attire wearing a white lab coat. Scrubs are not appropriate attire for clinical and academic activity outside of the operating room … when fellows must leave the [operating room] OR in scrubs, white lab coats should be worn."[4]

Surgical residents follow the example set by their attending surgeon mentors. When surgical residents wear scrubs to the outpatient clinic, they should be told to change; only properly attired, surgical residents and attendings should see patients. In this way, the resident quickly learns never to wear greens to the outpatient clinic except in unusual circumstances. In addition, surgical greens or "pajamas" do not belong in the hospital cafeteria or in such places as the supermarket; they should be restricted to the preoperative holding area, the operating room, and the postoperative recovery unit.[4] A whole set of issues regarding infection control are in alignment with these recommendations as well. "Greens" should never be worn outside the operating room unless covered by a gown or white coat and only for a short time to respond to an emergency or talk to a family member after surgery. Most hospitals require those that work in areas where OR attire is permitted (ER, ICU, endoscopy suites) require a different color of scrubs to maintain the culture of infection prevention.

Although patients expect surgeons to wear what they want on surgical rounds and in the outpatient department, the clothes must be clean, neat, a proper fit, and include a clean, pressed, and unstained white coat.[2,4] Unless an unusual emergency arises, patients also expect properly groomed hair, including facial hair. Again, the attending must set an example for this, and convey that professional behavior, including proper attire, not only respects the patient but shows self-respect as well.

Mechanism for Teaching:
Faculty should define proper physician attire for new residents. Proper attire should be modeled; everyone from faculty to department and program leaders should set the tone.

Assessment:
Physician attire propriety should be regularly assessed and documented each clinical rotation throughout the training years. Proper physician attire is expected at all levels of residency training.

First Patient Encounter
Appropriately attired, the house officer is ready to meet the patient. Upon introduction, the house officer should clearly identify themselves with their name and level of training, as well as the relevant attending physician.[5] Clarify how to pronounce the patient's name as well as their age and, in a sympathetic fashion, sensitivities about marital status, gender identity, sexual orientation, and so on. This reduces the chance of making embarrassing mistakes during later presentation on attending rounds.[6]

Take a detailed patient history with the same concern for privacy as you would show for a family member. Application of the William Osler, MD, principles of a careful history and physical examination, especially one in which the patient is comfortable in conveying information, will greatly determine the success of the treatment.[7] Especially during the first encounter, professionalism means showing compassion for the patient, which in turn portrays a sense of integrity and respect for others.[8] The resident should recognize and adjust to patient idiosyncrasies.[9] Although most of the history will focus on the patient's complaint, its accuracy and value can be augmented by questions such as, "Were you sick or hospitalized for any other problems?" or "Can you tell me about any operations that you have undergone?"

The relevant data from the history and physical examination, laboratory tests, and imaging studies are critical information for the attending surgeon. The resident must have the patient history ready for the attending surgeon even in potential emergencies, such as acute appendicitis; calling the attending without this kind of information shows that the house officer is not prepared.

The Physical Examination
After taking the history, the resident does a focused physical examination guided by the patient's complaints and history. Residents should wash their hands in full view of the patient before the exam. (Although some residents may choose to wear gloves, some physicians find that gloves alter the tactile ability and prefer handwashing alone.) Ask the patient to be an active participant during the exam. When examining the abdomen, the physician might ask, "Could you pull up your gown so that I can take a look at your stomach please?" During a breast exam, the resident should cover the other breast and then ask the patient, "Could you show me exactly where you feel this bump?" Using a single bedsheet, a clean bath towel, or a combination to cover areas not under immediate examination defers to possible patient

modesty and sensitivity to exposure.[7] Preventing unnecessary body exposure and respecting the patient's privacy while conducting the physical exam can help develop a good relationship between the house officer and the patient.

Occasionally, the resident should ask a colleague of the opposite sex to be present when examining a sensitive area of the patient's body, especially if this would make the patient more comfortable. Take cues from the patient. For example, if a woman patient requests a female physician, male residents should honor the entreaty without taking offense. Likewise, a male inguinal hernia patient who seems anxious about seeing a female surgeon should be offered the opportunity to see a male surgeon. Residents should have the opportunity during office visits to learn from the attending how to maturely respond to patient needs.[9]

During the training years, emphasis is often put on being thorough, such as when conducting a full physical. However, few American surgeons do complete physical examinations once they finish medical school; for example, they rarely do fundoscopic exams or exams of the auditory canal. The emphasis should be on a "focused" physical examination based upon the historical presentation and the patient's complaint. However, a focused examination of a patient with abdominal pain should also explore the possibility that the patient may have cervical lymphadenopathy, a breast mass, or lower extremity vascular disease, all of which can be readily identified in the history. If the symptoms warrant and the patient allows, the examiner can extend the focused examination.

Some traditional or "routine" parts of the physical examination are unnecessary. For example, although the authors were taught that a rectal examination was part of a complete examination that should be performed on all injured patients, over time we have learned to question that rule. What logic is there in performing a rectal examination on a 22-year-old patient who presents with a gunshot wound to the left shoulder involving the left axillary artery? Clearly, this decision can be deferred to a more appropriate time when permission to do this invasive examination can be granted.

Studies support this call for caution. Digital rectal exams provided no additional diagnostic information in most injured patients and were useful only when specifically related to the patient's history or complaints, according to Shlamozitz and colleagues.[10] Likewise, Esposito and colleagues showed that the digital rectal exam should only be performed for specific injuries.[11]

Certainly, the rectal exam has value in some clinical situations. Shresta and colleagues reported that when performed on patients presenting with gastrointestinal bleeding, the rectal exam decreased the likelihood of prescribing unneeded medical therapy and the need for endoscopic examination. They concluded that the exam should be considered in patients with altered mental status and a history of gastrointestinal bleeding.[12] But, in general, exams, especially those that may be considered intrusive or even abusive, such as digital rectal exams or pelvic exams, should be done only for a specific clinical reason.

Mechanism for Teaching:
The aforementioned information should be part of the initial instructions provided to all new residents. They can be taught as part of standard teaching conferences and by the example shown by the attending.

Assessment:
Residents should be assessed during daily attending-resident rounds, teaching conferences, and regularly scheduled sessions in which faculty and resident assessments of each other are reviewed and documented in writing.

Decorum During Rounds

During attending rounds, when residents and students may be present, physicians should show concern and respect for patient feelings and dignity. For example, patients should not be presented as if they were lab specimens, such as, "This is a 47-year-old small bowel obstruction" or even "This 47-year-old patient presented with small bowel obstruction." Rather, they should be presented as real people with real complaints; for example, "Mrs. Smith is 47 years old, and she presented with abdominal pain, which was later determined to be caused by small bowel obstruction." Maintaining patient rapport throughout the hospitalization can establish a positive relationship between the house officer and the patient. Respect patient privacy and do not use the patient's name during a formal presentation at a teaching conference.

Mechanism for Teaching:
From the moment they enter the program, residents should learn to follow the principles of decorum and respect for diversity during patient rounds, grand rounds, presentations, and other regularly scheduled teaching sessions to help them learn how to become a "doctor."

Assessment:
Residents should be assessed for decorum and sensitivity to diversity during the resident-attending patient care and teaching rounds.

Understanding the Patient

Empathy

Residents should be concerned for a patient's psychological well-being during the stress of illness. Residents should treat all patients as though they are family members, understand and be sensitive to their sufferings, and recognize the importance of their privacy. In a word, they should have empathy—the ability to relate to another person's pain as if they themselves were experiencing it. In fact, the definition of empathy includes the concept that the physician suffers with the ill patient.[13] The compassionate, caring resident or practicing surgeon may even exceed normal patient support by doing such things as providing taxi fare when other transportation options are unavailable.

Compassion should be apparent to the patient, but it must not interfere with the needed care.[14-16] For example, sorrow for the unfortunate patient with an incurable illness should not interfere with the surgeon's technical interventions to palliate that disease. While compassionate residents want to do their best for the patient, they should develop the humility to know when their technical skills cannot effectively palliate the patient's underlying disease.

Patients treated with empathy have improved outcomes, better compliance with physician recommendations, more satisfaction with their care, better communication with the health care team, and a clearer understanding of their disease process.[17,18]

Diversity, Cultural Awareness, and Humility

Residents must be able to recognize biases related to race and gender and ensure those beliefs do not interfere with their patient relationship. This emotional intelligence or self-awareness is vital to becoming an excellent surgeon. The mature doctor needs to relate to all circumstances and must not be negatively biased by age, gender, race, region of national origin, economic status, or sexual orientation. Being cognizant of a patient's cultural background and the potential areas of vulnerability that are part of that background is an essential part of the awareness and humility that is necessary for the resident to develop a satisfactory level of emotional interchange. When these goals are accomplished, the patient care process will become easier and more effective.

To overcome potential language barriers, the resident must find someone with the necessary language skills to effectively communicate with the patient.[19] Almost all health care institutions provide immediate access to translators, in part due to federal law aimed at reducing the communication gap because of language barriers.[19] When a translator cannot completely resolve the communication problem, it may help to find an individual of the same cultural background, such as the patient's friend or family member, to help with interpretation.

Patients Accepting Their Disease

The acceptance of a complex or chronic disease follows a well-recognized pattern described for cancer patients by Kubler-Ross in the 1970s. All significant medical problems can follow this model of acceptance, which includes denial, anger, bargaining, acceptance, and depression. This is important for the physician to recognize as their reaction to, and interaction with the patient will in part be determined where the patient is in this process of acceptance. How a physician supports a patient and shows empathy will often change over time, as the perception of their disease changes over time. Understanding of this model can also help the physician understand a patient's behavior, which may change quickly from anger and frustration to resolve and/or disengagement. The skilled physician is able to use this model to demonstrate a caring attitude and anticipate a patient's needs at different times during their journey with illness.

Patient Comfort and Safety

Pain Management

Management of patient pain is another affective domain issue. The physician must warn the patient that most people who undergo a major operation will have some pain. They should acquaint the patient with multimodal pain protocols that may include opioid drugs, nonopioid drugs, nerve blocks, and so on. They also must educate the patient about the dangers of prescription pain medications, such as opioids.

The resident should explain to the patient that the goal of the pain medicine will be to take the edge off severe pain without sedating them to the point where they cannot participate in the recovery process. Over-sedation makes it difficult for the patient to perform the activities needed for recovery, such as deep breathing, coughing, and frequent walking. Likewise, the patient should know that the intelligent administration of pain medicines prevents serious complications such as adynamic ileus and urinary retention.[20]

The resident needs to teach the patient about a balanced pain management regimen designed to prevent long-term dependence on narcotics.[21] For example, patients taking opioids before a major operation are more likely to engage in prolonged opioid use after surgery,[22] and protracted use contributes to addiction and associated long-term health risks. Develop a "contract" with the patient that explains the use of narcotics and analgesia may be extended for a specific period of time if a plan is in place to transition to nonnarcotics. This concept of a contract can be highly effective by engaging the patient to achieve defined endpoints and helping him or her prepare for the transition to nonnarcotic therapy.

The recent epidemic of patients impaired or killed by opioid misuse highlights the dangers of administering excessive pain medicines.[21] In the 1990s, pain was identified as the fifth vital sign, and that helped lead to the overuse of narcotics and sedation. Pain management remains important, but alternate approaches have been developed.

Each state has developed information on narcotic use and narcotic prescriptions to help physicians identify when addicted patients seek narcotics from multiple different physicians.[20] Likewise, the medical profession has responded to the opioid crisis by identifying alternatives for effective postoperative pain management. These strategies de-emphasize the use of narcotics and, for each operative procedure, show how to limit narcotics at discharge to avoid excess medications.[22,23]

Today, pain management planning starts before the operation, is guided by multidisciplinary protocols (with anesthesiologists and geriatricians), and functions through electronic health record (EHR)-enabled tools and order sets. Smartphone applications given to patients at discharge allow them to monitor their pain medicine usage with their physician and to substantially lower their narcotic use. Similarly, it is best practice to teach patients to return unused medications to avoid excess availability. Using the information in published care plans such as the American College of Surgeons Safe and Effective Pain Management after Surgery brochure (*www.facs.org/-/media/files/education/patient-ed/safe_pain_control_adult.ashx*) can assist residents as they work to implement safe and effective pain control strategies for their patients.

Mechanism for Teaching:
Attending physicians must emphasize the importance of pain management and appropriate patient education. Pain management techniques and medications should be part of daily teaching on rounds and in regular conferences. Likewise, the provision of discharge medications should be guided by hospital-developed programs that predict the average dose and duration of medicine needed for specific operations. Smartphone applications should be given to the patient at discharge to help them monitor and lower their pain medicine use with their physician. Finally, to identify patients receiving multiple narcotics prescriptions from different physician groups, the resident should be taught the necessary procedures in each state to access patient pharmaceutical records.

Assessment:
Use a written examination to assess the resident's knowledge of appropriate pain management. Every patient the resident encounters with an attending is an opportunity to discuss, co-manage, and learn optimal pain management techniques, including monitoring the patient's inhospital and discharge medicines.

Patient Safety
A physician's professional responsibility for patient safety extends beyond teaching the patient the risk/benefit ratio of a particular treatment or operation. Quality and safety are distinct and essential goals of surgical care. Patient safety aligns with the Hippocratic Oath pledge "to do no harm." Specific elements have been developed such as deliberate pauses, checklists, call outs for a hard stop to any procedure if a dangerous situation arises, and specific procedures to abate risk from known complications (for example, neuropraxia from inadequate padding, poor grounding of electrocautery units, and so on). The modern surgical procedure incorporates a series of patient safety events, which start in the preoperative holding area and occur with stepwise and sequential timeouts, end-of-procedure debriefs, and organized protocol-driven hand-offs to the post-anesthesia care unit or intensive care unit.

Throughout residency, the curriculum needs to enhance the resident's understanding of the patient's vulnerability to procedural risks. For instance, to protect the patient the resident should know the difference between bipolar and monopolar electrocoagulation and the distinction between high energy "cut" energy transfer with little lateral energy exchange and the lower energy "coagulation" with wide lateral energy transfer. Likewise, the resident must appreciate how energy transfer can "arc" and injure normal tissue when the coagulator tip is too close to an instrument, such as a clamp or retractor.

Another example of protecting the patient is to avoid electrocautery in an environment of high oxygen concentration (scalpel incision is preferred over electrical incision in this setting). This is especially true when performing an open tracheostomy on a critically ill patient who is on high oxygen concentration (greater than 60 percent oxygen). In this way, most operating room fires can be avoided.

Another safety issue relevant to both patients and care team members is the proper procedure in handling "sharps," such as needles, pins, and scalpels, to protect operating team members. The resident must learn to pass the scalpel with the blunt handle first into an appropriate receptacle with the blade facing the floor. Using blunt tip needles for closure when appropriate is another example of a safety precaution. Similarly, contaminated tissues must be passed with precision to avoid cross-contaminating the patient and/or surgical team members.

Providing the appropriate level of supervision is part of ensuring patient safety. Every day, residents at various levels perform technical procedures without direct supervision. Such procedures include placing peripheral or central lines, inserting Foley catheters, performing abdominal and thoracic ultrasound after injury, instituting diagnostic peritoneal lavage, and so on. Before granting the resident permission to independently perform such treatments, the resident should demonstrate competence to the supervising physician. This principle extends throughout training so that the attending physician knows when direct supervision is unnecessary. The types of treatment that a resident performs without direct supervision will increase with the level of training if the resident is identified as competent and awarded autonomy. This process requires that the supervising physicians have sufficient opportunity to determine the resident's competence. Thus, the program director needs to ensure resident assignments are long enough to allow the attending or supervising physician to make this assessment.

There are many other examples of how modern surgery incorporates patient safety. The basic principle is to achieve high reliability through systems-based care, transparency, teamwork, nonpunitive analysis of errors, structured tools and checklists, patient safety reports, preoccupation with failure, root-cause analysis, the examination and interpretation of registry data, and best practices, which are discussed in detail throughout the ACS *Optimal Resources in Surgical Quality and Safety* manual.

Mechanism for Teaching:
Teaching the principles of patient safety and high reliability should be conducted with the overarching intent to incorporate them into the organization's culture. To achieve this goal, efforts are driven and implemented at all levels through structured learning, often involving the use of simulation (CRM training, TeamSTEPPS, and so on), and provided by regular reinforcement at conferences and during patient care activities.

Assessment:
Assessment of resident skills in this area should be made by written examination and by intra-operative observations and simulation-based assessments.

Patient Communications

Communications with Patients, Families, and Referring Physicians

The affective domain also relates to communicating effectively with others, including patients, patient families, health care team members, and others involved in caring for the patient. "Doctor" connotes teacher; the mature physician helps educate the patient and the patient's friends and family members about the rationale for the treatment. This includes teaching the patient and family about the risk/benefit ratio of all planned interventions. The doctor should also help the patient understand the cost of care by providing information and data about treatment. The physician should fully disclose and interpret the facts relevant to the patient's condition to assist in decision-making. Such conversations help establish a relationship in which the physician and patient have confidence in each other and the information being communicated. As a result of a good relationship, the patient is less likely to bring a liability action.[24,25] The communication should be bidirectional. The physician should always be open to asking the patient if any additional facts need to be investigated.[26]

Residents must also develop mature, professional communications with the referring physician. In fact, a request for consultation is the highest honor a physician can show to another physician and should be treated with the greatest respect.

Conversations between physicians must remain professional, especially because they are often overheard by patients or other health care team members. For example, it is inappropriate for a surgical resident to report to a colleague that the intoxicated and uncooperative car crash patient was "B52'd" (a derogatory term for heavy sedation); rather, it would be better and more respectful to say that the patient required sedation and restraints.

Informed Consent

After the completion of the history, physical examination, and review of images and tests, the patient may be a candidate for operative intervention. This will require an operative consent that, like the history and physical, will focus on the procedure and its risks and benefits.[27] A formal program to teach residents how to obtain informed consent, including didactic material and role playing, can highlight the important aspects of an informed consent, according to Koller and colleagues.[28] The informed consent process documents the indications, contraindications, planned procedure, alternative forms of therapy, most common consequences, and complications of the procedure (which may include death). It should also describe the procedure's limitations.[28] The informed consent is not the paper form signed by the patient and the physician shortly before the operation, but rather the detailed discussion between the physician and the patient in the outpatient setting, which is documented in the outpatient medical record by the surgeon performing the operation (the preoperative note).[29] It should describe the planned approach, its rationale, and, if applicable, why an alternative approach is not recommended; an example might be an open versus laparoscopic surgical procedure. Handwritten diagrams are often useful for the patient and document the discussion as well. Again, this discussion does not appear on the piece of paper signed by the physician and the patient prior to going into the operating room.[29] It should occur and be documented before the day of surgery to avoid stressors that may interfere with the patient giving adequate informed consent, such as anxiety and preoperative medications. A letter should be sent to the referring physician that includes the outpatient note as part of the record of the office visit.[28,29]

The greater the magnitude of the operative procedure, the more complex the preoperative informed consent process and the higher the cognitive skill level required to conduct that process.[27] For example, a first-year resident may be capable of obtaining a meaningful informed consent for drainage of a periareolar breast abscess or a heroin injection abscess of the calf but should not be asked to obtain one for a planned pancreaticoduodenectomy.[27] Training the surgeon to become skillful at obtaining an informed consent should begin in medical school and extend through residency.

Residents must also learn to comply with hospital guidelines and health insurer requirements, which includes a documented process to ensure complete transmittal of information.[28] Physicians sometimes fall short, such as not providing adequate information regarding the risks of operation and long-term follow-up, according to McNair and colleagues. The physician needs to be proactive and thorough in providing this information, especially because patients may feel insecure asking questions about long-term follow-up and complications.[30]

Increased time must be spent to obtain informed consent from patients whose underlying disease and associated comorbidities means the procedure carries more risks and complexities.[27,28] The best way to judge morbidity and mortality objectively is by using the ACS National Surgical Quality Improvement Program (ACS NSQIP®) risk calculator. When objectively calibrated, a specific operation can be accurately assessed for risk and this information shared directly with the patient. The surgical resident must inform the patient with significant comorbidities of the risks to them of certain types of procedures, and what they might do to minimize those risks and the ACS NSQIP Surgical Risk Calculator is an excellent tool for this purpose. For example, in a patient who has cholelithiasis in association with Child's class C cirrhosis from alcohol has a greater than 25 percent risk of mortality associated with an elective cholecystectomy. This patient would be advised to adopt a very low-fat diet to reduce the risk of a gallstone obstructing the cystic duct or passing into the common duct. Similar examples may be given for many diseases normally treated by operation but not recommended if comorbidities pose unacceptable risks.

Mechanism for Teaching:
The ability of the resident to obtain an informed consent is dependent on their knowledge and technical skills relating to the procedure in question. A risk assessment done using the ACS NSQIP Surgical Risk Calculator should be part of every operation's consent process. This material may be taught during weekly conferences and supplemented by recordings of simulation exercises with patient actors. Residents at all levels need to see patients in the outpatient setting to observe the attending's informed consent discussion with a patient. Such role modeling is critical in teaching the process of obtaining an informed consent. Residents in academic institutions should be taught the differences between an informed consent for an operation and a consent to participate in a research study.

Assessment:
A resident's proficiency in obtaining an informed consent may be assessed through the use of simulation and direct observations by an attending physician or a senior resident. The frequency of using the ACS NSQIP Surgical Risk Calculator can also be measured as an objective assessment.

The Immediate Preoperative and Postoperative Periods
When a patient is scheduled for a surgical procedure, a formal outpatient discussion should include the initial patient assessment, the indication for surgery, preoperative risk factors and risk mitigation strategies, preoperative testing, preoperative anesthesia assessment, prehabilitation, and preoperative education. When the patient arrives in the preoperative holding area, the surgeon should provide safety assurance by marking the surgical site, answer last-minute questions, and help relieve the patient's stress. As an extra measure of security, the surgeon should be present as the patient goes to the OR and stand by as the patient is anesthetized.[5,31] After the operation, the surgeon should visit the patient in the recovery room before discharge or transfer to an inpatient bed.[5,31] By observing the surgeon model professionalism, the resident learns how the presence of the surgeon allays the patient's anxieties and eases the patient's transition throughout the episode of care.

Mechanism for Teaching:
Fulfilling the "doctor" role of patient support and encouragement is most efficiently taught by faculty example, including role modeling, but it also must be included in the introductory documents for new residents.

Assessment:
Assessment of these traits is best made by observing the resident during the patient transition and discussing them in regularly scheduled feedback sessions.

Avoiding Conflict and Stress

Physician-Patient Conflict
Many factors may lead to physician-patient conflict.[32] Some start with the physician, who may be experiencing feelings of "burnout" or fatigue, insecurity about responding to a patient's question, a negative bias toward the patient's disease process such as intravenous drug use, or stress from too many urgent tasks. These factors can lead to short-tempered or combative behavior and may be exacerbated by overwork and sleep deprivation. By remaining aware of these issues, the resident can avoid these internal conflicts, which are not in the patient's best interest. As role models, physicians are accountable for their behavior not only to their patients but also to their profession and position in society. No matter

the circumstances, physicians must learn to express empathy and avoid frustration with patients; this is especially true if the physician is not ready to receive or provide psychological support or lacks knowledge about their patient's underlying condition.

Other factors come from patients, such as anger about treatment, desire for drugs to feed an existing habit, or a short temper, which may lead them to lose control in encounters with physicians. Sometimes a previous difficult experience with another physician may trigger a negative encounter.[33] In such cases, the physician must stay composed, be a good listener, recognize there may be many reasons for the patient's frustrations, and assure the patient that every effort is being made to help them get better. Physicians should discuss other approaches to solving the patient's unease, including offering alternative modes of therapy. If alternatives are inappropriate, the physician should explain why a therapy that is undesirable to the patient should be continued.[9] The negative physician-patient encounter is common in patients with malignant disease;[34] in such cases, the physician who understands the stages of grief discussed previously can help gauge where the patient is in their acceptance of their illness.

Occasionally the patient is unhappy with some aspect of the physician-patient relationship. The mature physician must anticipate that a minor disagreement could rapidly escalate into a tense, heated discussion, which could, in turn, lead to a written patient complaint to the medical institution's administration or even to litigation.

To handle these situations, residents need to develop emotional intelligence. Unlike innate intelligence, emotional intelligence can be learned, enhanced, and expanded with introspection. To best serve their patients, the resident's exceptional intelligence required for admission to medical school and surgical residency must be balanced with the humility and self-awareness that is characteristic of emotional intelligence.

As residents mature, they must continue to hone their ability to handle negative interpersonal encounters. Once the young resident recognizes that a patient is upset, they should engage senior residents or attendings and tell the patient that any miscommunication or hurt was unintended. If they are unable to successfully manage the situation, the more senior resident should quickly bring the situation to the attention of the attending surgeon. The attending surgeon should show restraint, humility, and understanding of the patient's frustration and reassure the patient that all health care team members are there for the patient's welfare. In this way, the attending helps defuse a contentious patient encounter and models appropriate behavior to the resident. If the best efforts fail and the patient is left unsatisfied, the surgical team must properly and politely refer the patient to another surgeon and make the hospital administration aware of the issue.

Mechanism for Teaching:
Weekly conferences should offer typical examples of physician-patient conflict and demonstrate how physician patience, thoroughness of communication, and empathy can help reduce this type of conflict. Formal training to recognize and avoid emotional triggers that precipitate confrontational behavior should be taught and modeled in the residency program. One leader who modeled admirable self-restraint is Abraham Lincoln, who during the stresses and strains of the American Civil War would place an angry letter in a drawer for 24 hours before sending it and sometimes had to go to the balcony of the executive office to release tension before continuing to discuss a volatile issue with his cabinet. Residents should know that reduction of patient conflict is associated with reduction in malpractice lawsuits.

Assessment:
The relationship between resident and patient can be addressed on the attending-resident rounds and documented in the written assessments presented to the residents.

Avoiding Stress and Burnout
The psychological and emotional welfare of the resident can affect not only the patient relationship but also the resident's personal and professional well-being. It is important to support the resident by providing an environment that physically and emotionally protects the resident's mental equanimity. The concept of psychological safety is intrinsic to a culture that is committed to quality and is ideally suited to be a component of the surgical residency training environment.

Long hours and lack of administrative respect and support for physicians leads to depression, poor relationships with colleagues and patients, and is worsened by self-isolation, according to Kane.[35] Problems related to work hours and bureaucracy lead to burnout, family problems, increased alcohol and drug use, and even suicide. The requirement to fill out EHRs contribute to development of depression and burnout, especially when it comes as residents near the 80-hour duty-hours limit.

There must be a balance between the resident's workload, including the enjoyment of providing successful treatment to patients and nonprofessional life events. For example, residents must be taught that self-care and leading a balanced life are essential throughout their careers to help them avoid depression and burnout. Team members and the hospital administration must support the individual and ensure adequate time and authentic opportunity to have a life outside the hospital to build productive relationships and prevent burnout without guilt or shame.[36]

A decrease in job satisfaction, which often starts in residency, leads to higher absenteeism and more medical errors among physicians, according to McCary and colleagues.[33] They found no effective interventions for residency burnout if residents start to lose their sense of accomplishment and self-worth. This dilemma must be offset by a valued reward system built into residency training. Limiting residents to an 80-hour workweek has helped but is insufficient by itself.

Albrecht emphasized the importance of having a supportive team with partners who share in the work and the glory of improving patient health.[36] In the OR, establishing a safe culture through crew resource training attenuates the fear to speak up or question an action that is not in the patient's best interest. This fear detracts from an optimal learning environment and overall patient safety. Effective teamwork values each member's talents and contributions and builds enough trust to permit team members to safely admit errors and near misses and to identify and help correct inadequate performance by colleagues. The team members should view each other as family members and share equitably in monetary gain and national recognition.

The program must also provide residents access to appropriate counseling, including psychological services. Similarly, the faculty must identify changes in resident self-care, including family problems or suspicion of substance abuse, and offer appropriate interventional services.

Mechanism for Teaching:
Teaching the signs and symptoms of burnout should occur at grand rounds and in other sessions with dedicated lectures and videos. Faculty should watch for signs of burnout and encourage and reward residents for successful tasks.

Assessment:
Potential burnout may be indicated by absenteeism, poor patient support, sloppy patient care, and physician-patient conflict. These traits often reflect the resident's need for intervention.

The Cognitive (Thinking) Domain

Resident education within the cognitive domain, or the development of mental skills and acquisition of knowledge, begins long before residency training and continues throughout the physician's career. Residents must learn that excellent surgeons are committed to lifelong learning. Although the acquisition of cognitive skills often varies within a residency program, the trainee is expected to acquire the requisite knowledge at each level of training. Successful approaches to acquiring and maintaining knowledge of the medical sciences are discussed in a subsequent section of this chapter.

Individual Responsibility versus Teamwork
Increasing awareness that health care teams are essential to achieving excellent patient outcomes has led to the inclusion of teamwork and team leadership skills as essential components of learning that are necessary for surgical residents to become excellent surgeons. Sustaining excellence requires ongoing commitment to being a successful team leader and, when necessary, a dependable team member. To achieve this goal the resident must be sensitive, have high emotional intelligence skills, and understand the important contributions made by each member of the health care team. Successful teams are built upon trust; this trust implies that each member is free to contribute opinions, point out potentially dangerous situations, and implement a "hard stop" when necessary, to prevent patient harm during a patient care activity. The best team leaders foster and support this type of trust.

Medical students and residents are taught to take personal responsibility for every patient they treat. Working a patient up, mitigating their perioperative risks, performing the technical procedure, and providing the postoperative care to include critical care were all considered a professional responsibility of a well-trained surgeon. Today, the complexity of a patient's illness and the need for multidisciplinary care has created challenges that are beyond the expertise of any one person. Appreciating the value of teamwork is critical to patient-centered care and requires leadership development and team training of residents. The care of a patient includes collaborating with consultant physicians (preoperative consultation, operating room collaboration, critical care, and aftercare). In addition, the patient's family and friends, referring physician colleagues, nursing personnel, and other patient care services such as physical therapy, respiratory therapy, social work, case management, and housekeeping services are essential to the well-being of patients and makes leadership capability and teamwork skills necessary characteristics of an excellent surgeon.

The most critical relationship for residents in all patient care settings is that with nurses, a relationship that starts in medical school. Like all effective team relationships, this requires authentic trust and mutual respect. Residents need to understand that nurses provide minute-to-minute patient care and are the true source of care continuity for patients. The best source of information as residents navigate the patient care situation is often the bedside nurse who will use knowledge and past experience to help solve a problem or offer critically important suggestions. Nurses are irreplaceable in the care of surgical patients and deserve the highest respect for their knowledge and role. The resident can also learn from health care professionals who provide the adjunctive services that contribute to successful patient care; examples include learning about drug interactions from a pharmacist, gaining knowledge on planning a nutritional strategy from a dietician, learning how to care for a colostomy from the stomal therapist, or the advantages and disadvantages of various ventilatory settings from the respiratory therapist.

Residents should commit to the development of a reputation as a collaborative surgeon; their relationship with nurses will determine if they are successful. The resident who gives an order to a nurse over the telephone with the attitude that "I am the doctor" instead of going to the bedside and discussing the case with the nurse will miss an opportunity to learn; after all, an experienced nurse has many years of taking care of multiple patients.[37] By going to the patient's bedside and discussing the case with the nurse, the resident demonstrates humility, introspection, and a willingness to learn. Residents should take advantage of opportunities to help, such as setting up a patient's breakfast tray when making early-morning rounds if nurses are busy with other activities. These behaviors will quickly gain the respect of the nursing staff. Residents should be continuously aware of the fact that nurses will remember instances when nurses are asked to perform tasks that are unreasonable or unpleasant activities the resident would not do themselves; they will definitely have negative memories of residents who do not promptly answer their pages.

A resident's reputation will also be affected by how they behave in front of other hospital personnel. Housekeeping service personnel will remember a resident who removes a chest tube or changes a dressing without proper disposal. On the other hand, the surgical resident who is willing to help the other team members to provide care will be rewarded by their respect. For example, residents who help move the patient onto the operating table and stay to help move the patient back to the stretcher, will be remembered and respected by OR personnel. The resident's home during their training is the hospital. The people who deliver the mail, provide environmental services, staff the cafeteria, provide security services, and so on are the resident's auxiliary family. Residents who enquire about personal well-being and joke with them appropriately will become known as an approachable, go-to surgeon, which will open doors for them to learn valuable behaviors and interpersonal skills. If residents maintain a strong reputation as they progress to the senior or chief resident levels, they will benefit as hospital personnel make an extra effort to care for their patients and for the residents themselves.

Additional Aspects of the Affective, Cognitive, and Psychomotor Domains

An excellent surgeon uses knowledge of medical science and motor skills in concert to provide effective and safe patient care. This requires a commitment to learning that includes the ability to read, to absorb information, and to be continuously curious. As the old saying goes, "a surgeon is a physician who operates." The mental focus needs to be centered on achieving the knowledge necessary to provide high-quality care in a "high-reliability" setting. The abiding question should be "how can I improve?" When reflecting on a patient care event pertinent questions include: "What went wrong? How could this be done better? What mistakes were made? What was successful?" Each patient care experience is an opportunity to identify modifications that will lead to improvement. When the resident learns to constantly focus on improvement, avoid complacency, and strive for excellence there will be increased professional satisfaction that will be sustained throughout a surgical career.

Filling Knowledge Gaps

The cognitive knowledge necessary to practice modern surgery cannot be learned simply by participating in the 80-hour workweek curriculum. Although residents must tend to self-care, a balanced lifestyle, family, and other personal issues, they must balance those needs against their responsibility to gain expertise in the cognitive knowledge of surgery.

Each resident needs to be aware of their knowledge gaps. Striving to recognize what you don't know is perhaps the best way to learn. An honest assessment of each resident as an adult learner leads to habits of study that can last a lifetime. One simple technique that residents can use is to carry a 3x5 card or another device with them every day and jot down terminology that is new, drugs they have not encountered, anatomy they have not learned, or any other gap of cognitive knowledge that presents during each day. If the resident disciplines themselves to look up appropriate answers to the several points accumulated during the day over the course of a residency, they will have learned a tremendous amount of new knowledge on top of their formal curriculum-based study. Acquiring knowledge in this way in the context of actual patients they are caring for often allows learning to be more durable. They can also be guided by the yearly in-training examination (ABSITE), which allows comparison of their core knowledge to their peers at the same training level and provides objective goals to attain.

To fill these gaps, the resident must seek resources designed to teach basic physiology and anatomy and apply that knowledge to the clinical setting of different disease processes that require surgical therapy. For example, courses designed to enhance cognitive skills include the ACS *Surgical Education and Self-Assessment Program (SESAP®)* and the SCORE curriculum, which should be used as departmental teaching aids. Detailed descriptions of available learning resources and approaches to using them are included in other chapters of this manual.

As there is a need to acquire higher levels of cognitive skills each year, residents will develop a sense of duty to continue learning—a sense of duty that should last throughout their surgical careers. For example, as the resident learns the principles of surgical investigation, they will develop an appreciation for the scientific value of reading journal articles throughout their careers. The concept of reading every day to improve surgical knowledge should become ingrained in their behaviors. Addressing knowledge gaps often will require residents to study during extracurricular hours at home. To fulfill their obligation and desire for lifelong learning, focused periods of reading during personal hours should become habitual.

Using Research to Facilitate Knowledge Acquisition

The affective and cognitive domains join together in creative problem-solving by performing scientific research. Learning the principles of surgical investigation can be enhanced by engaging in defined research activities during residency training. Although basic laboratory research is essential for medical progress, a multitude of opportunities exist to use other techniques such as observational studies (chart reviews, database analyses), outcomes research, and systematic reviews of the literature as a means of increasing knowledge. Becoming familiar with the research process teaches the resident to be a creative thinker and to evaluate the scientific value of a journal article. Residents should learn how to gather and analyze data and make their data and analysis the subject of a formal presentation and/or a peer-reviewed publication. They should have the opportunity to experience the joy and satisfaction of investigating a scientific problem, discovering some previously unknown information, or finding a new way of managing a surgical condition. Research teaches residents the value of keeping an open mind and to understand that there is more than one way of doing things. Research can also teach residents not to see what they "believe" and to be careful not to allow their cognitive bias to skew their scientific analyses. Creative and critical thinking are essential for surgeons, and research helps teach both.

The Psychomotor Skills Domain

As residents acquire psychomotor (technical) skills, they must take advantage of opportunities to practice and enhance these abilities. For example, a new resident might begin by learning a simple but important activity such as suturing a laceration. In this example, the resident might begin by considering the location of the laceration, whether there is involvement of structures such as peripheral nerves, blood vessels, and so forth, whether tissue damage or ischemia will require debridement, and what repair options will provide the best functional and cosmetic result (for example, simple suture, mattress suture, staples, tissue glue). For more complex wounds, considerations would include the need for flap closure, flap design, techniques for tissue handling, achieving hemostasis, and interventions to reduce the risk of infection and improve the healing process (such as negative pressure wound therapy). The resident will be expected to master certain psychomotor skills by the end of each year of training.

A useful approach may be to consider ways of learning something new. For example, what are the strategic steps required to accomplish the task, how is each step located in the performance sequence, what criteria define successful completion of each step, and what is needed to measure and confirm the outcome? Residents will need to learn new skills as they develop and should remain open to acquiring new techniques and new skills that benefit patients.

Record Keeping

The basic documentation for each new patient should include a focused history and physical examination, a plan for preoperative preparation, documentation of completed preparation in a preoperative note (standard indications, contraindications, alternative forms of therapy, common complications, and confirmation that a conversation occurred with the patient about all of the above), an operative note, daily progress notes (ICU and Floor), interim summaries, and discharge notes. As the adoption of electronic health records (EHRs) has become a fact of life in surgical practice there are certain precautions that residents should practice (for instance, avoid cute or unprofessional references, do not copy/paste yesterday's note into today's note). Entries into the record should be relevant to the care of the patient and may include new clinical/laboratory/imaging findings and how these may influence the care process. Dictated notes should use acceptable English and briefly describe patient conversations and patient treatment plans. The introduction of the EHR with its redundancies does not eliminate the need for these simple tasks. More experienced residents should teach less-experienced residents and the medical students about proper documentation. Compliance with EHR requirements should not preclude a summary of the past 24 hours and plans for the next day; these brief notes should be used to select and write therapeutic orders.

Specific medical record entry practices, which may vary from program to program, should be included in regularly scheduled training sessions with written manuals that offer examples of record entries. The medical record is a legal document and entries must be clear and relevant. For example, a resident who comments, "He was treated with a banana bag," instead of describing the components of the intervention should be counseled by the attending physician and informed that such comments are unprofessional and unnecessary.

Conclusion

In this chapter we have reviewed basic concepts and practices that contribute to the acquisition of the necessary affective, cognitive, and psychomotor professional skills to provide safe, high-quality patient care. This information, along with additional research and innovation, will help ensure that residents become surgeons who are known for professionalism.

References

1. Rosenberg IK, Lucas CE, Pitts CC. Surgery: an integral part of core curriculum. *J Surg Res*. 1972;12:220-227.
2. Kamata K, Kuriyama A, Chopra V, et al. Patient preferences for physician attire: a multicenter study in Japan. *J Hosp Med*. 2020;15:204-210.
3. Petrilli CM, Saint S, Jennings JJ, Caruso A, Kuhn L, Snyder A, Chopra V. Understanding patient preference for physician attire: a cross-sectional observational study of 10 academic medical centers in the USA. *BMJ Open*. 2018;8:e021239.
4. Jennings JD, Ciaravino SG, Ramsey FV, Haydel C. Physicians' attire influences patients' perceptions in the urban outpatient orthopaedic surgery setting. *Clin Orthop Relat Res*. 2016;474(9):1908-1918.
5. Xu KT, Borders TF, Arif AA. Ethnic differences in parents' perception of participatory style of their children's physicians. *Med Care*. 2004;42:328-335.
6. Cooper-Patrick L, Gallo JJ, Gonzales JJ, Vu HT, Powe NR, Nelson C, Ford DE. Race, gender, and partnership in the patient-physician relationship. *JAMA*. 1999;282:583-589.
7. Osler W. *A Way of Life*. 1929. Oxford University Press, American Branch. New York.
8. Ferguson WJ, Candib LM. Culture, language, and the doctor-patient relationship. *Fam Med*. 2002;34:353-361.
9. Silverman DD. Physician behavior and bedside manners: the influence of William Osler and the Johns Hopkins School of Medicine. *Proc (Bayl Univ Med Cent)*. 2012;25:58-61.
10. Shlamozitz GZ, Mower WR, Bergman J, Crisp J, DeVore HK, Hardy D, Sargent M, Schroff SD, Snyder E, Mortan MT. Lack of evidence to support routine digital rectal examination in pediatric trauma patients. *Pediatr Emerg Care*. 2007;23:537-543.
11. Esposito TJ, Ingraham A, Luchette FA, et al. Reasons to omit digital rectal examination in trauma patients: no fingers, no rectum, no useful additional information. *J Trauma*. 2005;59:1314-1319.
12. Shrestra MP, Borgstrom M, Trowers E. Digital rectal examination reduces hospital admissions, endoscopies, and medical therapy in patients with acute gastrointestinal bleeding. *Am J Med*. 2017;130(7):819-825.
13. Zinn W. The empathic physician. *Arch Intern Med*. 1993;153:306-312.
14. Hirsch EM. The role of empathy in medicine: a medical student's perspective. *AMA J Ethics*. 2007;9(6):423-427.
15. DasGupta S, Charon R. Personal illness narratives: using reflective writing to teach empathy. *Acad Med*. 2004;79:351-356.
16. Platt FW, Keller ZF. Empathic communication: a teachable and learnable skill. *J Gen Intern Med*. 1994;9:222-226.
17. Halpern J. What is clinical empathy? *J Gen Intern Med*. 2003;18:670-674.
18. Canale SD, Louis DZ, Maio V, Rossi G, Hojat M, Gonnella JS. The relationship between physician empathy and disease complications. *Acad Med*. 2012;28:1243-1247.
19. Goode T, Sockalingam S, Brown M, Jones W. Linguistic competence in primary health care delivery systems: implications for policy makers. Washington DC: National Center for Cultural Competence, Center for Child Health, and Mental Health Policy. 2001.
20. Lucas CE, Vlahos AL, Ledgerwood AM. Kindness kills: the negative impact of pain as the fifth vital sign. *J Am Coll Surg*. 2007;205(1):101-107.
21. Chaparro LE, Smith SA, Moore RA, Wiffen PJ, Gilron I. Pharmacotherapy for the prevention of chronic pain after surgery in adults. *Cochrane Database Sys Rev*. 2013; 2013(7):C008307.
22. Mudumbai SC, Oliva EM, Lewis ET, Trafton J, Posner D, Mariano ER, Stafford RS, Wagner T, Clark JD. Time-to-cessation of postoperative opioids: a population-level analysis of the veterans affairs health care system. *Pain Med*. 2016;17:1732-1743.
23. Trasolini NA, McKnight BM, Dorr LD. The opioid crisis and the orthopaedic surgeon. *Arthroplasty*. 2018;33(11):3379-3382.
24. Birshup BB, Oppenberg AA, Coleman MM. Strategic risk management: reducing malpractice claims through more effective patient-doctor communication. *Am J Med Qual*. 1999;14:153-159.
25. Ha JF, Longnecker N. Doctor-patient communication: a review. *The Ochsner Journal*. 2010;10:38-43.
26. Barrier PA, Li JT, Jensen NM. Two words to improve physician-patient communication: what else? *Mayo Clin Proc*. 2003;78:211-214.
27. Meredyth NA, deMelo-Martin I. (Under)valuing surgical informed consent. 2020. *J Am Coll Surg*. 230:257-282.
28. Koller SE, Moore RF, Goldberg MB, et al. An informed consent program enhances surgery resident education. *J Surg Educ*. 2017;74:906-913.

29. Ledgerwood A, Lucas KA, Lucas CE. The convergence of trauma, medicine, and the law. In: *Trauma, 6th Edition*. EE Moore, DV Feliciano, KL Mattox (Eds). McGraw-Hill, New York, NY. 2008:1169-1180.
30. McNair AJK, MacKichan F, Donovan JL, Brookes SJ, Avery KML, Griffin SM, Crosby T, Blazeby JM. What surgeons tell patients and what patients want to know before major surgery: a qualitative study. *BMC Cancer*. 2016;16:258-265.
31. Isaacson A. A surgeon on the other side of the operation. February 10, 2020. Available at: https://www.kevinmd.com/blog/2020/02/a-surgeon-on-the-other-side-of-the-operation.html. Accessed March 25, 2021.
32. Lorenzetti RC, Jacques CHM, Donovan C, Cottrell S, Buck J. Managing difficult encounters: understanding physician, patient, and situation factors. *Am Fam Physician*. 2013;86:419-425.
33. McCary LW, Cronholm PE, Bogner HR, Gallo JJ, Neill RD. Resident physician burnout: is there hope? *Fam Med*. 2008;40(9):526-632.
34. Peteet JR, Meyer FL, Miovic MK. Possibly impossible patients: management of difficult behavior in oncology outpatients. *J Oncol Pract*. 2011;7(4):242-246.
35. Kane L. Medscape. Medscape national physician burnout & suicide report 2020: the generational divide. Available at: https://www.medscape.com/slide-show/2020-lifestyle-burnout-6012460. Accessed: January 15, 2020.
36. Albrecht R. Duty and what really matters – professionalism and self. *J Trauma Acute Care Surg.* 2019;87:1007-1011.
37. Yeston, NS. Veni, Vidi, Existitus. *J Am Coll Surg*. 2014;218(6):10911094.

AMERICAN C
SURGEONS A
OF SURGEON
COLLEGE OF
AMERICAN C
SURGEONS A
OF SURGEON
COLLEGE OF
AMERICAN C
SURGEONS A

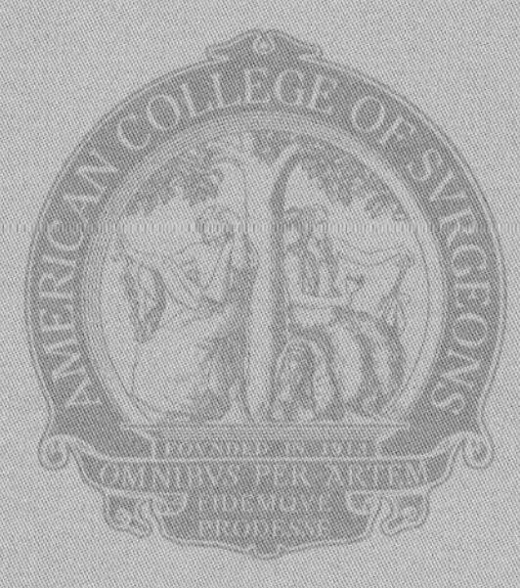

CHAPTER 6
Curriculum: Technical Surgical Skills

Lead Author

Fabrizio Michelassi, MD, FACS, MAMSE, ESA(Hon), SIC(Hon)

Co-Authors

Demetrios Demetriades, MD, PhD, FACS, MAMSE

David V. Feliciano, MD, FACS, MAMSE

Ernest E. "Gene" Moore, MD, FACS, MCCM, FACN, FISS, MAMSE

Mohsen M. Shabahang, MD, PhD, FACS, MAMSE

Nathaniel J. Soper, MD, FACS, MAMSE

Dimitrios Stefanidis, MD, PhD, FACS, FASMBS, FSSH

Consultant

J. David Richardson, MD, FACS, MAMSE

CHAPTER 6

Curriculum: Technical Surgical Skills

Executive Summary

This chapter describes the optimal resources and the ideal curriculum needed to teach residents in surgery training programs the technical surgical skills for the performance of essential general surgery procedures. It seeks to answer the following questions:

- What preparatory courses are available to medical students who intend to pursue surgical residency?
- What fundamental surgical skills should residents develop while in training?
- Can residents receive certification in surgical skills?
- What resources are available to teach these skills outside of the operating room (OR)?
- How do we expose residents to surgical technique in the perioperative phase of care?
- How do we assess the technical skills of trainees?
- How do we prepare residents to perform complex surgical procedures autonomously?

Introduction

The chapter is divided into six sections as follows:

- Preparatory courses. Training surgical residents is a complex process because they not only need to develop into specialists with detailed knowledge of disease processes, but they must also acquire technical skills. This section will focus on the utility of preparatory courses prior to entering residency.
- Fundamental technical skills. Surgeons differ from other medical professionals in that they must learn an additional but fundamental set of technical skills. Surgical educators should focus on providing trainees with discrete skills they can hone to improve technical performance.
- Available resources to teach technical skills outside the operating room. Simulation and fresh tissue dissection labs (such as animal labs or human cadaver labs) have become integral parts of surgical education and training. These labs provide learners with uniform training experiences through standardized interventions. They also enable learners to better understand a procedure and acquire skills in a safe environment without placing patients at risk, allowing them to learn how to prevent errors by practicing error-prone techniques. This approach, which has been shown to be effective in helping learners acquire and improve surgical skills, complements what occurs in the clinical environment. As a result, all modern surgery residency skills curricula incorporate simulation and/or dissection labs.
- Teaching surgical technique in the perioperative period. Surgical residents need to intellectually understand the tasks associated with surgical procedures, integrate the techniques required to perform those tasks with their learning, and, finally, acquire the requisite skills to perform tasks with automaticity resulting in reduction of cognitive load. This three-step approach is an ideal method to enhance teaching of clinical operative procedures. Often, real-life factors can complicate or prevent one or more of these suggested steps from occurring. These steps can be modified depending on time pressures, the postgraduate year (PGY) level and previous experience of the surgical resident, the faculty surgeon's prior exposure to the individual resident, and the complexity of the operation.
- Assessing the technical skill of trainees. The information obtained from assessing technical skills can be used to inform residents of their progress toward the achievement of the appropriate level of performance and proficiency. These technical skill assessments must be valid, reliable, and reproducible.
- Ensuring competency of trainees in common and high-risk procedures for autonomous practice after training. To learn surgical procedures, residents must see how fundamental skills are integrated into an actual surgical procedure. Four examples that are based on the frequency of occurrence and the degree of technical difficulty are depicted at end of this chapter.

Preparatory Courses before Residency Training (Boot Camp)

Residents' level of technical skills upon entering surgical training is an important foundation upon which further skill acquisition is built. In a multidisciplinary 2015 study by Minter and colleagues, incoming first-year residents felt unprepared to begin training. This finding does not surprise most program directors, especially those with years of experience in training residents. In fact, a joint statement by the American Board of Surgery (ABS), the American College of Surgeons (ACS), the Association for Surgical Education (ASE), and the Association of Program Directors in Surgery (APDS) from 2014 states that a preparatory course is essential to improve skills acquisition by residents. Data show that such courses increase the confidence of the first-year resident.

Although the content of the course may vary, it must include focus on cognitive, clinical, technical, and non-technical skills and employ the use of simulation as appropriate. For example, a preparatory course might span four weeks with time devoted to simulation-based training and assessment and clinical time allocated to general surgery, trauma, specialty surgery, and critical care. During the clinical time, the learner must be held accountable for working up, admitting, and discharging a specified number of patients.

The faculty and resident teams also must understand the purpose of the curriculum. Unlike an acting internship, in which the purpose may be to expose the learner to a large volume of clinical material, a preparatory course is intended to enable the trainee to acquire the ability to perform the duties of a junior resident. In addition to the clinical portion, time should be reserved to discuss the disease processes inherent in certain common surgical conditions, such as gallbladder disease, appendicitis, or small bowel obstruction. The simulation portion (see later in chapter) must include laparoscopic skills, venous access procedures, suturing, and radiologic interpretations; some also may expose the learners to robotic technology through simulation. A cadaveric laboratory offers the learners a chance to dissect tissue, gain operative skills, and become comfortable with complex anatomy. Finally, a preparatory course must ensure each learner participates in low-complexity operations, such as lipoma removal, inguinal hernia repair, or cholecystectomy. The ACS Division of Education offers the ACS/APDS/ASE Resident Prep Curriculum ("Boot Camp"), which has 30 defined modules that incorporate many of these critical areas of content into a structured curriculum.

Fundamental Technical Skills

Surgeons need to acquire and demonstrate multiple competencies in order to perform at the highest skill level. The Accreditation Council for Graduate Medical Education (ACGME) has defined six competencies that apply to all medical specialties: patient care, medical knowledge, practice-based learning and improvement, interpersonal and communication skills, professionalism, and systems-based practice. Other organizations, such as the Royal Australasian College of Surgeons, have further defined competencies specific to surgical practice, including collaboration and teamwork, communication, health advocacy, judgment and decision-making, management and leadership, medical expertise, professionalism, scholarship and teaching, technical expertise, and cultural competence and cultural safety.

To focus and simplify training efforts, surgical technical performance can be broken down into fundamental, unique, and independent components. This approach provides a strong skills foundation for residents, enabling them to use these discrete basic skills to perform numerous procedures.

Table 1. ACS essential technical skills for entering PGY1

- Practice universal precautions routinely
- Administer a local anesthetic
- Insert and maintain nasogastric tubes
- Insert and maintain urinary catheters
- Assess the presence of peripheral blood flow using handheld Doppler instruments
- Perform venipuncture and insert peripheral intravenous catheters
- Perform an arterial stick and obtain an arterial sample
- Scrub, gown, and glove properly for operative procedures and bedside procedures
- Maintain appropriate sterile technique in the clinic, emergency department, intensive care unit (ICU), OR, and patient's room
- Use proper techniques for skin preparation and the draping of the incision site
- Remove sutures and staples
- Perform minor surgical procedures under supervision (for example, incision and drainage of superficial abscesses; minor excisions; and skin suture using simple, subcutaneous, and mattress sutures and/or staples)
- Understand potential complications of these procedures as they relate to patient safety

Numerous programs recognize the benefits of this approach. An example is the *ACS Fundamentals of Surgery Curriculum*®, which is a highly interactive, case-based, online curriculum that addresses the essential content areas that all surgical residents should acquire early in their training. Although this curriculum does not include technical skills, the ACS Essentials for Medical Students and PGY1 Residents defines fundamental technical skills that medical students should have upon entering surgical residency (Table 1) and those that surgical interns should acquire in their first year of training (Table 2).

Table 2. ACS essential technical skills at completion of PGY1

- Describe concepts of atraumatic tissue handling
- Perform as first assistant
- Obtain hemostasis of small vessels in the operative field
- Identify common surgical instruments and suture materials and their proper uses
- Perform basic surgical maneuvers (suture of skin, soft tissues, and fascia; knot tying)
- Demonstrate appropriate techniques of dissection, handling of tissues, and wound closure
- Under supervision, perform basic surgical procedures such as anoscopy, breast biopsy, digital amputation, burr hole, excision of skin lesions, thoracentesis, paracentesis, spinal tap, and more
- Manage central venous lines and gastrostomy and jejunostomy feeding tubes
- Insert, maintain, and remove drains and chest tubes
- Insert and manage tubes and drains placed operatively or percutaneously
- Perform orotracheal intubation
- Manage surgical airways (cricothyroidotomy, open and percutaneous tracheostomy)
- Immobilize extremities and spine immobilization
- Insert indwelling arterial and venous lines
- Demonstrate appropriate methods of routine and reverse isolation procedures
- Maintain appropriate sterile technique in the emergency department, ICU, office, and at the patient's bedside
- Describe potential complications of procedures and how they relate to patient safety

Similarly, the ACS/APDS Surgery Resident Skills Curriculum involves the use of simulation for the teaching of basic technical skills to surgical residents through 16 modules of Phase I of the curriculum (Table 3).

Table 3. ACS/APDS Surgery Resident Skills Curriculum, Phase I modules

- Module 1: Asepsis and instrument identification
- Module 2: Knot tying
- Module 3: Suturing
- Module 4: Skin flaps
- Module 5: Skin grafts
- Module 6: Urethral catheterization
- Module 7: Airway management
- Module 8: Chest tube insertion
- Module 9: Central line insertion
- Module 10: Surgical biopsy
- Module 11: Laparotomy opening and closure
- Module 12: Basic laparoscopy skills
- Module 13: Advanced laparoscopy skills
- Module 14: Hand-sewn bowel anastomosis
- Module 15: Stapled bowel anastomosis
- Module 16: Arterial anastomosis

Other programs, all of which are discussed in detail later in this chapter, have gone a step further and focus on defining specific fundamental skills. For example, the Fundamentals of Laparoscopic Surgery (FLS) course defines and offers training in four basic skills that underlie successful laparoscopic performance, including laparoscopic suturing and knot tying, cutting, endo-loop application, and a transfer task to promote bimanual dexterity. Similarly, the Fundamentals of Endoscopic Surgery (FES) program incorporates endoscopy-specific basic skills such as scope navigation, loop reduction, targeting, mucosal evaluation, and retroflexion. More recently, the Fundamentals of Robotic Surgery (FRS) program has been developed to train and assess seven basic robotic skills (Table 4).

Table 4. Fundamental technical skills for basic robotic surgery as defined in the FRS

- Task 1: Docking/instrument insertion
- Task 2: Ring tower transfer
- Task 3: Knot tying
- Task 4: Railroad track
- Task 5: Fourth arm cutting
- Task 6: Puzzle piece dissection
- Task 7: Vessel energy dissection

Many courses across the spectrum of medical school and early training are available. Based on our collective expertise and a literature review, we propose the fundamental technical skills listed in Table 5. This list may not be exhaustive, but it does include the most important basic skills that define technical performance in surgery. Focusing training on these skills will help prepare surgical trainees to apply them in a variety of procedures and settings.

It also is important to define skill categories applicable to the practice of surgery. These categories may include several of the basic skills listed in Table 6, but their psychomotor requirements are distinctly different. Hence, a basic skill mastered in one category may not always transfer to another category. For example, a surgeon who has mastered suturing and knot tying in open surgery may not have mastered these skills in laparoscopy, which is a different surgical technique. Surgeon educators need to ensure that residents learn these basic skills in all skill categories relevant to their training.

Table 5. Fundamental technical skills in surgery

- Handling of instruments and devices (including stapling, docking of robotic arms, and so forth)
- Dissection
- Exposure and retraction
- Respect for tissue/tissue handling
- Suturing
- Knot tying
- Cutting
- Debridement
- Clamping
- Application of a loop/snare around a structure
- Injection and aspiration
- Tube/catheter/trocar insertion and manipulation (urinary, nasogastric, endotracheal, intravascular, and laparoscopic)
- Application and use of surgical energy (including using foot pedals)
- Taking a biopsy (direct, percutaneous)
- Use of ultrasound
- Scope navigation/manipulation (camera, endoscope, bronchoscope, and so on)*
- Tissue transfer between hands – bimanual dexterity
- Perceptual skills (the ability to recognize anatomic spatial relationships, surgical planes, depth perception, 2D- to 3D-image conversion/spatial orientation, and more)

** Endoscope manipulation consists of further subskills as defined by the FES program (such as loop reduction, targeting, mucosal evaluation, and retroflexion), which are described later in this chapter.*

Table 6. Technical skill categories

- Open surgery skills
- Laparoscopic skills
- Robotic skills
- Endoscopic skills
- Endovascular skills
- Microsurgery skills

Resources to Teach Technical Skills Outside the Operating Room

Simulation

A variety of simulations and simulators are used in surgery today. These include low- and high-fidelity simulators for technical training as well as cognitive case-based simulations, standardized patients (SPs), virtual reality (VR), and immersive environments. To teach technical skills, surgical educators may rely on low-fidelity part-task trainers, box trainers, and high-fidelity VR procedural simulators. Low-fidelity simulators, when appropriate, can be effective training tools with a low cost. High-fidelity simulators can better approximate clinical practice and procedure variability and are more appealing to the learner. At the same time, the limited realism of existing VR platforms may blunt user enthusiasm, and their high cost has limited adoption. Nevertheless, VR simulators, unlike low-fidelity models, typically provide numerous easy-to-obtain, objective performance metrics that benefit performance assessment and support provision of feedback to the trainee.

Following is an explanation of the effective simulation programs and their relevance to surgical educators.

Fundamentals of Laparoscopic Surgery

FLS is a comprehensive, web-based educational program that includes hands-on skills training and assessment, and is designed to teach the physiology, fundamental knowledge, and technical skills required in basic laparoscopic surgery. FLS was designed for surgical residents, fellows, and practicing physicians to learn and practice laparoscopic skills and to assess and document those skills using a standardized platform and objective metrics. The FLS test measures cognitive knowledge, case/problem management skills, and manual dexterity. The FLS program content is a joint educational offering of the ACS and the Society of American Gastrointestinal Endoscopic Surgeons (SAGES) and is accredited for Continuing Medical Education (CME) credits. The program includes five tasks (peg transfer, cutting circle, endo-loop application, intracorporeal, and extracorporeal suturing and knot tying). FLS certification has been required for completion of general surgery training since 2009 and for gynecology in 2021. There is strong supporting evidence for the use of FLS for training and high stakes assessment. Details can be found at *www.flsprogram.org*.

Fundamentals of Endoscopic Surgery

FES is a comprehensive tool designed to teach and assess the fundamental knowledge, clinical judgment, and technical skills required to perform basic gastrointestinal (GI) endoscopic surgery. FES was created by SAGES and is designed for medical and surgical residents, fellows, practicing general surgeons, gastroenterologists, and other physicians to learn and demonstrate basic endoscopic skills required to perform flexible endoscopy. Like FLS, it includes an online curriculum, a high-stakes cognitive test, and a standardized technical skill assessment. Unlike FLS, the test is based on a VR simulator that is unavailable for practice (FLS uses a realistic box trainer for both practice and testing). FES certification has been a requirement for graduating general surgery residents since 2018. Details can be found at *www.fesprogram.org*.

Fundamentals of Robotic Surgery (FRS)
FRS is an education, training, and assessment program for basic robotic surgical skills that the Institute for Surgical Excellence (ISE) developed with input from an international multispecialty group with representation from the major surgical specialties in the U.S. that perform robotic-assisted surgical procedures. FRS offers a proficiency-based curriculum of basic cognitive, technical, and team skills to train and assess surgeons to perform robot-assisted surgery safely and efficiently. Learners must complete an online curriculum on how to perform basic robotic surgery, and learners must pass a knowledge test. Learners can develop basic robotic technical skills by training on a simulator that incorporates seven tasks chosen through expert consensus. Specific expert performance levels and metrics have been defined for proficiency-based training. The curriculum also offers team training modules and assessment tools for effective implementation. Evidence of the effectiveness of this program has been published previously. Details can be found at *www.frsurgery.org*.

Advanced Trauma Life Support
The Advanced Trauma Life Support® (ATLS®) program teaches a systematic, concise approach to the early care of injured patients. ATLS was developed by the ACS Committee on Trauma (COT) for physicians and other qualified health care professionals, and was first introduced in the U.S. and abroad in 1980. ATLS offers participants a safe, reliable method for immediate management of the injured patient and the basic knowledge necessary to complete the following tasks:

- Assess the patient's condition rapidly and accurately
- Resuscitate and stabilize the patient according to priority
- Determine if the patient's needs exceed a facility's capacity
- Arrange appropriately for the patient's interhospital transfer (who, what, when, and how)
- Assure that optimal care is provided and that the level of care is maintained throughout the evaluation, resuscitation, and transfer process

ATLS provides a scaffold for evaluation, treatment, education, and quality assurance. Details can be found at *www.facs.org/quality-programs/trauma/atls*.

ACS/APDS Surgery Resident Skills Curriculum, Phases I & 2 — Core Surgical Skills
The ACS Division of Education, in collaboration with the APDS, developed the ACS/APDS Surgical Skills Curriculum to address simulation-based skills training of general surgery residents outside the OR across all five years of training. This proficiency-based skills curriculum is web-based, inexpensive, and accessible to all. The curriculum includes the use of a variety of simulations to achieve specific learning objectives and was developed and launched in three phases; Phases I and II address core surgical skills, and Phase III addresses teamwork skills.

Phase I includes 16 modules that address basic surgical skills and tasks, and Phase II includes 15 modules that address surgical procedures. Each module in Phases I and II includes objectives, assumptions, suggested readings, descriptions of steps for specific skills and common errors, a video of an expert performance, recommendations for guided practice, and information on clinical skills station setup and use. A number of modules also include tools for the verification of proficiency to assess the readiness of individual residents for the OR. An instructor's guidebook provides descriptions of station design, information on supplies, vendors, products, and laboratory setup, as well as information on recommended teaching times. Details can be found at *www.facs.org/education/program/resident-skills*.

Fundamental Use of Surgical Energy
The Fundamental Use of Surgical Energy (FUSE) program is aimed at teaching surgeons the safe use of energy in the OR. SAGES developed FUSE in response to the approximately 400 fires and 40,000 thermal injuries that happen yearly in U.S. ORs. It includes an online curriculum that addresses the principles of energy and safe use of related devices in the OR and a high-stakes assessment for certification. Although a distinct skills curriculum is not part of the program, the program provides examples of potential problems encountered during energy use to help surgical trainees and surgeons retain the concepts. Details are available at *www.fusedidactic.org*.

Animal Models
ACS Advanced Trauma Operative Management Course
The Advanced Trauma Operative Management (ATOM®) course uses a porcine model to teach operative techniques for penetrating trauma, mainly to the abdomen and, to a lesser extent, the chest. ATOM addresses many didactic requirements of the advanced procedures in the ACS/APDS Surgery Resident Skills Curriculum. The course includes operative techniques in the following areas:

- Trauma laparotomy, damage control procedure
- Spleen
- Liver (major hepatic trauma, hepatic vascular isolation)
- Diaphragm
- Pancreas and duodenum
- Colon injury
- Urinary system (bladder, nephrectomy, and ureter repair)
- Cardiovascular system
- Abdominal aorta and major branches, Mattox maneuver
- Inferior vena cava
- Cardiac injury

The course simulates realistic tissue handling, bleeding, and some abdominal organs that are similar to human anatomy. In addition, each chapter includes "Tips from the Masters" written by leading trauma surgeons. Yet the differences in anatomy between pigs and humans makes it impossible to reproduce surgical procedures in some anatomical areas. Specifically, the anatomic differences prevent adequate teaching of management of the following: vascular injuries in the neck or extremities; neck procedures, such as cricothyroidotomy; tracheoesophageal injuries; and pulmonary or intrathoracic vascular trauma. In addition, the anatomy of some intraabdominal organs varies so much from human anatomy that reproducing surgical procedures in these anatomical areas does not carry the same level of technical challenge as in humans. Details can be found at *www.facs.org/quality-programs/trauma/education/atom.*

Cadaveric Models

Advanced Surgical Skills for Exposure in Trauma

Advanced Surgical Skills for Exposure in Trauma (ASSET) is a one-day course that uses human cadavers to train mid-level and senior surgical residents, trauma surgical fellows, and trained surgeons. The low student-to-faculty and low cadaver-to-student (one body for four students) ratios allow closer faculty instruction and interaction with students and more intensive hands-on surgical exposures.

ASSET helps in training residents to surgically expose the neck, chest, abdomen, pelvis, and upper and lower extremities. Students gain confidence in performing surgical exposures, especially in difficult anatomical areas.

The ASSET course requires the following:

- Cadaver lab, according to state, regional, and local regulations
- Appropriate refrigerator facility to house cadavers, well-equipped operating rooms, and appropriate surgical instruments
- Availability of fresh/fresh frozen human cadavers (tested for infectious diseases)
- Adequate audio-visual (A/V) equipment in the lab for slides and video projections
- A qualified ASSET course director
- One qualified ASSET instructor (or instructor candidate) per cadaver
- An on-site coordinator to help the course run smoothly and to complete necessary paperwork

Details can be found at *www.facs.org/quality-programs/trauma/education/asset.*

Perfused and Mechanically Ventilated Fresh Cadavers

This system uses fresh human cadavers and is the highest-fidelity surgical simulation model. It involves insertion of catheters in the femoral artery and femoral vein, which are connected to a cardiac centrifugal pump. The trachea is intubated, and the lungs are mechanically ventilated. With this model, dermal and microvascular perfusion occur, and the skin and soft tissues bleed when incised, the arteries pulsate, and the heart can be set to beat at a desired rate. This model allows training in central venous catheterization with or without ultrasound guidance and is ideal for surgical vascular exposures and open or endovascular procedures. The model provides high-quality training in lung resections because the lung parenchyma bleeds or leaks air when incised.

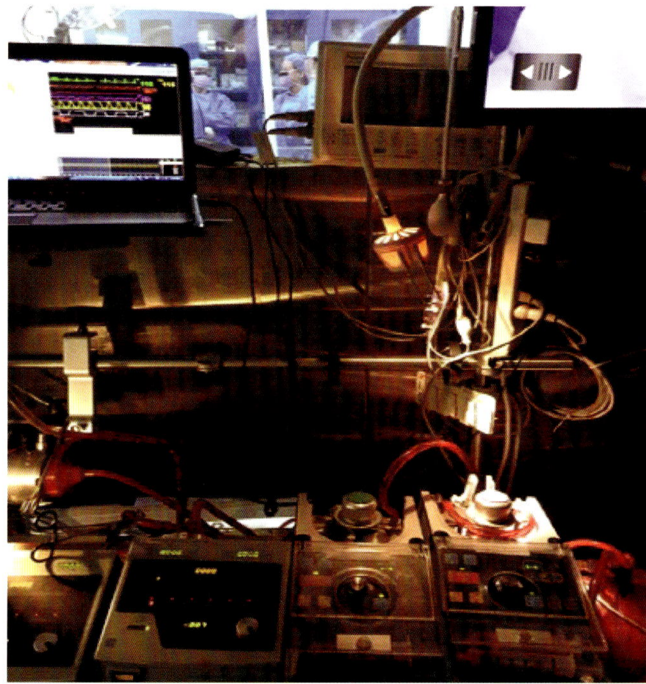

Vascular perfusion system. Source: ACS Image Library.

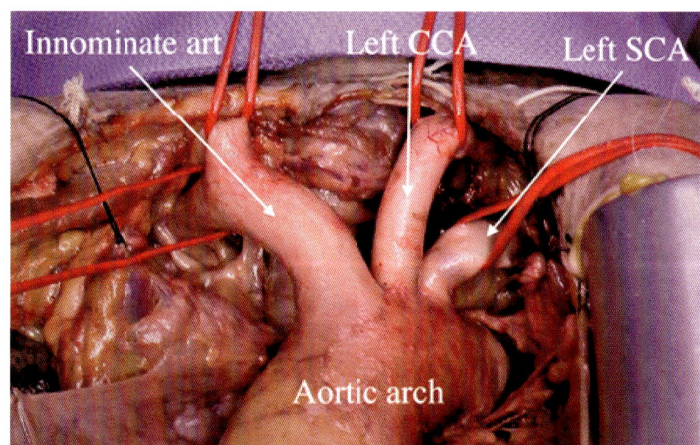

Aortic arch and branches in a perfused cadaver model. Source: ACS Image Library.

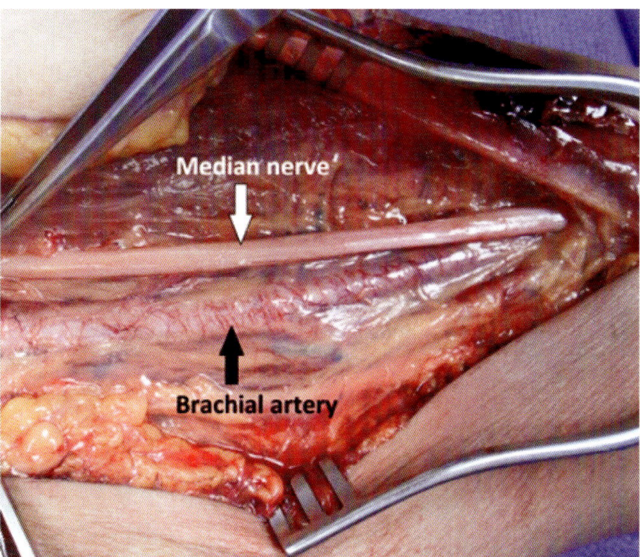

Alive-looking tissues and neurovascular structures. Source: ACS Image Library.

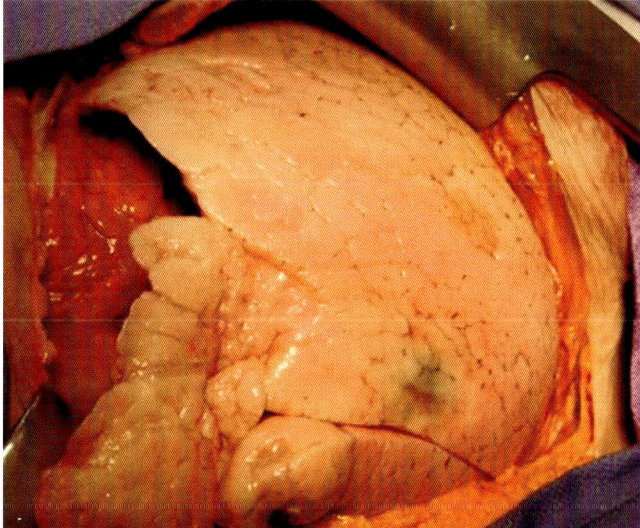

Lung appearance with mechanical ventilation and in fresh, perfused cadaver vascular perfusion. Source: ACS Image Library.

The system can be calibrated to simulate various hemodynamic conditions, such as various degrees of shock and the physiological response to therapeutic interventions, which allows the development of simulation programs that include operative decision-making, team training, needs assessments, cognitive task analysis, and validated assessment tools.

The perfused and mechanically ventilated fresh cadavers require the following:

- Cadaver lab, according to state, regional, and local regulations
- Appropriate refrigerator facility to house cadavers, well-equipped operating rooms, and appropriate surgical instruments
- Availability of fresh human cadavers (tested for infectious diseases)
- Adequate A/V equipment in the lab for slides and video projections
- A lab technician trained in basic cardiac perfusion techniques

The ASSET course and the perfused and mechanically ventilated fresh cadavers are extremely valuable for trauma and acute care surgery fellows and desirable for general surgery residents. Regionalization of this valuable educational resource may address the complexity and costs of required resources and the difficulties in procuring cadavers. Details are available at *www.keck.usc.edu/surgery/training-education/surgical-skills-simulation-and-education-center/*.

Basic Endovascular Skills for Trauma
The Basic Endovascular Skills for Trauma (BEST) workshop uses simulator-based training and serves as an introduction to resuscitative endovascular balloon occlusion of the aorta (REBOA). The appropriateness and indications for REBOA are addressed in a consensus statement and emphasize the importance of adequate training before undertaking this procedure. BEST workshops require plastic simulation models and a BEST instructor.

For more in-depth training, the trainee may attend the BEST course, which teaches the use of REBOA to temporize life-threatening hemorrhage below the diaphragm. It allows hands-on training with perfused cadavers, including ultrasound-guided common femoral arterial (CFA) access, percutaneous, and open cannulation of the CFA and CFA repair. BEST courses require a perfused cadaver model and a course director. Details can be found at *www.facs.org/quality-programs/trauma/education/best*.

Other Training Opportunities
As suggested previously in Chapter 4, surgical residency programs should develop a relationship with the medical examiner's office so that residents can participate in autopsies with anatomic pathologists and learn anatomy on fresh cadavers. There is usually a schedule that allows residents to participate in their off time or by formal agreement between the resident program director and the medical examiner's office. This exercise is a tremendous opportunity for residents to learn anatomic relations and critical dissection planes that are difficult to comprehend.

Teaching Surgical Technique

The use of preparatory courses and simulation programs needs to take into account the principles of massed versus distributed learning. Moulton has demonstrated that learning in large segments may be less effective than that done over a longer period in small segments. Therefore, in addition to an effective preparatory course and simulation session, programs need to distribute education and training over a longer period of time.

Much of the literature on perioperative teaching divides technical learning into three phases:

1. The cognitive phase where the learner intellectualizes the task, usually in the preoperative period. This phase includes study by the learner, such as video-based teaching, discussing the operation with faculty, and practicing on an inanimate model or cadaver, as discussed previously.
2. In the integration or associative phase, techniques are further refined and movements are made more efficient under supervision and guidance provided by an expert. This phase occurs in the intraoperative phase of technical learning. Postoperative review and discussion between the resident and faculty will help identify deficiencies or opportunities for improvement.
3. The mastery-based learning or autonomous phase is when technical proficiency becomes more automatic and the skills can be performed with minimal supervision and guidance. This phase requires reflection, self-awareness, practice, and further intraoperative experience. Figure 1 schematically represents the progression of these steps.

Preoperative Preparation

The faculty surgeon should know the level of training of the resident assisting with or performing the operation to confirm whether the operation is appropriate for the resident given the overall curriculum of the surgical residency program; the resident has specialized skills training, such as the FLS or introduction to robotic surgery; and the resident has previously performed the operation in an animal laboratory or with a simulator.

In the preoperative cognitive phase of the operation, the learner and instructor must collaborate to maximize task engagement. This responsibility can be achieved by setting goals based on performance or learning. The former focuses on the achievement of outcomes measured by metrics; the latter on the learning process and mastery of content. Gardner and colleagues have demonstrated that establishing learning goals will lead to better metacognition and higher-order mental processes. Preoperative teaching also can detect and document any gaps in the technical skills of the learner. The combination of preparation, establishment of learning goals, and understanding the needs of the learner will maximize effectiveness of the cognitive phase of technical learning.

A purposeful discussion between the faculty surgeon and the resident should occur before the planned operation, either in person or virtually. The discussion should focus on the pertinent surgical anatomy and relevant anatomic variants, as well as the portions of the operation where dissection poses a distinct risk of injury. These issues should be viewed through the prism of the patient's unique history and characteristics;

Figure 1. Phases of technical learning for perioperative teaching

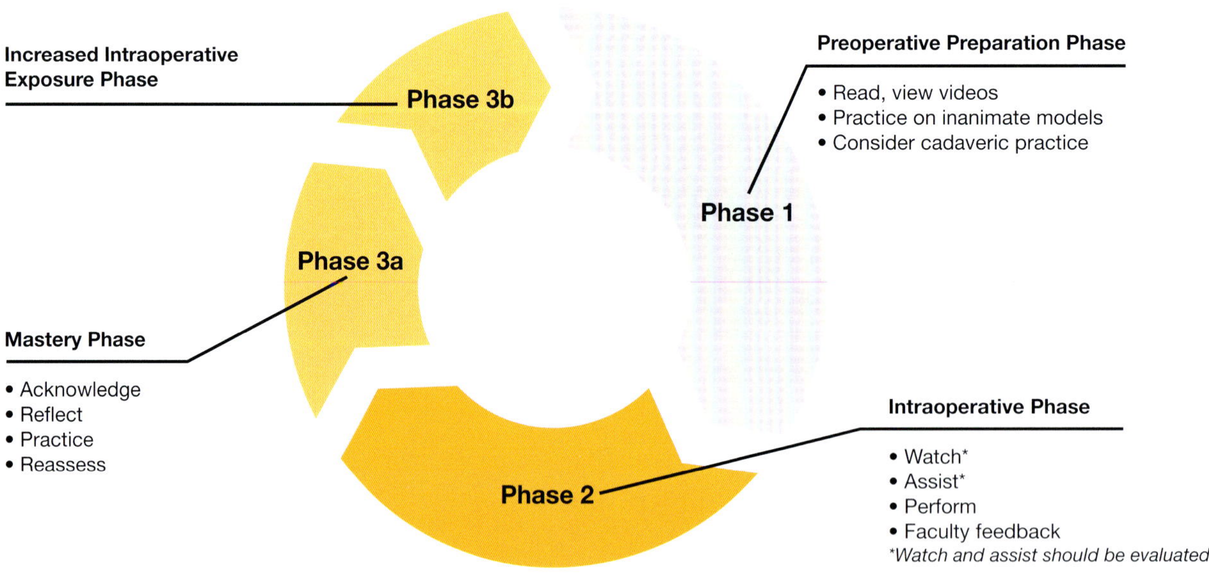

that is, body habitus, previous operations, previous bouts of inflammation, existing imaging studies, and so on. The faculty should ascertain the trainee's previous experience with the specific operation and familiarity with the various steps in the operation. When multiple surgical approaches (open, laparoscopic, robotic, endoscopic, natural orifice) are available, the most appropriate one and an alternate should be decided upon. A review of the positioning of the patient on the OR table and relevant positioning safety precautions should be highlighted (for example, protection of the axilla or the peroneal nerve). Specific technical steps (in order of the operation), including the faculty surgeon's "tricks of the trade," are beneficial elements of this interaction.

Teaching in the OR

The intraoperative phase of technical teaching is demanding for both the teacher and learner. The surgeon is trying to ensure the operation proceeds smoothly and without errors while simultaneously teaching technical skills to the learner. There may be a gap between the level of autonomy expected by the learner and the level the surgeon is willing to give. This misalignment increases the stress level in the OR. Studies show that the best intraoperative teaching is done when the faculty surgeon uses every aspect of the case for the purposes of teaching. At the same time, the best acquisition of intraoperative skills occurs when the learner has prepared themselves appropriately and is in an OR environment that offers encouragement, not excessive criticism.

In view of all of these factors, the attending surgeon should bear in mind that the way to minimize mistakes while teaching in the OR is to maximize verbal teaching; this means pausing the operation to describe the bigger picture to the learner, questioning the resident on each step of the operation, and verbalizing specific commands. Finally, the instructing surgeon must monitor the learner's performance and assess their entrustability in order to determine the level of autonomy to grant. What makes this part of perioperative teaching extremely demanding and challenging is the need for simultaneous performance of all of these tasks: keep the patient safe, use every opportunity to teach, assess the level of autonomy one can grant, and offer encouragement. The premise that a teaching hospital must reinforce is that teaching operative care takes additional time. Planning for and accepting this premise is critical in today's training environment where the emphasis on efficiency may detract from teaching time. A program, its leaders, and the institutional leadership need to invest in the next generation of surgeons by ensuring adequate time to teach.

The operation should be broken down into major steps, and the faculty member should strive to gain a sense of the trainee's comfort level throughout these steps. Ultimately, trainees make the most technical progress when they are allowed to operate in their own "zone of proximal development," just beyond their comfort level, during the various stages of an operation.

Actual supervision and teaching in the OR should be appropriate to the level of the resident and based on the concept of graduated responsibility over a five-year training program in general surgery. Basic questions on applied anatomy are appropriate for a junior surgical resident or medical student in the classroom but often inappropriate for a chief resident performing a complex operation under supervision. In addition, teaching comments should be integrated into the workflow of an operation so as to not unduly prolong any procedure. With unanticipated operative findings or complications, a faculty member may take over from the resident for a specific portion to move through the difficulty or to maintain patient safety.

A resident surgeon may be more receptive to reflection after the critical part of the operation is completed; therefore, this occasion is often an excellent time for the faculty surgeon to teach the importance of the finishing steps of a major operation. These steps would include: 1) survey of the operative cavity and removal of foreign bodies, 2) placement of drains, 3) insertion of oral or percutaneous feeding tubes, 4) confirmation of hemostasis, 5) irrigation of the operative field, 6) optimal technique for closure of the incision, 7) management of the subcutaneous tissue and skin of the incision, and/or 8) coverage of the open abdomen. In addition, a discussion of what went right or wrong might be appropriate when the procedure is directly in mind.

Postoperative Review

The postoperative phase is the best time for a review session with the trainee to provide feedback on performance and set goals for the future. The faculty surgeon should emphasize teaching points that were made during the operation and answer any questions the resident has on operative technique or flow of the operation. When necessary, the faculty surgeon should recommend further textbook or atlas review and/or additional practice in the laboratory (cadaver or animal) or simulation center. Time pressures, however, often prevent a detailed postoperative review in person at the conclusion of the operation. This is when the dictation function within the System for Improving and Measuring Procedural Learning (SIMPL) system (discussed later) or a locally developed evaluation tool may be used to maximum benefit, detailing both the positive and negative aspects of the trainee's performance. Any formal evaluation that the faculty member submits should be discussed with the trainee during the postoperative review.

Assessing Technical Skill of Trainees

Accurate assessment of performance is paramount for optimal acquisition and maintenance of surgical skill. It is important to distinguish between summative and formative assessments, which surgeon educators often confuse. Summative assessments, which are often high stakes, evaluate learning at the end of an assignment or rotation by measuring learner performance against a standard or benchmark. In contrast, formative assessments, which are typically low stakes, are used to monitor the learning process and the learner's progress. These assessments help learners focus their efforts on areas where they need to improve and guide instructors on how to focus their teaching to address their students' needs. If formative assessments are conducted frequently, there typically will not be any surprises on summative assessments.

Performance assessment is a staple of competency-based training. Such outcome-based training often is synonymous with proficiency-based training or mastery learning. It relies on frequent and accurate assessments that determine whether the trainee has achieved predefined training goals, and it offers remediation pathways for residents who have yet to achieve these goals. Given that training goals must be specific to be effective, competency-based evaluation must include frequent and accurate assessments.

Assessments of technical skill in surgery typically rely either on expert assessment tools or on objective metrics, such as task time and errors. Many assessment tools and metrics have been used to assess technical performance of surgeons and surgical trainees; these measures have variable evidence of validity and reliability. Given the multitude of existing tools, surgical educators are encouraged to search the literature for tools relevant to the skills or procedures they want to assess.

Validated Organized Assessment Tools

Some of the most commonly used and better studied assessments, which can be used for both formative and summative purposes, are described herein. For all of the tools but the last one, experts provide their ratings in each skill domain using a 5-point behaviorally anchored Likert scale.

Objective Structured Assessment of Technical Skill
Objective Structured Assessment of Technical Skill (OSATS) assesses technical skill in six domains (respect for tissue, time and motion, instrument handling, knowledge of procedure, flow of operation, and overall skill) and has been studied extensively across many common surgery domains and for a variety of skills.

Global Operative Assessment of Laparoscopic Skills
Global Operative Assessment of Laparoscopic Skills (GOALS) is specific to laparoscopic surgery and a derivative of the OSATS scale with ample evidence of validity. It assesses laparoscopic skill in five domains, including depth perception, bimanual dexterity, efficiency, tissue handling, and autonomy.

Global Evaluative Assessment of Robotic Skills
Global Evaluative Assessment of Robotic Skills (GEARS) is specific to robotic surgery and is derived from GOALS. It assesses robotic skill in six domains: depth perception, bimanual dexterity, efficiency, force sensitivity, robotic control, and autonomy.

Global Assessment of Gastrointestinal Endoscopic Skills
Global Assessment of Gastrointestinal Endoscopic Skills (GAGES) includes a version of the tool specific to upper endoscopy (GAGES-Upper Endoscopy) and a version specific to colonoscopy (GAGES-Colonoscopy). These tools comprise four common skill domains, including scope navigation, ability to maintain clear endoscopic visibility, use of instrumentation, and thoroughness of examination, in addition to a unique skill set focused on the quality of examination (such as intubation of the esophagus for upper endoscopy, reversal of scope, use of inflation pressure to position scope, and so on).

Global Rating Assessment Device for Endovascular Skills
Global Rating Assessment Device for Endovascular Skills (GRADES) tool is specific to endovascular skill and assesses skill in six domains: efficiency, wire and catheter manipulation, use of the device, image quality, image safety (including fluoroscopy, contrast use), and autonomy.

University of Western Ontario Microsurgical Acquisition/ Assessment Instrument
This tool is specific to microsurgery skill and assesses skill in eight domains: respect for tissue, time in motion, instrument handling, suture training, flow of operation, knowledge of procedure, final product, and overall performance.

System for Improving and Measuring Procedural Learning
In System for Improving and Measuring Procedural Learning (SIMPL), the roles of the faculty teacher and resident can vary throughout the steps of the operation from "show and tell" to "supervision only." Between these two extremes, most operations will be orchestrated by the faculty member as "active help" or "passive help" levels of guidance and assistance. Details can be found at *www.simpl.org*.

Other Specific Assessment Metrics

Numerous assessment tools have been developed for technical performance assessment, similar to the ones presented previously, including checklists and global rating scales. However, skill ratings obtained through these tools are subjective and influenced by rater biases, including central tendency bias, leniency or severity bias, and halo and horn effects. They introduce undesired rating variability that limits the reliability of these performance assessments. Rating variability can be reduced through the use of expert raters and rater training, but it cannot be entirely eliminated. However, rater training requires significant resources, and the use of expert raters is costly. The incorporation of more objective metrics of surgical performance may help minimize assessment bias and reduce the need for expert raters.

The following performance assessment metrics have been proposed; some have been widely adopted, whereas others have not.

Task Time and Errors

These metrics are the most studied and frequently used performance metrics in surgical simulation. Measurement of task time is very reliable, with little room for variation. Errors are discrete and well defined for each task and minimize assessment bias by allowing little room for interpretation. The FLS and several of the ACS/APDS skill modules incorporate these metrics.

Motion Tracking

Tracking of surgeon hand and instrument movements has been reproducibly shown to distinguish among levels of surgical expertise. Instrument motion metrics automatically recorded during robotic prostatectomy have been associated with surgeon expertise and patient urinary continence outcomes after surgery. A variety of motion tracking methods exist, with sensors embedded either at the instruments or attached to the surgeon's hands.

Metrics of Respect for Tissue

Respect for tissue is a staple of surgical performance and a domain of many skill assessment tools, such as the OSATS. Nonetheless, expert ratings of respect for tissue are subjective, influenced by several rater biases, and are not directly quantifiable. Therefore, it is necessary that we develop objective metrics to assess respect for tissue. Studies have suggested that force-based metrics are better indicators of performance than metrics based on time to task completion or instrument and hand position.

Metrics of Automaticity

One of the main characteristics that distinguishes experts from less-accomplished performers is automaticity, or the ability to engage in activities without using significant attentional resources. Many habitual or highly practiced motor acts can be performed automatically, allowing the performer's capacity for attention to be engaged in other activities. Assessing automaticity can be accomplished through the use of a secondary task that is performed concurrently with the primary task and competes for the same attentional resources. A visual-spatial secondary task for performance assessment on simulators has previously been shown to be more sensitive in detecting subtle performance differences between skilled individuals and individuals who exhibit the traditional metrics of time and accuracy. Application of this metric during skills training has further been shown to lead to superior skill acquisition compared with proficiency-based training.

Eye Tracking

Eye tracking quantifies the point of gaze and motion of the eye during a specific scene or event and is thought to reflect visual attention and cognitive intention during task execution. Eye tracking technology, typically assessed through stationary cameras or cameras integrated within eyeglasses, monitors visual attention by recording corneal reflection of infrared lighting to detect pupil positioning. Furthermore, eye tracking assessments can also allow for assessment of dwell time (that is, a surrogate assessment of stimulus importance), fixation frequency, and pupil dilation (a measure of concentration and cognitive effort). Research using eye tracking assessments in surgery has shown that experts focus more accurately on relevant task-related stimuli and focus longer on anatomic targets than do trainees. Research shows that novices tend to focus more on their instruments than on anatomic targets. Thus, use of eye tracking analysis appears to be an effective method to discriminate between surgeons of varying skill levels.

Metrics of Artificial Intelligence (AI)

Machine learning algorithms applied to visual data have recently been successfully implemented to obtain insights relevant to surgical skill. These deep learning algorithms are applied to procedural videos and use multilayered neural networks with a hierarchical computational structure to recognize data patterns. By combining deep learning classification and anomaly detection algorithms to analyze video data, AI metrics have been shown to correlate with human ratings of performance based on the GOALS assessment tool. The use of AI for performance assessment in surgery is growing rapidly and will complement skill assessment in the future.

Procedure Certification for Residents

The main goal of certification is to ensure that a candidate is competent in essential elements required of their specialty. The main goal of the certification process is to support delivery of safe and effective patient care by affirming that a candidate has achieved the requisite level of knowledge, skills, and judgment as defined by the profession. Surgery resident board certification in the U.S. includes a Qualifying Examination, a multiple-choice examination to assess surgical knowledge and its application to surgical practice; and the Certifying Examination, an oral examination that focuses on assessment of diagnostic and management skills, problem solving, and judgment. Unfortunately, technical skills, which are the hallmark of surgery and have been shown to be associated with patient outcomes, are not directly assessed during these examinations and the outcomes of the exams do not correlate with technical skill and operative performance. To ensure adequate technical skills, residents have to fulfill case number requirements and are assessed by faculty and the program director at individual residency programs. The indirectness of this approach limits technical skill assessment; a more objective and direct approach is needed.

To address this gap, professional societies are using simulation to assess technical performance and develop high-stakes certification programs more objectively. Examples include the FLS examination, the FES examination, the European Board of Vascular Surgery Technical Skill Examination, and the Colorectal Objective Structured Assessment of Technical Skill (COSATS). The first two are required for graduation from general surgery residency programs and have been described previously in this chapter.

The European Board of Vascular Surgery Examination is a technical skills examination consisting of three vascular surgery tasks on simulated bench-top models with demonstrated evidence for construct validity, interrater reliability, and good internal consistency. Since 2004, this technical skill examination has been incorporated into the board certification process. A limitation of this examination is the lack of rigorous methodology for standard setting.

The COSATS Examination was developed by the American Society of Colon and Rectal Surgeons (ASCRS) and is a multiple station examination conducted on simulation models. Candidates rotate through eight stations and are asked to perform technical tasks specific to the practice of colon and rectal surgery. Although this program can identify failure of specific skills acquisition, its role in the certification process remains unclear.

Procedure certification will become more objective in the future, but before adoption any high-stakes assessment used for certification purposes must be supported by high-validity evidence. Further, valid standard-setting methodologies are needed to set reliable passing scores. Incorporating simulation in such assessments can help standardize the assessment process and make it reproducible. The cost of these examinations is an obstacle to implementing them on a wide scale.

Ensuring Competency of Trainees in Common and High-Risk Procedures for Autonomous Practice after Training

Ideally, each procedure that is taught as part of a training program needs the following elements:

- Formal objectives
- Formal assumptions
- Specific resources
- Simulation laboratory modules for practice
- A list of the necessary equipment/instrumentation necessary to safely complete the procedure
- A specific description of the procedure, including a description of strategic decisions to make during a procedure
- An outline of challenges, pitfalls, and unusual complications and solutions
- Strategies for trainee assessment

A complete curriculum for procedure skills training is beyond the scope of this manual. However, to organize procedures in a way to give detail to these eight elements, we will give an example of each of the most challenging principles and procedures to learn. The authors offer four types of procedures for consideration:

- A frequent procedure of intermediate technical difficulty (cholecystectomy)
- An infrequent procedure of intermediate technical difficulty (cricothyrotomy)
- An infrequent procedure of high technical difficulty (resuscitative thoracotomy)
- A frequent procedure of high technical difficulty (pancreaticoduodenectomy)

Each of these four types of procedures will be presented according to the eight elements described.

- Objectives:
  - Objectives point to the critical elements that need to be considered for this type of procedure, the factors that may complicate the decision-making, the elements to be considered in ordering the steps of the procedure, critical elements to comprehend the anatomic considerations, and specific technical goals incumbent within that procedure, including intraoperative assessment procedures.

- Assumptions:
  - Includes critical knowledge unique to the procedure, which one assumes is appreciated and acquired before undertaking the operation. Topics listed will deal with important factors related to diagnosis and staging of primary disease, patient risk assessment, needed equipment, and ancillary resources such as specialized anesthesiology support and radiologic capabilities.

- ACS resources/suggested reading:
  - ACS educational offerings, atlases, and publications will be included.
  - Textbook content and important journal articles will be listed.

- Description of simulation laboratory module:
  - Available simulation resources will be listed.
  - Cadaver laboratory and animal laboratory resources along with comments related to feasibility and expense will be described.

- Equipment and instrumentation considerations:
  - Important equipment items and specialized instrumentation recommended by expert surgeons will be listed.

- A specific description of procedure, including strategic decisions to make during a procedure:
  - A step-by-step description of the procedure with technical steps that are key to procedural success and avoidance of complications will be included.

- Challenges, pitfalls, and unusual complications:
  - Unusual situations that arise because of anatomical variations, unexpected involvement of adjacent organs, and imperfect preoperative disease staging will be listed. Advice from expert surgeons on steps to manage these challenges will be included.

- Trainee assessment:
  - Methods for assessing trainee performance will be included. These will specifically deal with criteria for determining successful operative performance and documenting readiness for autonomy.

A Frequent Procedure of Intermediate Technical Difficulty: Open and Laparoscopic Cholecystectomy

OBJECTIVES

- Choose appropriate approach based on patient's disease (acute cholecystitis versus recurrent attacks of biliary colic), condition, and history of prior abdominal surgery.
- Recognize when top-down approach during either open or laparoscopic cholecystectomy is needed.
- Recognize the "Critical View of Safety" during dissection.
- Perform safe clipping or ligation of cystic artery and duct.
- Perform accurate cystic duct cholangiogram, if needed.

ASSUMPTIONS

- Incidence of anatomic variants and long-term morbidity of iatrogenic ductal injury are underappreciated by surgical trainees (Figures 2 and 3).

Figure 2. Biliary tract and arterial variants

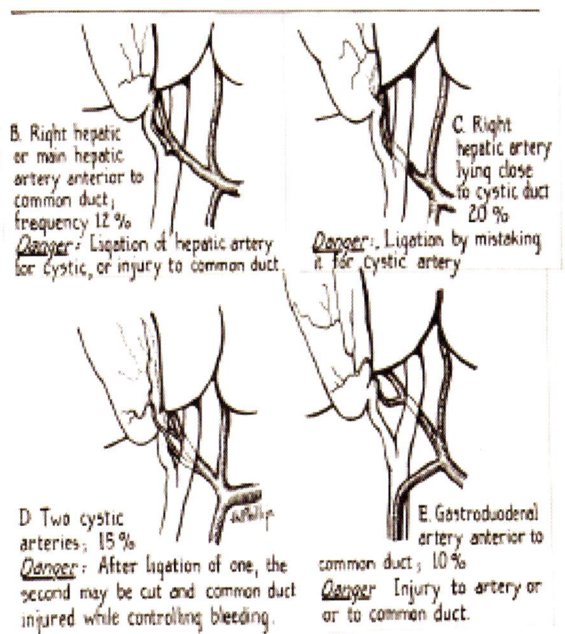

Source: Edwards EA, et al. *Operative Anatomy of Abdomen and Pelvis*. Philadelphia: Lea & Febiger; 1975.

Figure 3

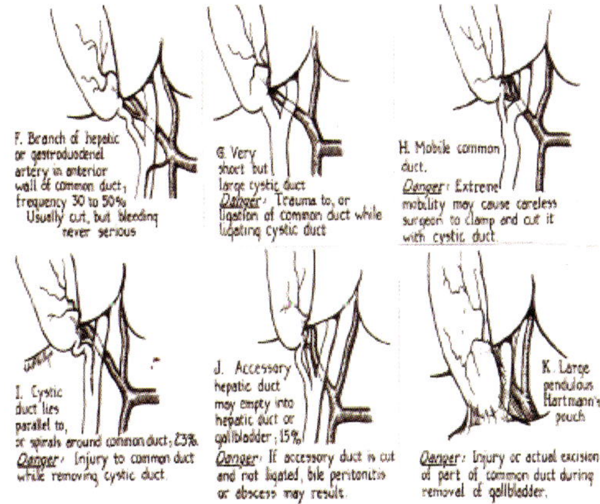

Source: Edwards EA, et al. *Operative Anatomy of Abdomen and Pelvis*. Philadelphia: Lea & Febiger; 1975.

ACS RESOURCES/SUGGESTED READING

American College of Surgeons. *ACS Multimedia Atlas of Surgery, Liver Surgery Volume*. Available at: https://learning.facs.org/content/acs-multimedia-atlas-surgery-liver-surgery. Accessed October 21, 2021.

American College of Surgeons and Association of Program Directors in Surgery. ACS/APDS Surgery Resident Skills Curriculum – Phase 2, Module 13. Available at https://learning.facs.org/content/acsapds-surgery-resident-skills-curriculum-phase-2. Accessed October 21, 2021.

Jensen MO. Liver, biliary system, pancreas, and spleen. In: *Surgical Anatomy for Mastery of Open Operations*. Philadelphia, PA: Wolters Kluwer; 2019.

Swanstrom LL, Soper NJ. Laparoscopic Cholecystectomy. In *Mastery of Endoscopic and Laparoscopic Surgery*. Philadelphia, PA: Wolters Kluwer; 2014.

DESCRIPTION OF SIMULATION LABORATORY MODULE

- Animal laboratory: Porcine model, expensive, effective
- Simulation from module from ACS/APDS Surgery Resident Skills Curriculum, Phase 2: Expensive, not widely available

EQUIPMENT AND INSTRUMENTATION CONSIDERATIONS

- Laparotomy (after incision): Kelly clamp, DeBakey tissue forceps, Metzenbaum scissors, peanut dissector, right angle clamp, clip applier, and cholangiogram equipment and supplies (catheter, three-way stopcock, water-soluble contrast)
- Laparoscopy: 4 ports (5-10 mm), 30-degree laparoscope with video camera, light source, 2 TV monitors appropriately positioned, CO_2 insufflator and tubing, "L" hook cautery, 2 atraumatic graspers (one with ratchet), Maryland dissector, clip applier, laparoscopic Metzenbaum scissors, cholangiogram material (same as above with Olsen clamp), endo-loop, and extraction bag

A SPECIFIC DESCRIPTION OF PROCEDURE

- Patient positioning
  - Supine with strap and footboard, arms at sides (allows for easy placement of self-retaining retractors) or at 90 degrees
- Laparotomy incision/access for laparoscopy
  - Laparotomy incision—Right subcostal versus upper midline based on patient's habitus and/or presence of upper abdominal scars. Mini subcostal if conditions are ideal.
  - Access for laparoscopy: Open blunt-tipped Hasson cannula versus percutaneous Veress needle; transumbilical or infraumbilical incision for entrance of 10 mm trocar through which CO_2 insufflation to <15 mm Hg pressure is performed; epigastric and right subcostal trocars inserted under direct view of 30-degree angled laparoscope with transillumination to avoid epigastric vessels.
- Exposure of gallbladder
  - Laparotomy: Appropriate multidirectional packing, including retraction of the costal margin and right lobe of liver superiorly, packing abdominal viscera from hepatic flexure inferiorly, medial exposure to demonstrate gallbladder fossa and portal triad and retracting gallbladder with Kelly clamps.
  - Laparoscopy: Position patient in reverse Trendelenburg position with left-sided rotation; retract right lobe of liver superiorly and grasp gallbladder with atraumatic graspers at fundus and infundibulum.
- Anterior and lateral caudal traction (to demonstrate cystic duct and underlying common bile duct) (Figure 4)

Figure 4. Caudal and lateral retraction

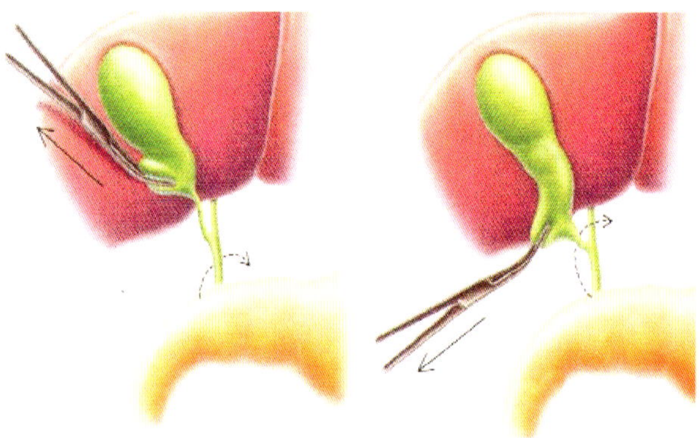

Source: Fried GM, et al. Cholecystectomy and common bile duct exploration. In: *ACS Surgery: Principles & Practice*. 6th edition. 2006.

- Laparotomy: Obtained by Kelly clamps on fundus and Hartmann pouch of gallbladder
- Laparoscopy: Obtained by right subcostal graspers at midclavicular and anterior axillary lines; if graspers unable to hold distended gallbladder, decompression with a needle-suction device is helpful

STRATEGIC DECISION

- Top-down versus bottom-up.
- Decide based on retraction ability of the gallbladder and clear separation of the cystic duct/cystic artery mesentery from the portal triad whether bottom-up is safe or whether, due to inflammation/infection/pancreatitis, the cystic duct and cystic artery should be exposed using a top-down approach.
- Adhesiolysis and exposing cystic duct and artery
  - Greater omentum adherent to fundus, body, and Hartmann pouch can often be removed at laparotomy with finger dissection or at laparoscopy by traction and dissection with a Maryland dissector. The L-hook can be used judiciously during this dissection, using low-wattage setting. Peritoneal adhesions or attachments to the neck of the gallbladder are dissected circumferentially to allow for widening of the cystic-common hepatic duct angle.
- Dissection to achieve the Critical View of Safety (Figure 5)

Figure 5. The Critical View of Safety is displayed after dissecting the gallbladder away from its hepatic bed, leaving two, and only two, structures entering the gallbladder

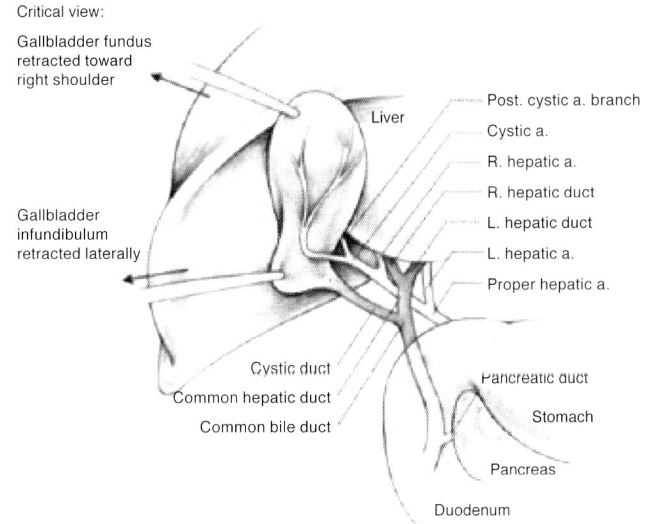

Source: Jensen MO. Liver, biliary system, pancreas, and spleen. In: *Surgical Anatomy for Mastery of Open Operations*. Philadelphia, PA: Wolters Kluwer; 2019.

  - Continue dissection until the Critical View of Safety is obtained; that is, the gallbladder has been separated from its bed, only two structures are entering into the gallbladder, and the base of the liver can be visualized through the dissected triangle of Calot. If this critical view cannot be achieved, consider top-down dissection to avoid injury to the common duct.

- At laparotomy, the cystic artery is divided between metal clips or 3-0 silk ties and the cystic duct is divided between metal clips or 3-0 absorbable ties. A very wide cystic duct is oversewn with interrupted 3-0 absorbable sutures. At laparoscopy, the cystic artery and duct are divided between metal clips. A very wide cystic duct is sequentially divided after placement of overlapping clips. Alternatively, the duct can be sharply divided and occluded with an endo-loop.
- Dissection of the gallbladder from the liver bed
  - With superior traction on the infundibulum superior to the divided cystic artery and duct, the gallbladder is dissected away from the liver bed using Metzenbaum scissors or cautery at laparotomy or an L-hook with electrocautery at laparoscopy. If bile is seen leaking from the liver bed, either caused by a divided duct of Luschka, or more likely a small superficial bile duct exposed in the hepatic parenchyma, this area may be oversewn with a 3-0 absorbable suture or cauterized.
- Laparoscopic extraction of the gallbladder
  - The freed gallbladder is placed on top of the right lobe of the liver with a grasper. The laparoscopic camera is placed in the epigastric port site, and the gallbladder is extracted through the umbilical port site using a grasper. A ruptured, thin-walled, or infected gallbladder is placed in a plastic bag attached to an external handle. Manipulation of the handle will seal the bag around the gallbladder and the entire system is removed with the umbilical port.
- Alternate maneuvers if unable to obtain Critical View of Safety
  - "Bailout": convert to cholecystostomy tube
  - Laparotomy: perform fenestrating or nonfenestrating subtotal cholecystectomy
  - Laparoscopy: Convert to laparotomy or perform subtotal cholecystectomy
    - This may allow for finger dissection of the tissues, identification of surgical anatomy, addressing of significant operative bleeding, managing an injury to the common hepatic or bile duct, or confirming suspicion of unanticipated gallbladder cancer or other intra-abdominal pathology. Alternatively, with advanced laparoscopic skills, a subtotal cholecystectomy can be performed, either fenestrating or nonfenestrating, with placement of a subhepatic suction drain for anticipated bile leakage postoperatively.
- Intraoperative cystic duct cholangiogram
  - Once the cannula is in place, proper final concentration of contrast (33 percent), proper positioning of patient with right side down (distal common bile duct isolated away from spine), low-volume injections, and head-up/head-down positions should lead to precise images. Visualization should include extrahepatic ducts, intrahepatic ducts, and contrast delivery into the duodenum.

CHALLENGES/PITFALLS/UNUSUAL COMPLICATIONS

- Failure to recognize anatomic variants: dual cystic arteries, aberrant right hepatic artery, short cystic duct, accessory right hepatic duct, and so on (both modes of operation)
- Misidentification of common bile duct for cystic duct (both)
- Blind application of clips/clamps/cautery for bleeding (both)
- Cholangiogram: indications, misreading of images, management of filling defects (both)
- Management of perforated gallbladder (both)
- Management of multiple stone spillage (both)
- Infundibular technique versus critical view of safety (laparoscopy)
- Over dissection of cystic duct-common bile duct junction (laparoscopy)
- Bleeding from port site, closure of port site(s) (laparoscopy)

TRAINEE ASSESSMENT

- With respect to perioperative assessment of the resident's skills, two primary systems may be used. As discussed above, GOALS assesses skills in five domains using a Likert scale. Alternatively, the SIMPL system can be used as a global assessment of the independence demonstrated by the trainee in performance of the operation. This is an app-based system that assesses the relative difficulty of the operation, the technical performance of the resident, and the degree of autonomy achieved by the resident during the majority of the operation. Importantly, a dictation function can also be used to give immediate formative feedback regarding technical details of the procedure or other aspects of the case deemed important by the attending surgeon.

An Infrequent Procedure of Intermediate Technical Difficulty: Cricothyroidotomy

OBJECTIVES

- Identify through palpation external landmarks for a cricothyroidotomy incision.
- Recognize the cricothyroid space.
- Learn stabilization of thyroid and cricoid structures in the midline to allow performance of a vertical or transverse incision over the cricothyroid membrane.
- Insert an appropriate-sized tracheostomy tube.

ASSUMPTIONS

- Although this is a lifesaving procedure, most surgeons have limited experience and training is therefore prerequisite. Training will increase the chances of success during an emergency.

ACS RESOURCES/SUGGESTED READING

ATLS Subcommittee, ACS COT, International ATLS working group. Advanced trauma life support (ATLS): the ninth edition. *J Trauma Acute Care Surg*. 2013;74(5):1333–1366.

Demetriades D, Chudnofsky CR, Benjamin ER. *Color Atlas of Emergency Trauma*. Cambridge University Press; 2021.

Demetriades D, Inaba K, Velmahos GC. In: *Atlas of Surgical Techniques in Trauma*. Cambridge, United Kingdom; New York, NY, USA: Cambridge University Press; 2020:7-15.

DeVore EK, Redmann A, Howell R, Khosla S. Best practices for emergency surgical airway: a systematic review. *Laryngoscope Investig Otolaryngol*. 2019;4(6):602-608.

Thal ER, Weigelt JA, Carrico CJ. *Operative Trauma Management: An Atlas*. New York: McGraw-Hill, Medical Pub. Division; 2002.

DESCRIPTION OF SIMULATION LABORATORY MODULE

- Demonstration of anatomic landmarks and palpation on self and colleagues is a primary skill that can be rehearsed repeatedly
- Simulation trauma man trainer: Affordable, effective, reusable, widely available (Figure 6)

Figure 6. Trauma man trainer (SIMULAB)

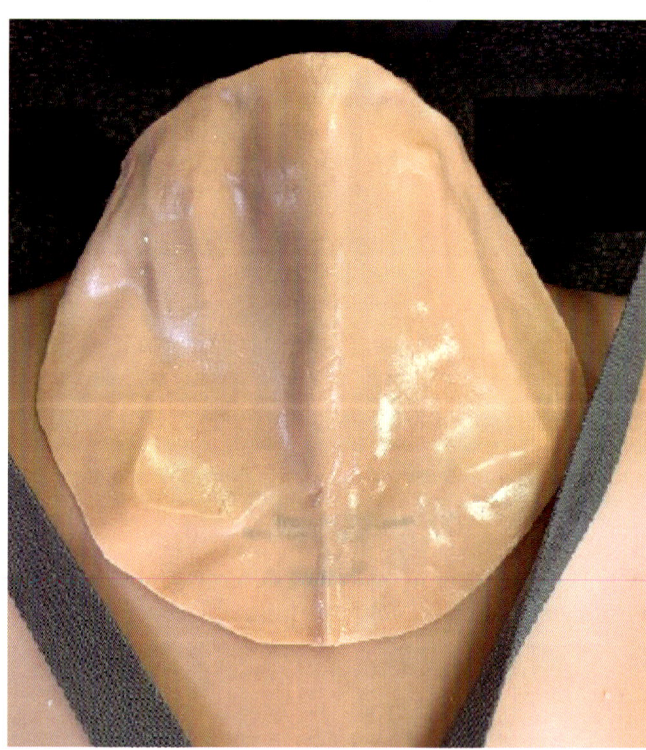

Source: Getty Images

- Cadaver model: Realistic; however, not widely available, expensive, not reusable, only in selected facilities (Figure 7)

Figure 7. Human cadaver model

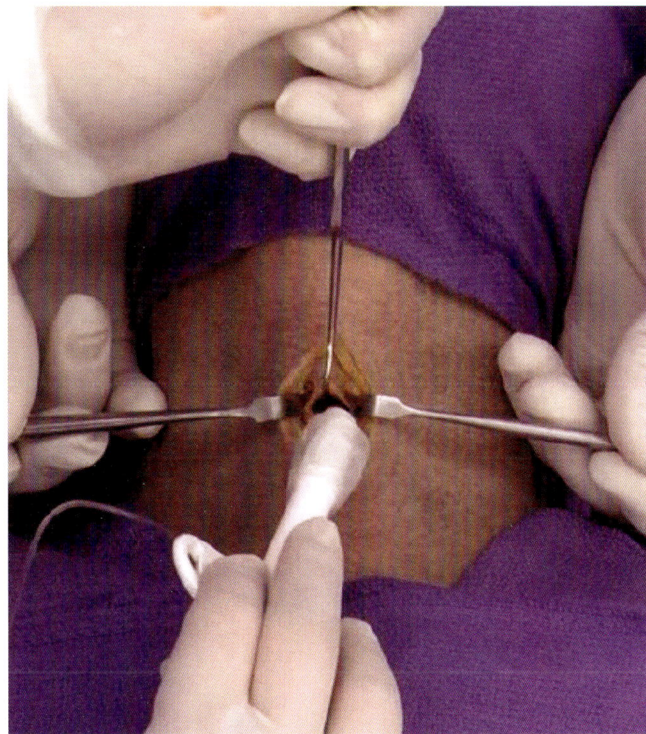

Source: Schellenberg M, Demetriades D. Cricothyroidotomy. In: Demetriades D, Inaba K, Lumb P, eds. *Atlas of Critical Care Procedures*. Cham, Switzerland: Springer; 2018.

EQUIPMENT AND INSTRUMENTATION CONSIDERATIONS

- Identify key instruments for the procedure (Figure 8)

Figure 8. Key instruments

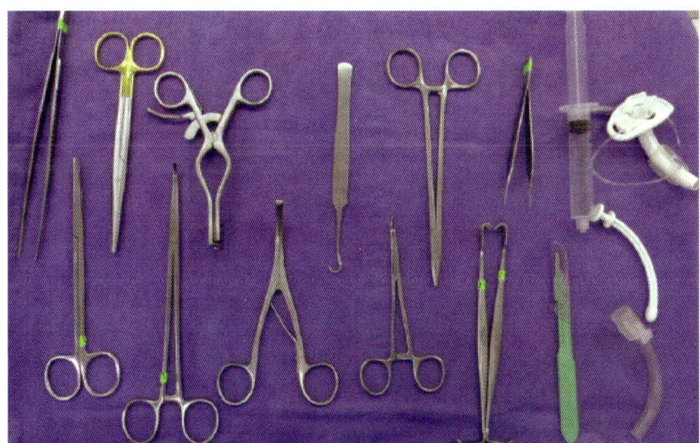

Source: Schellenberg M, Demetriades D. Cricothyroidotomy. In: Demetriades D, Inaba K, Lumb P, eds. *Atlas of Critical Care Procedures*. Cham, Switzerland: Springer; 2018.

A SPECIFIC DESCRIPTION OF PROCEDURE

- Key steps:
  - Appropriately position the head and neck.
  - Identify external landmark for cricothyroid space.
  - Perform a vertical incision at the appropriate site.
  - Perform a transverse incision in the cricothyroid space.
  - Immobilize the trachea with a tracheostomy hook.
  - Cannulate cricothyroid opening and gently leverage tip side to side and down.
  - Confirm position of tracheostomy tube with CO2 return.
  - Secure tracheostomy tube to the skin.
  - Treat any wound or tract bleeding with pressure on the wound and tube together and do not remove tube.
- Strategic considerations:
  - Are surface landmarks readily palpable versus excessive subcutaneous tissue making palpation difficult?
  - Decide tracheostomy tube size to facilitate cannulation or occasional use of endotracheal tube when a neck is particularly thick.
  - Have a clear plan for how to confirm appropriate placement; ensure bag valve mask (Ambu bag) and CO2 detector readily available.

CHALLENGES/PITFALLS/UNUSUAL COMPLICATIONS

- Insertion of the tracheostomy tube too high or too low
  - Prevention: (1) learn to directly palpate cricothyroid membrane between thyroid prominence and cricoid prominence or (2) identify the external surface landmark with the 4-fingers technique (small finger in the suprasternal notch, tip of the index finger at cricothyroid space) (Figure 9).

Figure 9. The 4-finger technique for identifying the cricothyroid space

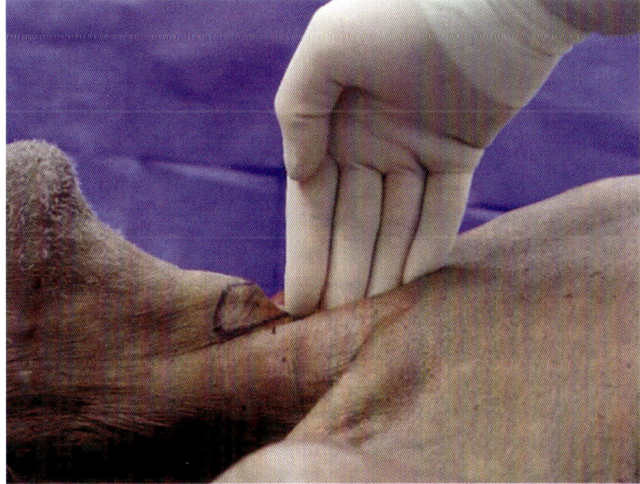

Source: Schellenberg M, Demetriades D. Cricothyroidotomy. In: Demetriades D, Inaba K, Lumb P, eds. *Atlas of Critical Care Procedures*. Cham, Switzerland: Springer; 2018.

- Injury to the anterior jugular vein, bleeding
  - Prevention: Stabilize airway so that blade does not drift laterally, perform a vertical skin incision.
- Insertion of the tracheostomy tube in the pretracheal space (high incidence in obese patients)
  - Prevention: Appreciate challenge in thick neck, immobilize trachea with tracheostomy hook (Figure 10), and anticipate occasional need for regular endotracheal tube.
- Accidental injury to the posterior tracheal wall
  - Prevention: Do not insert the tracheostomy tube in an anteroposterior direction. After trachea is entered, follow a path towards the carina and twist back and forth slightly to facilitate smooth descent of the tube and balloon.

Figure 10. Use of tracheal hook to immobilize the trachea

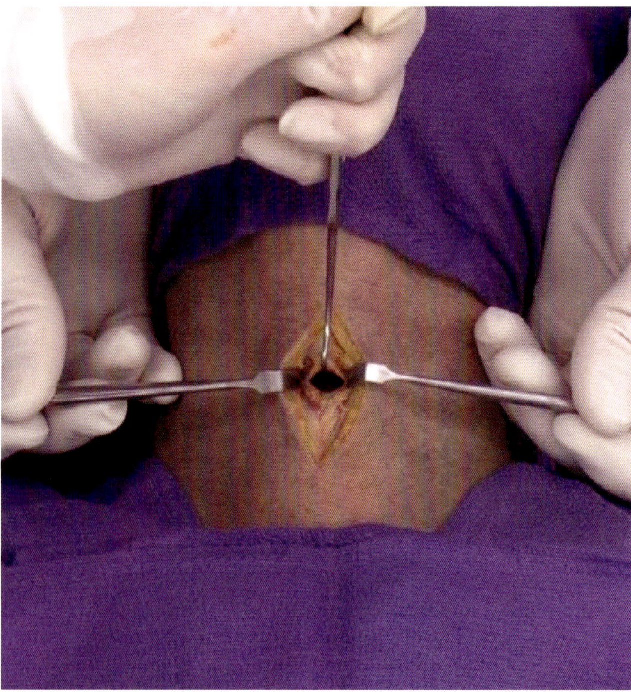

Source: Schellenberg M, Demetriades D. Cricothyroidotomy. In: Demetriades D, Inaba K, Lumb P, eds. *Atlas of Critical Care Procedures*. Cham, Switzerland: Springer; 2018.

TRAINEE ASSESSMENT

OSATS Scoring System:

1. Positioning of the head

Failed to perform	0
Performed but insufficiently	1
Performed appropriately	2

2. Identification of cricothyroid space

Failed to perform	0
Performed with some difficulty	1
Performed appropriately	2

3. Use of the tracheal hook to immobilize trachea

Did not use hook	0
Used hook, after experiencing difficulty	1
Used hook, immobilized trachea effectively	2

4. Progression of the procedure

Disorganized	0
Organized but hesitant	1
Organized and deliberate	2

Evaluation:

Score 0, in any of the 4 observations:
Failure, Remediation, Repeat Procedure

Score 1, in any of 4 observations:
Pass, Verbal Remediation

Score 2, in all of the 4 observations:
Pass

An Infrequent Procedure of High Technical Difficulty: Resuscitative Thoracotomy

OBJECTIVES

- The physiologic rationale for resuscitative thoracotomy (RT) is to restore life-sustaining perfusion to the cerebral and myocardial circulation in a patient in imminent or actual cardiopulmonary arrest.
- The primary objectives for performing RT include:
  - Decompression of pericardial tamponade
  - Control of cardiac or intrathoracic hemorrhage
  - Placement of a thoracic aortic cross clamp to enhance cerebral and myocardial perfusion
  - Placement of a pulmonary clamp with aspiration of the left heart for air embolism
  - Open cardiac massage
- Guidelines for RT are based on the duration of cardiopulmonary resuscitation (CPR) mechanism of trauma (blunt versus penetrating), and location of injury (compressible versus noncompressible bleeding). These capabilities vary institutionally based on available resources.
- The ultimate goal is to resuscitate a critically injured patient for definitive operative management resulting in a functional neurologic outcome.

ASSUMPTIONS

- Most general surgery residents have limited experience with RT unless they have trained in a program that includes a large urban trauma center. This lack of expertise is compounded by the fact that many of the recent generation of trauma surgeons lack experience with this procedure.

ACS RESOURCES/SUGGESTED READING

Burlew CC, Moore EE. Emergency Department Thoracotomy. In: Feliciano DV, Mattox KL, Moore EE eds. *Trauma, 9th ed.* New York, NY: McGraw-Hill; 2021.

DESCRIPTION OF SIMULATION LABORATORY MODULE

- Simulation trauma man trainer: Affordable, effective, reusable, widely available
- Cadaver model: Realistic, not widely available, expensive, not reusable, only in selected facilities
- Large animal model: Realistic, relatively expensive, not reusable

EQUIPMENT AND INSTRUMENTATION CONSIDERATIONS

- Identify key instruments for the procedure. Prior to patient arrival in the emergency department, all necessary equipment should be oriented for sequential use during the RT (Figure 11).
  - Betadine-soaked 4x4 gauze to prep the anterior chest
  - Laparotomy pads
  - 10-blade scalpel
  - Curved Mayo scissors
  - Fianchetti chest retractor (rib spreader)
  - Toothed forceps
  - Satinsky vascular clamps (large and small)
  - Lebsche knife and mallet
  - Needle holder
  - Sutures
    - 3-0 Prolene on a MH needle
    - 3-0 silk ties
    - 2-0 silk sutures
    - Teflon pledgets - 1x2 cm in size
    - Internal defibrillator paddles
    - 10 cc syringe with 18-gauge needle

A SPECIFIC DESCRIPTION OF PROCEDURE

Patient positioning: The patient should be supine with the left arm extended up over the head.

- Thoracic incision (Figure 12)
- A left anterolateral thoracotomy is the standard incision because it provides rapid access for pericardiotomy, descending thoracic aortic cross-clamping, and open cardiac massage.
  - The incision is made at the fifth intercostal space at the inframammary line.
  - In women, the breast is retracted cephalad to prevent entry at a lower intercostal space.
- Bilateral anterolateral "clamshell" thoracotomy is achieved via extension into the right hemithorax for patients with penetrating wounds to the right chest, access to the posterior heart, the transverse arch, and left ventricle in the event of air embolism.

Figure 11. Prior to patient arrival in the emergency department, all necessary equipment should be oriented for sequential use during the resuscitative thoracotomy

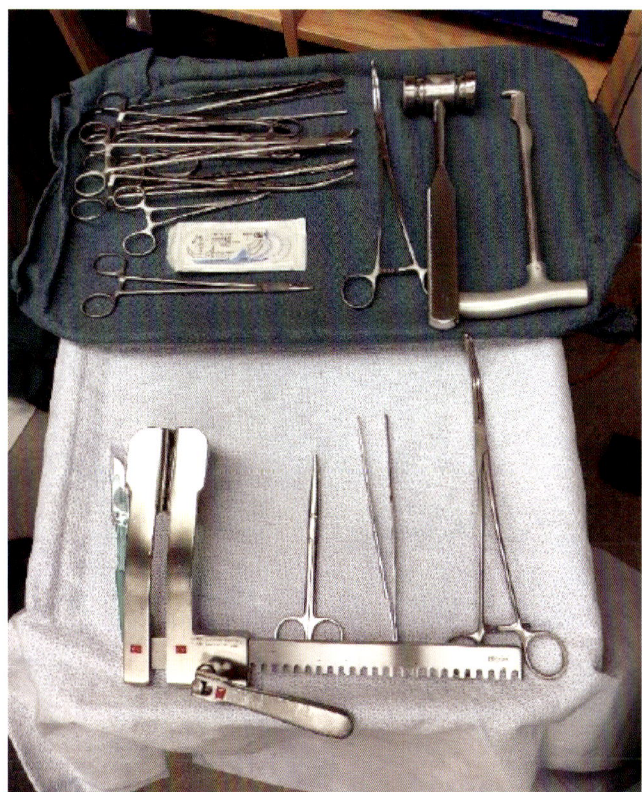

Source: Getty Images

Figure 12. The resuscitative thoracotomy incision is made at the 5th intercostal space at the inframammary line, starting at the right side of the sternum and curving toward the patient's axilla; this incision follows the rib cage's natural curvature

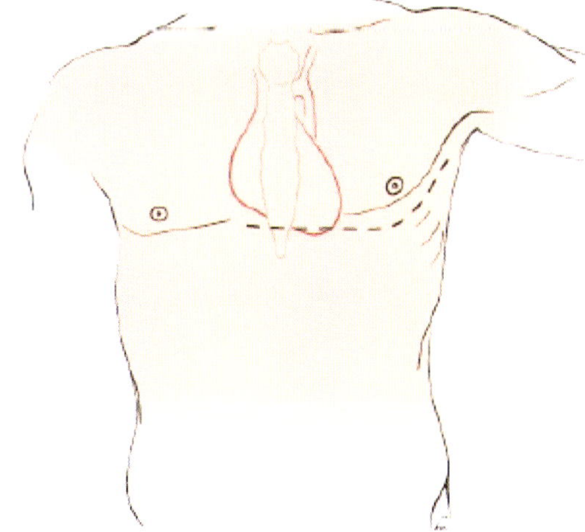

Source: Feliciano DV, Mattox KL, Moore EE. *Trauma*. Ninth Edition. McGraw Hill; 2021.

- If a bilateral thoracotomy is thought to be likely, start the incision on the patient's right side of the sternum to facilitate transection of the sternum with the Lebsche knife or access to transect the costal marginal cartilage without an additional skin incision.
- The skin incision is extended in the inframammary fold, passing beneath the nipple, gently curving toward the patient's axilla. The orientation of the incision should mirror the rib's natural curvature.
- The subcutaneous fat and chest wall musculature are sharply divided with a 10-blade to expose the ribs and associated intercostal space.
- The intercostal muscle is divided along the superior margin of the rib using with the curved Mayo scissors.
  - Avoid the intercostal neurovascular bundle by placing the scissors on top of the rib and follow the curve of the rib from medial (sternum) to lateral (axilla).
- The Finochietto retractor (rib spreader) is inserted with the handle up and toward the bed (Figure 13).
  - Extension across the sternum is possible without moving the rib spreader. If additional exposure is needed, the Lebsche knife is used to transect the sternum; extend into the right hemithorax, incising soft tissue with the knife and opening the intercostal space with scissors.
- Hold the Lebsche knife tightly against the underside of the sternum when dividing the sternum to prevent an iatrogenic cardiac injury.

Figure 13. The Finochietto rib spreader is positioned with the handle and cross-bar toward the bed

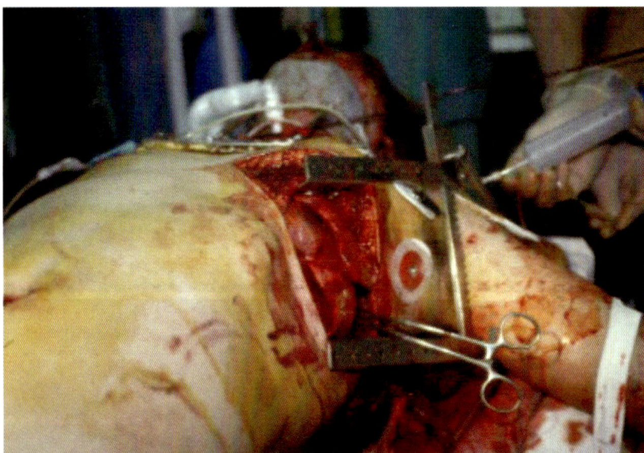

Source: Feliciano DV, Mattox KL, Moore EE. *Trauma*. Ninth Edition. McGraw Hill; 2021.

- After transecting the sternum, the internal mammary vessels should be identified and suture ligated with 2-0 silk after control of the thoracic bleeding. Failure to do this may cause postoperative bleeding which was not detectable in a patient in shock.
- Once a bilateral anterolateral "clamshell" thoracotomy is complete, move the rib retractor to a midline position to separate the chest wall for maximal exposure, or insert a second Finochietto (Figure 14).

Figure 14. If a clamshell thoracotomy is performed, the rib retractor should be moved to a midline position or a second rib retractor is placed on the right side to further separate the chest wall for maximal exposure

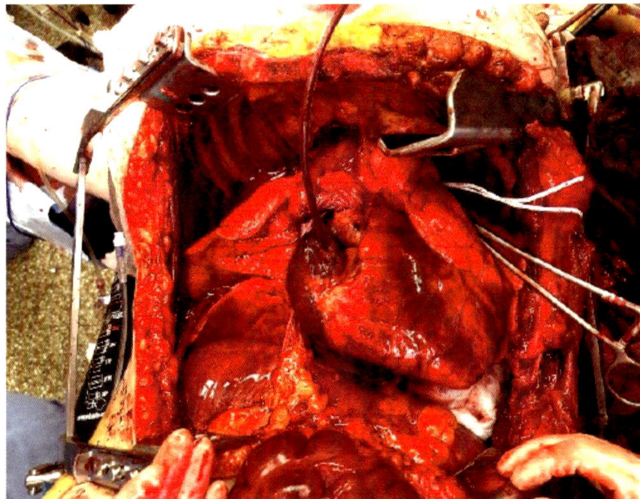

Source: Feliciano DV, Mattox KL, Moore EE. *Trauma*. Ninth Edition. McGraw Hill; 2021.

- Pericardotomy
  - After performing the resuscitative thoracotomy, the first step is to open the pericardium to exclude tamponade and facilitate open cardiac massage, unless an active bleeding site is identified upon entering the chest.
    - The pericardium is opened at the cardiac apex for decompression, bearing in mind the incision should be anterior to the phrenic nerve (Figure 15).
    - Elevate the pericardium with toothed forceps as the pericardium is tough, and open sharply with scissors.
    - In the event of tense pericardial tamponade, a scalpel can be used to enter the pericardium.
  - The small pericardial opening is extended using curved Mayo scissors.
    - Incise from the open aperture at the apex toward the sternal notch, staying anterior to the left phrenic nerve.
  - Evacuation of blood from the pericardial sac releases tamponade and the heart becomes directly visible.

Figure 15. When opening the pericardium, start at the apex and extend the opening toward the great vessels, staying on the anterior surface, avoiding the more laterally located phrenic nerve

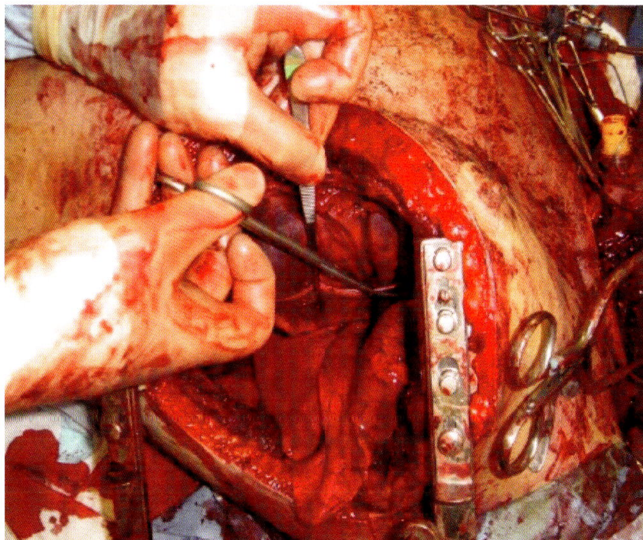

Source: Feliciano DV, Mattox KL, Moore EE. *Trauma*. Ninth Edition. McGraw Hill; 2021.

- Cardiorraphy
  - With the heart delivered out of the pericardium by rotating the heart into the left hemithorax, enhanced visualization of the cardiac chambers facilitates repair of the injury.
    - Identify cardiac wounds and apply digital control of bleeding.
    - Perform cardiac repair with 3-0 Prolene suture or stapler.
    - Aspirate air from the left ventricle if air embolism is suspected.
    - Initiate bimanual open cardiac massage (Figure 16).
  - Administer intracardiac epinephrine for a slow ventricular rhythm, and amiodarone for recurrent ventricular fibrillation.
    - Lift the heart up slightly with your left hand to expose the more posterior and muscular left ventricle, injecting the epinephrine with your right hand.
    - Avoid the coronary arteries during injection.
  - Defibrillate the heart, 30 joules.
    - To ensure the paddles stay on the surface of the heart in close apposition, another clinician may need to press the button on the paddles which is located at the back of the handle.

Figure 16. Internal cardiac massage is performed with wrists apposed and a hinged clapping motion of the hands

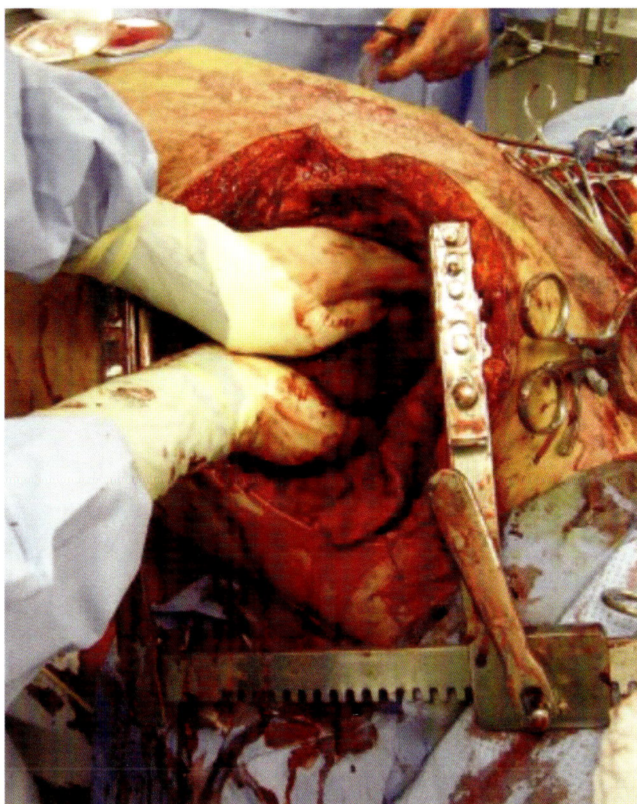

Source: Feliciano DV, Mattox KL, Moore EE. *Trauma*. Ninth Edition. McGraw Hill; 2021.

- Thoracic aortic occlusion
  - The descending thoracic aorta is occluded to maximize coronary and cerebral perfusion when the systolic blood pressure (SBP) is <70 mm Hg. The procedure is often performed following pericardiotomy and evaluation of the heart. However, aortic cross-clamping is done immediately upon entry into the chest for patients with presumed intra-abdominal, pelvis, or extremity injury with major blood loss.
    - Apply the cross-clamp to the thoracic aorta inferior to the left pulmonary hilum just above the diaphragm to minimize the risk of spinal ischemia.
    - Elevate the left lung anteriorly and superiorly.
    - Run your left hand along the posterior chest wall to the spine.
    - Digitally palpate the aorta on top of the spine as the first structure encountered by your fingers when moving up over the spine.
    - Digital occlusion of the aorta against the spine may be sufficient to optimize cerebral and coronary blood flow until the patient's blood volume can be replaced.
      - You will feel the aorta proximal to your digital cross-clamp begin to fill.

        - With ongoing transfusion, slowly allow some distal perfusion and track the patient's blood pressure with an arterial line tracing.
    - A large vascular clamp (Satinsky or DeBakey) is placed once the aorta is clearly identified. A Satinsky clamp is side-biting and will include the aorta and avoids damage or avulsion of the aortic branches, which are at risk when using a DeBakey clamp across the entire aorta (Figure 17).
        - Use your thumb and fingertips to bluntly isolate the descending aorta from the surrounding tissue.

Figure 17. Following dissection of the aorta away from the investing mediastinal pleura, a Satinsky clamp is placed just above the diaphragm for complete, hands-free occlusion

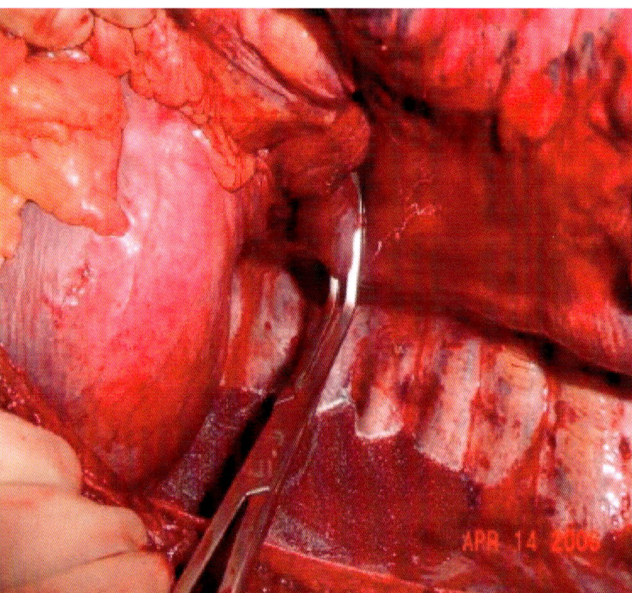

Source: Feliciano DV, Mattox KL, Moore EE. *Trauma*. Ninth Edition. McGraw Hill; 2021.

        - Dissecting the thoracic aorta using direct vision is ideal but rarely feasible. If possible, first incise the mediastinal pleura and then bluntly separate the aorta from the prevertebral fascia posteriorly and the esophagus anteriorly.
        - If blunt fingertip dissection proves difficult, the aorta may be held away from the spine with the fingertips of your left hand while using the Satinsky clamp with your right hand to make an opening in the investing mediastinal pleura between the aorta and the spine. Once the clamp enters between the aorta and spine, place your left hand's thumb and index finger through the opening to encircle the aorta completely.
        - Encircling the aorta ensures complete clamping but may avulse small vascular branches.
        - With your left index finger around the aorta, place the bottom jaw of the Satinsky clamp on its tip and guide it through the opening in the mediastinal pleura beneath the aorta.
        - Once around the aorta, close the Satinsky clamp for complete, hands-free occlusion.
- Pulmonary hilar control (Figure 18)
  - Pulmonary hilar control is occasionally required to prevent propagation of an air embolism and exsanguination due to a hilar injury or major hemorrhage from a central lung parenchymal injury.
    - The pulmonary hilum is encircled with your thumb and forefinger of your left hand by cupping along the lateral border of the heart inferiorly and moving cephalad. Your thumb should be anterior to the hilar structures and fingers posterior.
    - Oppose your thumb and forefinger to encircle the hilar structures; pull toward you to develop a column of structures amenable to clamping.
    - Place a large Satinsky clamp or DeBakey vascular clamp across the hilar structures.
  - Following hilar control, air embolism is aspirated from the apex of the left ventricle and the aortic root. If visible in the coronary vessels, air may be aspirated with a 27-gauge syringe.

Figure 18. After encircling the pulmonary hilum with thumb and forefinger, pull toward yourself to develop a column of the pulmonary hilar structures amenable to clamping with a large vascular clamp

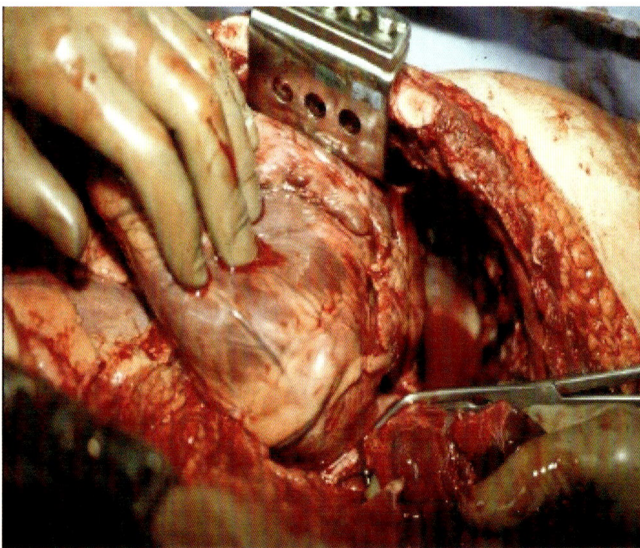

Source: Feliciano DV, Mattox KL, Moore EE. *Trauma*. Ninth Edition. McGraw Hill; 2021.

- Thoracotomy closure
  - Closure of the thoracic incision proceeds in multiple layers:
    - Place two chest tubes, anterior and posterior, under direct vision of the pleural space, ensuring the posterior tube lays in the posterior hemithorax, providing gravity-dependent drainage.
    - If the sternum was transected, reapproximate the sternal edges with two sternal #5 wires placed in a simple interrupted fashion.

        › Re-approximate the ribs using pericostal sutures of #1 PDS, taking care to avoid the intercostal vessels while encircling the ribs. A rib approximator may be used to close the space while tying the sutures.
        › The musculature is closed in two layers with running 0-PDS sutures.
        › Skin is closed with skin staples.
        › If available, subcutaneous pain catheters may also be placed during closure.
- Strategic decisions
    - Initial decision regarding unilateral thoracotomy – is adequate visualization possible?
    - Initial rapid evacuation of blood with laparotomy pads instead of suction.
    - Immediate assessment of source of shock: bleeding versus exsanguination versus tamponade. Prioritize pericardial decompression versus immediate hemorrhage control. For major arterial injury versus lung parenchymal injury, consider subclavian injury and apical compression. If pulmonary parenchymal bleeding is uncontrollable by direct pressure, consider direct hilar compression early.

CHALLENGES/PITFALLS/UNUSUAL COMPLICATIONS
- Multiple bleeding sites.
- Forgetting to ligate internal mammary arteries before closure.
- Inadvertent injury to the heart, lung, or aorta during initial control.
- Preoccupation with opening the pericardium when bleeding is paramount.
- Failure to compress or clamp the aorta to increase afterload and perfuse carotids and coronaries.
- Failure to position and open the Finochietto properly, which can cause inadequate opening of the chest and poor visibility.

TRAINEE ASSESSMENT
OSATS Scoring System:
1. Equipment tray
    0 Missing essential instrument
    1 Disorganized
    2 Well organized

2. Left anterolateral thoracotomy
    0 Arm at side
    1 Incision too high/low
    2 Correct

3. Clamshell thoracotomy
    0 Cross too high/low
    1 Insufficient extension
    2 Correct

4. Pericardiotomy
    0 Traverses phrenic nerve
    1 Inadequate extension
    2 Correct

5. Cardiorraphy
    0 Ligates coronary artery
    1 Ineffective control of bleeding
    2 Effective control of bleeding

6. Thoracic aortic clamping
    0 Clamps the esophagus
    1 Avulses intercostal arteries
    2 Correct position

7. Pulmonary hilar clamping
    0 Inferior to superior
    1 Incomplete closure
    2 Complete occlusion

Assessment: 0–6 Failure
7–11 TACS surgeon
12–14 Trauma surgeon

A Frequent Procedure of High Technical Difficulty: Pancreaticoduodenectomy (Whipple Procedure)

OBJECTIVES
After reading this section, the reader will be able to:
- Break down a complex procedure into sections that make teaching the operation more manageable and comprehensible.
- Describe pancreaticoduodenectomy in terms of dissection, resection, and reconstruction.
- Analyze the intricacies of each step of the operation.

ASSUMPTIONS
- The assumption underlying the following description is that a complex procedure is difficult to learn and often difficult to perform even for the experienced surgeon. To facilitate learning and teaching, the procedure should be broken down into stages with specific steps and critical skills so that the learner can master everything required to perform the operation successfully. Each step can be used in other operations. For instance, the Kocher maneuver is commonly used in many operations. Identification and ligation of a specific artery is also commonly used. Similarly, reconstruction anastomosing specific structures such as the pancreas, common bile duct, or stomach to small intestine is a common general surgery procedure. Thinking of each step of a pancreaticoduodenectomy as a sum of many straightforward surgical procedures allows the learner to break the operation down into a manageable sequence with very defined endpoints.

- The initial part of the operation is assessment of resectability and reassessment occurs at several points until the resection is accomplished or aborted.

ACS RESOURCES/SUGGESTED READING

American College of Surgeons. ACS Video Library. Available at: https://www.facs.org/education/division-of-education/publications/videolibrary. Accessed October 21, 2021.

Cameron J, Sandone C, Cameron JL. *Atlas of Gastrointestinal Surgery* (2nd Edition). Shelton, CT, USA: People's Medical Publishing House; 2006.

DESCRIPTION OF SIMULATION LABORATORY MODULE

- Cadaveric model: A fresh cadaver allows for the instructor and learner to perform the operation from beginning to end. Learner should be put in the position of the operating surgeon to allow for the evaluation of their comprehension of the operation and technical skills.

EQUIPMENT AND INSTRUMENTATION CONSIDERATIONS

- As this procedure is complex with multiple steps, the equipment needs can be divided into several categories. The surgeon must think of the tools they want to use in each of these categories:
  - Tools for dissection and reconstruction
  - Energy devices used for dissection
  - Stapling devices used in the operation

Figure 19. Kocher maneuver

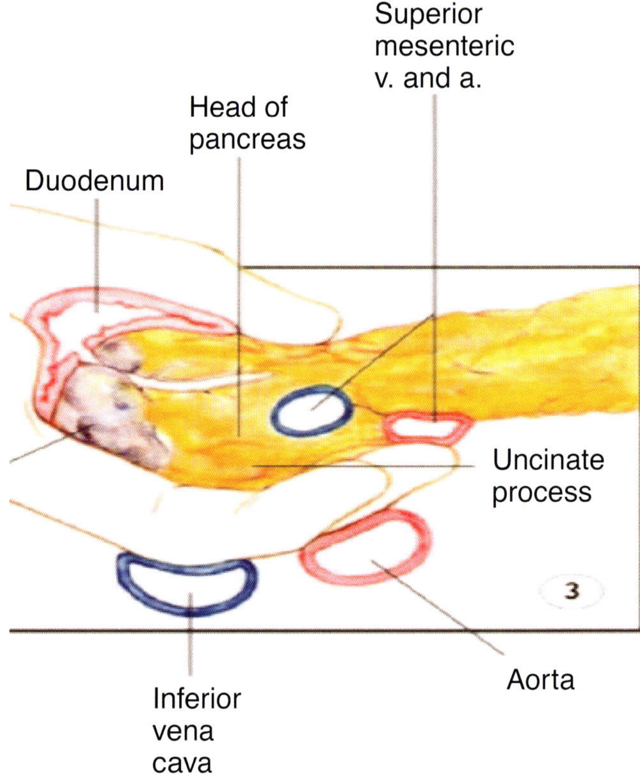

Source: Cameron JL, Sandone C. *Atlas of Gastrointestinal Surgery, Volume One*. Second Edition. Hamilton, Ontario: BC Decker Inc; 2007.

A SPECIFIC DESCRIPTION OF PROCEDURE

- Dissection (clockwise direction)
  - Upon entering the abdomen, examine all peritoneal surfaces and the liver for metastases. Any possible metastasis should be biopsied before proceeding.
  - Retract greater omentum superiorly and observe to transverse mesocolon for any obvious adherence.
  - Enter the lesser sac through the gastrocolic ligament.
  - Follow the middle colic vein and/or right gastroepiploic vein to find the superior mesenteric vein (SMV).
  - Develop a plane between the pancreas and SMV, if easy.
  - Ligate the right gastroepiploic vein.
  - Perform an extensive Kocher maneuver carefully getting a hand behind the head of the pancreas until the superior mesenteric artery (SMA) is palpable.
  - Adherence to the vena cava may preclude further dissection (Figure 19).
  - Perform cholecystectomy. Dissect the peritoneum overlying the gallbladder. Dissect the gallbladder dome down. Ligate the cystic duct and the cystic artery.
  - Check for replaced right hepatic artery lateral to the common hepatic duct (CHD).
  - Dissect the common hepatic artery (usually located under large lymph nodes) up to the bifurcation into the proper hepatic artery and gastroduodenal artery (GDA).
  - Dissect all lymph nodes along the celiac trunk, common hepatic artery, and porta hepatis. Remove all peripancreatic nodes. At this point, distinction between the structures in the porta hepatis should be clear.
  - Ligate the GDA using a vascular stapler or suture ligature close to the superior edge of the pancreas (Figure 20).
  - Dissect the portal vein (PV) and develop a plane between the PV and the posterior aspect of pancreas, careful to stay anterior throughout.
  - Connect the dissection plane posterior to the pancreas and anterior to the PV/SMV by dissecting cranial to caudad to the pancreas (Figure 21). The plane should develop appropriately and if not, then tumor invasion and resectability have to be considered or PV resection considered. Once complete, pass a Penrose or umbilical tape around the neck of the pancreas.

Figure 20. The GDA courses anterior to the pancreas

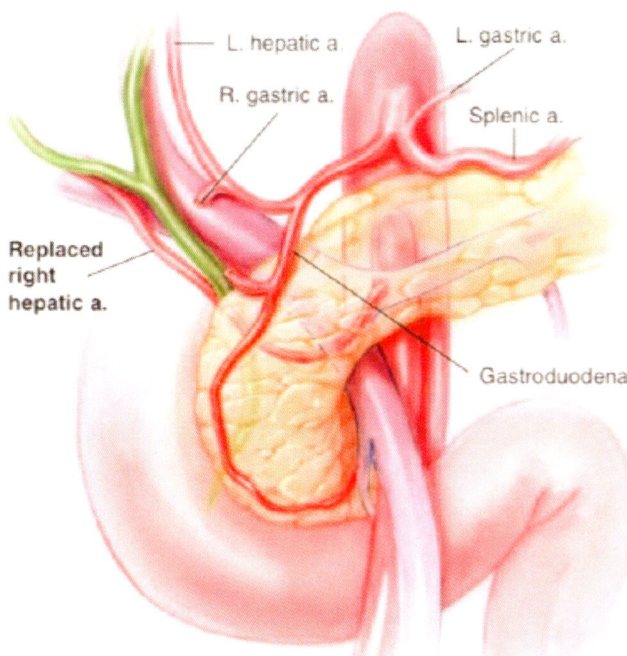

Source: Cameron JL, Sandone C. *Atlas of Gastrointestinal Surgery, Volume One*. Second Edition. Hamilton, Ontario: BC Decker Inc; 2007.

Figure 21. A plane is developed between the posterior surface of the pancreas and the junction of the SMV and PV

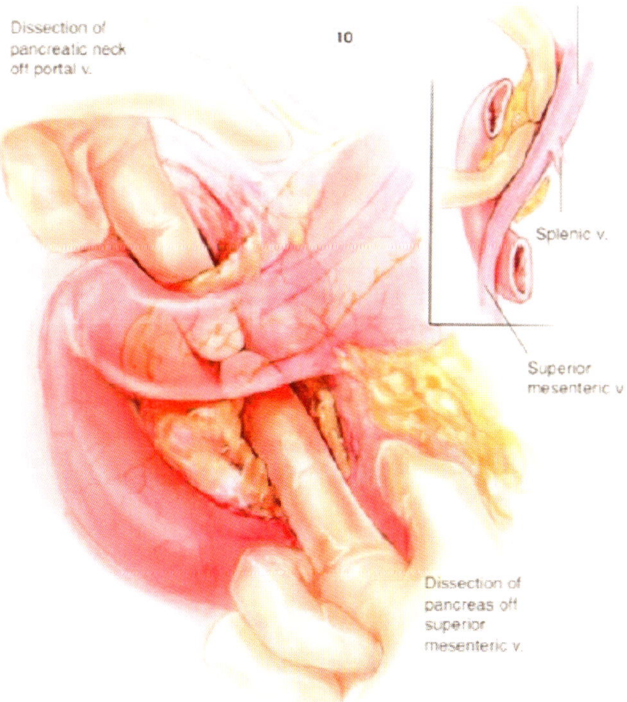

Source: Cameron JL, Sandone C. *Atlas of Gastrointestinal Surgery, Volume One*. Second Edition. Hamilton, Ontario: BC Decker Inc; 2007.

- Resection (counterclockwise direction)
  - Transect the first portion of the duodenum (pylorus-preserving) or stomach (between the incisura and a point opposite on the greater curvature – non-pylorus preserving) using a GIA stapler.
  - Transect the CHD proximal to the cystic duct stump. Obtain hemostasis as the feeding arteries located at the 3 o'clock and 9 o'clock will most likely bleed.
  - Transect the jejunum about 5 to 10 cm beyond the ligament of Treitz. Dissect the ligament extensively freeing up the third and fourth portion of the duodenum. Take care not to injure the inferior mesenteric vein which is located lateral to the ligament. At this point, the fourth portion of the duodenum and the first two inches of the jejunum can be moved to the right of the SMA and SMV.
  - Transect the neck of the pancreas over the Penrose drain using cautery. Take care to coagulate the vessels superior and inferior to the pancreas.
  - Dissect the retroperitoneal margin of the pancreas off the SMV and SMA. Begin by ligating branches from the pancreas coming into the SMV (there are usually 2 to 3 branches; one is superiorly located and one is more inferior). Once the SMV has been dissected, retract it medially (Figure 22). The uncinate process can then be dissected off of the SMA using clamps/ties or a thermal energy device. Note that the inferior pancreaticoduodenal vessel will be transected in this dissection. Label the specimen (Figure 23).

Figure 22. The pancreas is dissected off the SMV by ligating branches that connect the vein and the pancreas

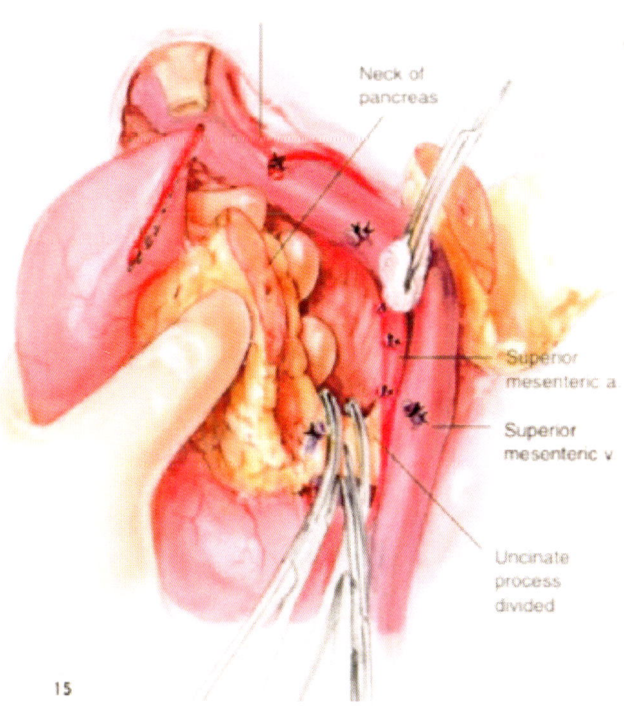

Source: Cameron JL, Sandone C. *Atlas of Gastrointestinal Surgery, Volume One*. Second Edition. Hamilton, Ontario: BC Decker Inc; 2007.

Figure 23. The Whipple specimen includes the duodenum/jejunum along with the head of the pancreas/uncinate process and the distal bile duct/gallbladder

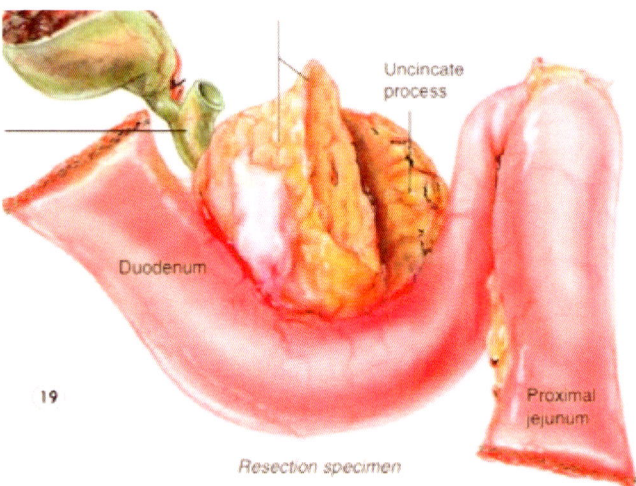

Source: Cameron JL, Sandone C. *Atlas of Gastrointestinal Surgery, Volume One*. Second Edition. Hamilton, Ontario: BC Decker Inc; 2007.

- Anastomoses (three anastomoses)
  - Pancreaticojejunostomy (two-layered retrocolic end-to-side): Pass the distal end of the jejunum through the mesocolon to the right of the middle colic vein. The side of the jejunum is placed lateral to the end of the pancreas. 4-0 silk sutures are used in an interrupted fashion for the posterior layer approximating the seromuscular layer of the bowel to the capsule of the pancreas. Make a small opening in the jejunum. 5-0 Dexon sutures are used in all four corners to approximate the full thickness of the intestine to the pancreatic duct. Once complete, 4-0 silk sutures are used to do the anterior layer of the anastomosis.
  - Choledochojejunostomy (single layer end-to-side): About 5 cm distal to the pancreaticojejunostomy, an opening is made in the jejunum. The CHD is approximated to the jejunum using 5-0 Dexon suture in an interrupted fashion completing the posterior layer first followed by the anterior layer.
  - Gastrojejunostomy (single layer side-to-side): 40 cm distal to the choledochojejunostomy, make an opening it the jejunum and the greater curvature of the stomach (or duodenum for pylorus-preserving; the length of this limb can be reduced to 25 cm in this case). The posterior layer is approximated using a 3-0 silk suture in a full thickness interrupted fashion. The same is done for the anterior layer.
- Completion (Figure 24)
  - The nasogastric tube is placed proximal to the gastric anastomosis.
  - The drain can be placed posterior to the pancreaticojejunostomy and choledochojejunostomy.

Figure 24. The completed reconstruction shows the pancreaticojejunostomy, hepaticojejunostomy, and duodenojejunostomy

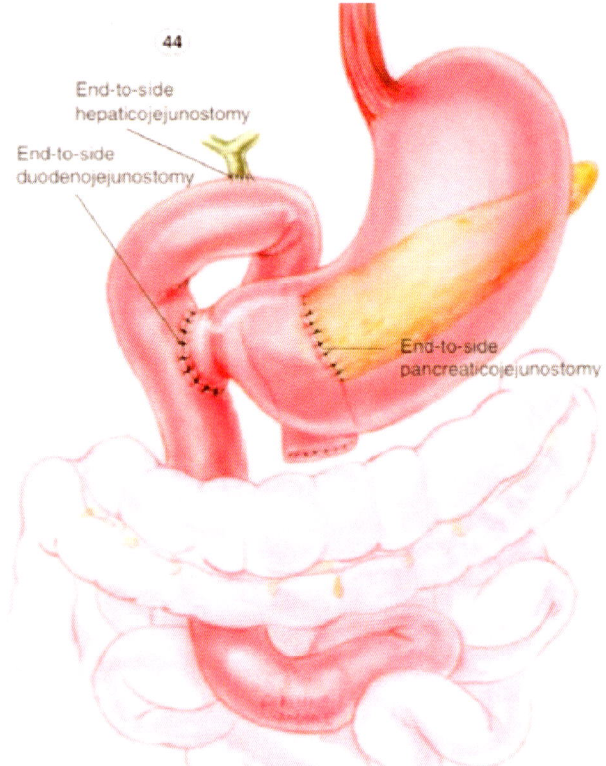

Source: Cameron JL, Sandone C. *Atlas of Gastrointestinal Surgery, Volume One*. Second Edition. Hamilton, Ontario: BC Decker Inc; 2007.

CHALLENGES/PITFALLS/UNUSUAL COMPLICATIONS

- The avoidance of significant hemorrhage during critical mobilization and dissection to free the tumor and judge resectability
- Encountering unusual anatomic variance (right hepatic artery) and unusual disease-specific variants (fatty pancreas, non-dilated common duct)
- Delayed complications (pancreatic leak and sepsis, vascular pseudoaneurysm and bleeding, delayed gastric emptying, and nutritional compromise)
- Dependence of successful complication management on institutional-specific rescue therapy

TRAINEE ASSESSMENT

For a complex operation like pancreaticoduodenectomy, it is difficult to develop an OSATS-like test. Instead, several areas of technical skills need to be evaluated.

- Knowledge of the overview of the operation as previously outlined
- Ability to perform steps previously listed
- Handling of tissue
- Efficiency of steps; as there are many steps involved in the operation, efficient transition between stages is essential
- Autonomy granted to resident as evaluated by the Zwisch model divided by the three stages of the operation

Conclusion

In this chapter, the authors reviewed the critical components of a process for teaching technical skills in surgical residency programs. Becoming an excellent surgeon starts with the understanding that the main objective of knowledge and skills acquisition is to provide safe and effective care to patients. Developing a learning mindset begins at a young age and evolves as the learner matures. Fundamental ingredients in this mindset include intense curiosity, willingness to reflect on every learning experience, and the ability to recognize knowledge gaps (knowing what one does not know) as well as opportunities for improvement.

The commitment to a lifelong pursuit of mastery learning is imbedded in the personality of every excellent surgeon. Internalizing the process of learning surgical science allows the resident to move on to add the necessary technical skills that will lead to autonomous independent practice. Technical skills are learned first in medical school where simple tasks such as venipuncture and bladder catheter insertion are taught, and successful learning is documented. As residency training progresses, increasingly complex skills are presented; learning can occur through formal didactic courses, simulation and cadaver labs, and one-on-one interactions between master surgeon educators and learners.

Examples of each resource are provided as are discussions of ways to implement and determine value. For each resident, the technical skills learning process culminates with perioperative and intraoperative experience first under supervision and then independently. Progress is monitored and recorded until the resident is deemed capable of independent practice. In this chapter, assessment methods are described as a necessary part of each learning episode. Acquiring knowledge, refining skills, and learning new skills continues throughout a surgeon's career.

The authors, who are all experienced surgical educators, also have described approaches that help residents acquire procedure-focused skills. A valuable way to learn a surgical procedure is to divide the operation into a sequence of steps and list the skills necessary to complete each step. An understanding of the challenges, pitfalls, and unexpected variants that may be encountered in individual patients must be acknowledged. In the included content, this approach is described using four selected procedures chosen because of complexity and frequency with which they will be encountered in residency training and practice.

We understand that variations in resource availability, case mix, and faculty composition will require each program to develop its own approach to teaching technical skills. Our hope is that this manual will help program directors and their faculties create their unique learning structures.

Suggested Readings

American Board of Surgery, American College of Surgeons, Association of Program Directors in Surgery, Association for Surgical Education. Statement on surgical preresidency preparatory courses. *J Surg Educ.* 2014;71(6):777-778.

American College of Surgeons. ACS Video Library. Available at: https://www.facs.org/education/division-of-education/publications/videolibrary. Accessed October 21, 2021.

ATLS Subcommittee, ACS COT, International ATLS working group. Advanced trauma life support (ATLS): the ninth edition. *J Trauma Acute Care Surg.* 2013;74(5):1333–1366.

Azari DP, Frasier LL, Quamme SRP, Greenberg CC, Pugh CM, Greenberg JA, Radwin RG. Modeling surgical technical skill using expert assessment for automated computer rating. *Ann Surg.* 2019;269(3):574-581.

Bohnen JD, George BC, Williams RG, et al. Procedural learning and safety collaborative (PLSC). The feasibility of real-time intraoperative performance assessment with SIMPL: early experience from a multi-institutional trial. *J Surg Ed.* 2016;73:e118-e130.

Burlew CC and Moore EE. Emergency Department Thoracotomy. In: Feliciano DV, Mattox KL, Moore EE eds. *Trauma, 9th ed.* New York, NY: McGraw-Hill; 2021.

Cameron J, Sandone C, Cameron JL. Atlas of Gastrointestinal Surgery (2nd Edition). Shelton, CT, USA: People's Medical Publishing House; 2006.

Carey JN, Minneti M, Leland HA, Demetriades D, Talving P. Perfused fresh cadavers: method for application to surgical simulation. *Am J Surg.* 2015;210(1):179-187.

Demetriades D, Chudnofsky CR, Benjamin ER. *Color Atlas of Emergency Trauma.* Cambridge University Press; 2021.

Demetriades D, Inaba K, Velmahos GC. In: *Atlas of Surgical Techniques in Trauma.* Cambridge, United Kingdom; New York, NY, USA: Cambridge University Press; 2020:7-15.

DeVore EK, Redmann A, Howell R, Khosla S. Best practices for emergency surgical airway: a systematic review. *Laryngoscope Investig Otolaryngol.* 2019;4(6):602-608.

Duran C, Estrada S, O'Malley M, et al. The model for Fundamentals of Endovascular Surgery (FEVS) successfully defines the competent endovascular surgeon. *J Vasc Surg.* 2015;62(6):1660-6.e3.

Edwards EA, MacArthur JD. In: *Operative Anatomy of Abdomen and Pelvis.* Philadelphia: Lea & Febiger; 1975:188-189.

Flinn J, Miller A, Pyatka N, Brewer J, Schneider T, Cao C. The effect of stress on learning in surgical skill acquisition. *Med Teach.* 2016;38:897-903.

Gardner A, Jabbour I, Williams B, Huerta S. Different goals, different pathways: the role of metacognition and task engagement in surgical skill acquisition. *J Surg Educ.* 2015;73(1):61-65.

Goh AC, Goldfarb DW, Sander JC, Miles BJ, Dunkin BJ. Global evaluative assessment of robotic skills: validation of a clinical assessment tool to measure robotic surgical skills. *J Urol.* 2012;187(1):247-252.

Grant AL, Temple-Oberle C. Utility of a validated rating scale for self-assessment in microsurgical training. *J Surg Educ.* 2017;74(2):360-364.

Huffman E, Anton N, Martin J, Timsina L, Dearing W, Breece B, Mann I, Stefanidis D. Optimizing assessment of surgical knot tying skill. *J Surg Educ.* 2020;77(6):1577-1582.

Jensen MO. *Surgical Anatomy for Mastery of Open Operations.* Philadelphia; Wolters Kluwer:2019; p. 147 in chapter entitled "Liver, Biliary System, Pancreas, and Spleen", pp. 146-174.

Kowalewski KF, Garrow CR, Schmidt MW, Benner L, Müller-Stich BP, Nickel F. Sensor-based machine learning for workflow detection and as key to detect expert level in laparoscopic suturing and knot-tying. *Surg Endosc.* 2019;33(11):3732-3740.

Law B, Atkins MS, Kirkpatrick AE, Lomax AJ. Eye gaze patterns differentiate novice and experts in a virtual laparoscopic surgery training environment. In: Proceedings of the 2004 symposium on eye tracking research & applications 2004; 41-48. ACM.

Mandavia DP, Newton EJ, Demetriades D. *Color Atlas of Emergency Trauma*. Cambridge University Press; 2003.

Martin JA, Regehr G, Reznick R, et al. Objective structured assessment of technical skill (OSATS) for surgical residents. *Br J Surg.* 1997;84(2):273-278.

Meyerson S, Sternbach J, Zwischenberger J, Bender E. Resident autonomy in the operating room: expectations vs. reality. *Ann Thorac Surg.* 2017;104:1062-1068.

Minter R, Amos K, Bentz M, Blair P, Brandt C, D'Cunha J, Davis E, Delman K, Deutsch E, Divino C, Kingsley D, Klingensmith M, Meterissian S, Sachdeva A, Terhune K, Termuhlen P, Mullan P. Transition to surgical residency: a multi-institutional study of perceived intern preparedness and the effect of a formal residency preparatory course in the fourth year of medical school. *Acad Med.* 2015;90(8):1116-1124.

Moulton C, Dubrowski A, MacRae H, Graham B, Grober E, Reznick R. Teaching surgical skills: what kind of practice makes perfect? A randomized, controlled trial. *Ann Surg.* 2006;244:400-409.

Shaker D. Cognitivism and psychomotor skills in surgical training: from theory to practice. *Int J Med Educ.* 2018;9:253-254.

Singapogu RB, Smith DE, Long LO, Burg TC, Pagano CC, Burg KJ. Objective differentiation of force-based laparoscopic skills using a novel haptic simulator. *J Surg Educ.* 2012;69(6):766-773.

Souba WW, Fink MP, Jurkovic GJ, et al. *ACS Surgery: Principles & Practice*, 6th ed., New York: WebMD Professional Publishing; 2006.

Swanstrom LL, Fried GM, Hoffman KI, Soper NJ. Beta test results of a new system assessing competence in laparoscopic surgery. *J Am Coll Surg.* 2006;202(1):62-69.

Thal ER, Weigelt JA, Carrico CJ. *Operative Trauma Management: An Atlas. New* York: McGraw-Hill, Medical Pub. Division; 2002.

Timberlake M, Mayo H, Scott L, Weis J, Gardner A. What do we know about intraoperative teaching? A systematic review. *Ann Surg.* 2017;266:251-259.

Trejos AL, Patel RV, Malthaner RA, Schlachta CM. Development of force-based metrics for skills assessment in minimally invasive surgery. *Surg Endosc.* 2014;28(7):2106-2119.

Vassiliou MC, Feldman LS, Andrew CG, et al. A global assessment tool for evaluation of intraoperative laparoscopic skills. *Am J Surg.* 2005;190(1):107-113.

Vassiliou MC, Kaneva PA, Poulose BK, et al. Global Assessment of Gastrointestinal Endoscopic Skills (GAGES): a valid measurement tool for technical skills in flexible endoscopy. *Surg Endosc.* 2010;24(8):1834-1841.

Winkler-Schwartz A, Yilmaz R, Mirchi N, Bissonnette V, Ledwos N, Siyar S, Azarnoush H, Karlik B, Del Maestro R. Machine learning identification of surgical and operative factors associated with surgical expertise in virtual reality simulation. *JAMA Netw Open*. 2019;2(8):e198363.

AMERICAN C
SURGEONS A
OF SURGEON
COLLEGE OF
AMERICAN C
SURGEONS A
OF SURGEON
COLLEGE OF
AMERICAN C
SURGEONS A

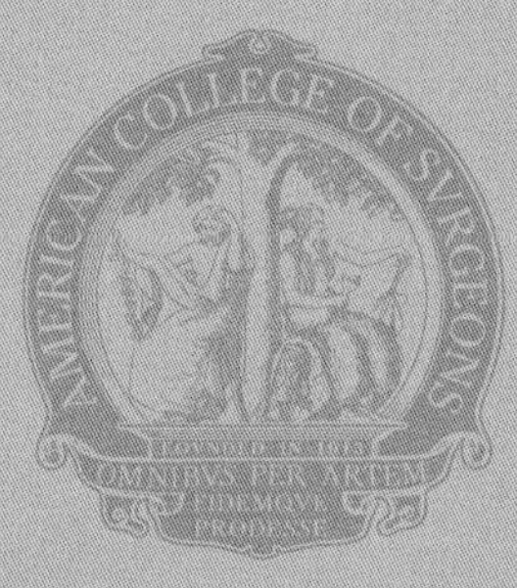

CHAPTER 7

Curriculum: Non-Technical Skills

Lead Author

Carlos A. Pellegrini, MD, FACS, FRCSI(Hon), FRCS(Hon), FRCSEd(Hon), FWACS(Hon), MAMSE

Co-Authors

Keith D. Lillemoe, MD, FACS, MAMSE

Mary H. McGrath, MD, MPH, FACS, MAMSE

Roy Phitayakorn, MD, MHPE (MEd), FACS

Douglas S. Smink, MD, MPH, FACS, MAMSE

CHAPTER 7

Curriculum: Non-Technical Skills

Executive Summary

This chapter is divided into five sections that answer the following questions:

Section 1: Non-Technical Skills
What is the definition of non-technical skills?
What are non-technical skills for surgeons?
How do you teach non-technical skills to surgeons?
How do you assess non-technical skills?

Section 2: Emotional Intelligence
What is emotional intelligence?
How do you teach emotional intelligence to surgeons?
How do you evaluate emotional intelligence?

Section 3: Professionalism
What is professionalism?
Why is it critical to support professionalism?
What are the key attributes and responsibilities of the professional?
Why is clinical ethics fundamental to professionalism?
What are the principles for teaching professionalism?
What are methods for teaching and learning professionalism?
What are methods for assessing professionalism?

Section 4: Interprofessional Education
How should health care professionals relate and what is interprofessional education?
Why is interprofessional education important?
What are the barriers to interprofessional education?
How do we teach interprofessional education?
How do we assess interprofessional education?

Section 5: Leading a Diverse Team
How do we lead a diverse team?
What are important issues of equity, diversity, and inclusion?
What is psychological safety and how do we provide it?

Non-Technical Skills

The Definition of Non-Technical Skills

Surgeons and surgeon educators commonly focus on technical skills and for good reason: sound surgical technique is essential to safely completing an operation. Technical skills range from the simple and straightforward, such as suturing and knot-tying, to the complex, such as fine dissection, creation of an anastomosis, and robotic or laparoscopic suturing. Multiple studies have shown the importance of technical skill in surgical outcomes, and as a result, technical skills should be taught and stressed in the development of a competent surgeon.

Nonetheless, technical skill is insufficient to develop surgical excellence. Typically, those whom colleagues identify as the best surgeons they have worked or trained with are distinguished by several qualities, some of which are non-technical. These may include decision-making, emotional intelligence (discussed in a later section), leadership, and teamwork.

These are examples of non-technical skills. They differ from technical skills in that they relate to how surgeons interact with colleagues and patients in clinical or nonclinical environments. They include cognitive skills, such as decision-making and situation awareness, and social skills, such as leadership, teamwork, and communication.

Although some surgeons might believe that these skills are innate and cannot be taught, evidence shows that they can be taught and can be improved, much like technical skills. Multiple taxonomies exist, with many similarities but subtle differences, enabling educators to both teach and assess non-technical skills. These taxonomies include Oxford Non-Technical Skills (NOTECHS) and NOTSS (Non-Technical Skills for Surgeons, described in detail below).

Non-Technical Skills for Surgeons (NOTSS)

NOTSS was originally developed in Scotland, and a new revision has been published recently in the U.S. in collaboration with the American College of Surgeons (ACS). The NOTSS taxonomy was developed and refined through direct observation, interviews, and focus groups with surgeons, in which they identified the core skills, outside of surgical technique, that define excellence in the field. Through multiple iterations, this process identified not only the key cognitive skills (situation awareness and decision-making) and social skills (communication and teamwork and leadership), but the process also identified specific behaviors. These behaviors provide surgeons and educators with examples of good and bad behavior that can guide learning and improvement.

Situation Awareness

The operating room (OR) is a complex environment. The surgeon must be aware of many aspects of the OR, ranging from the operating team, to the surgical equipment, to the patient; this includes self-awareness. Who is in the OR? What are their abilities? What are the patient's vital signs? What is the surgical anatomy? Are there any deviations from normal? What vital or delicate structures are adjacent to the area of dissection? What is the surgeon's internal level of comfort or knowledge? Is the surgeon aware of his or her limitations?

Most importantly, the surgeon needs to be aware of the operative field, which requires an understanding of normal anatomy, as well as any abnormalities because of the patient's unique physiology or disease. The surgeon should be particularly aware when approaching major blood vessels or other vital structures. Moreover, the surgeon needs to see the larger picture, such as the patient's physiologic state and hemodynamic stability. For example, if there is hypotension or coagulopathy, the surgeon must reflect that in the operative plan. Finally, the surgeon needs to be aware of the team members and their capabilities: How familiar are they with the procedure or with the required equipment? Which team members are present in the OR and who is working outside the room? To be an effective leader, the surgeon should also assess the tenor of the operating team to determine comfort or anxiety levels and act accordingly.

Surgeons rely on the other members of the operative team to help identify important information and share it with the team. Ideally, the surgeon creates a psychologically safe environment (described later in this chapter), where all members of the team feel comfortable sharing information relevant to patient safety. Once shared, the surgeon must process and understand the information and project what will happen next. Situation awareness is necessary for a surgeon so that the surgical team makes sound decisions, safely progresses through the operation, and achieves maximum patient benefit.

Decision-Making

In many ways, decision-making distinguishes great surgeons from competent ones. When to operate, what operation to perform, and how to progress through that operation are all components of surgical decision-making. To make sound decisions in the OR, the surgeon must be aware of the situation and process the inputs from this awareness. If a change in course is required, the surgeon should notify the surgical team and then implement the necessary modifications.

There are many types of decision-making:

- *Analytical.* The surgeon identifies multiple courses of action, analyzes each to its endpoint, and selects the one that indicates the best outcome. Although effective, this type of decision-making is time-consuming and sometimes too slow to respond to an OR event.
- *Rule-based.* The surgeon follows a predetermined rule; in other words, "if X occurs, we will do Y." This works well for simple decisions, like which antibiotic to give at the beginning of a procedure, but it can be too restrictive for the complex decisions during an operation.
- *Recognition-primed.* Used by most experts, in this decision-making method the surgeon recognizes a situation based on past experience and proposes a workable solution most likely to be appropriate and successful. If the initial solution is ineffective, the surgeon quickly develops and pursues an alternate solution; if the alternative solution fails, a third is developed and pursued, and so on. Recognition-primed decision-making tends to be the fastest and most effective approach, but is heavily reliant on experience.
- *Creative.* Sometimes, a surgeon encounters a rare or unique problem for the first time. This rules out decision-making based on rules or recognition. The surgeon must adjust and use creativity to address the situation. This type of decision-making typically takes the most time and mental effort, and should be reserved for the rarest surgical challenges when traditional techniques have failed.

Communication and Teamwork

Ideally, the participants in an operation perform as a high-functioning team; this requires strong communication and teamwork.

Many health care institutions work to establish a culture of high reliability, which emphasizes systems-based care, transparency, teamwork, nonpunitive analysis of errors, and best practices. The ACS *Optimal Resources for Surgical Quality and Safety,* the "Red Book," describes the specific tools that surgeon leaders can use to cultivate a culture of patient safety and high reliability, including patient safety reports, open discussion of errors, root-cause analysis, and the examination and interpretation of registry data. Ultimately it is the surgeon champion who is responsible to successfully implement these tools and to ensure across-the-board compliance with safe practices that lead to reliable outcomes, according to the Red Book. Organizations such as The Joint Commission and the Agency for Healthcare Research and Quality (AHRQ) also recognize the need for health care institutions to consistently strive to ensure patient safety, improve quality of care, and reduce errors. These principles have value for surgical teams that seek to provide the best care for all patients.

Communication is an essential aspect of teamwork. The surgeon plays a critical role in OR team function by participating in and encouraging the exchange of information among team members, which creates a shared understanding, also referred to as a "shared mental model." When this approach is used, every team member is on the same page and understands the indications and thought process leading to the procedure, the challenges, and the task at hand. In most instances, the surgeon determines the next step during an operation, typically according to a preconceived plan (as described in Chapter 6). By communicating this plan to the other team members and seeking their opinions, the surgeon coordinates team activities, ensuring that all members work toward common goals.

Communication is key to a high-functioning OR team and is a core component of every non-technical skill element. Communication allows free exchange of information, ensures mutual trust, and enhances team member awareness of an operation's progress and challenges. Surgeons and their teams should practice closed-loop communication, in which a request is directed at an appropriate team member, who then acknowledges it and responds by completing the requested action. Closed-loop communication allows the surgeon and other members to focus on the task at hand rather than wondering if a request has been received.

Leadership

Leadership is necessary for a team to be effective and in the OR this responsibility typically falls on the surgeon. There may be times during an operation when leadership is passed to the anesthesiologist or the OR nurse, but most of the time, the surgeon is the team leader. It may be challenging for the surgeon to provide leadership while performing the technical aspects of a procedure, but it can and must be accomplished.

Leadership can be taught like any other non-technical skill. One aspect of a surgeon's leadership is to set and maintain high standards, such as a commitment to patient safety; starting with preparation for the procedure and extending through the safety pause, every aspect of the operation, and completion of the case. Certain aspects of an operation may be challenging for team members. The surgeon can exert leadership by supporting the team members and encouraging them to speak up if they have concerns or questions. This support includes teaching; an important role of every surgeon is to educate trainees and other members of the operative team. Finally, the team members typically turn to the surgeon when the procedure becomes more challenging or they are under pressure, such as during a trauma case. Surgeon leaders must cope with this pressure, remaining calm to reduce tension and enable the team to perform at its best.

Teaching Non-Technical Skills to Surgeons

Traditionally, it was thought that non-technical skills, such as leadership or situation awareness, were not teachable, but rather were innate personality characteristics. Other surgical skills, like decision-making, were believed to be gained only by experience. More recently, the surgical community has learned that, just like technical skills, non-technical skills can be intentionally taught and acquired. Some of the more effective and novel methods of training non-technical skills include simulation and coaching.

Simulation

Practice is used to hone almost every skill-based discipline, including music, athletics, and the military. K. Anders Ericsson espouses deliberate practice, the concept of mastering a skill through repeated practice with regular feedback through progressive levels of difficulty. In surgery, the ideal method of deliberate practice uses simulation, allowing repetition at increasing levels of complexity and feedback while enabling the learner to fail without harming patients.

Simulation is now increasingly used in surgery to instill non-technical skills, especially those required for effective teamwork, communication, and leadership. One of the leading curricula for team training, Team Strategies and Tools to Enhance Performance and Patient Safety (TeamSTEPPS), was developed specifically for health care teams, and it includes simulation as a training option. Applied to the OR, TeamSTEPPS has been shown to increase efficiency and enhance patient safety. In addition to TeamSTEPPS, other simulation-based team training programs have proven to enhance non-technical skills like communication and teamwork.

Coaching

More recently, coaching, typically by a surgeon-peer, is gaining acceptance as an effective form of professional development. In these programs, the surgeon coaches are respected members of a department or society; they receive training in important aspects of coaching, such as goal setting, listening, collaborating, and creating action plans. Surgeon coaches are paired with a resident and through either direct observation or video review, the pair discusses performance and identifies areas for improvement. Studies show that when setting personal goals, most residents in coaching sessions identify non-technical skills as an area of focus, and most coaching conversations center on non-technical skills.

Resident-as-Teacher
Residents play a vital teaching role for more junior residents and medical students on surgery rotations. Just like other non-technical skills, instruction and practice can improve teaching. Many residency programs and institutions have residents-as-teacher curricula directed at important educational skills such as communication, exchanging feedback, and delivering a lecture or presentation. Even when they practice outside of a university setting, surgeons frequently are called upon to teach trainees or colleagues, so it is vital to develop their teaching skills. The ACS Residents as Teachers and Leaders course is a valuable resource for learning the necessary skills to become an effective teacher.

Assessment of Non-Technical Skills
In addition to training, assessment of non-technical skills is important for resident development. Trainees benefit from constructive feedback. Although the assessment of non-technical skills may seem subjective, reliable assessment tools with objective scoring rubrics are available. For instance, the NOTSS taxonomy includes an assessment tool for each of its elements—situation awareness, decision-making, communication and teamwork, and leadership. In addition to giving an objective score, these assessment tools focus on the positive and negative behaviors of the surgeon or surgical trainee, thus providing valuable feedback to guide development.

Emotional Intelligence

What Is Emotional Intelligence?
The term emotional intelligence (EI) was introduced in 1990 to describe a person's ability to understand his or her emotions and the emotions of others, and then use this knowledge to guide one's thinking and actions.[1] From a neurobiological perspective, human lesion and functional neuroimaging studies indicate that EI refers to an emotional network of the brain that includes the anterior cingulate cortex, insula, amygdala, and ventromedial prefrontal cortex.[2] In clinical medicine, physicians use this process to improve relationships with patients, work on an interprofessional team, and manage conflict with their colleagues.

Why Surgeons Should Develop EI
For surgeons, EI may be especially useful in high-stakes, emotionally charged situations such as intraoperative emergencies or military medicine where the clinical goals, roles, and responsibilities are constantly shifting.[3] After an adverse event, EI may decrease the likelihood of litigation.[4] In general, higher EI has been linked to improved caring, empathy, job satisfaction, resilience, self-support, psychological adjustment, and decreased burnout and stress.[5-10] Unlike innate intelligence (IQ), EI can be learned, practiced, and improved to enhance day-to-day interactions and leadership skills.

Research studies typically think of EI as either an emotion-related cognitive ability (ability EI) or as a reflection of one's disposition and self-perception (trait EI).[11,12] Ability EI comprises four main abilities including emotional understanding and management, emotional perception, expression, and using one's emotions to control oneself and/or influence others.[13] Trait EI is similar to but distinct from personality traits and includes well-being, self-control, emotionality, and sociability.[14]

For example, imagine that a surgeon is in the midst of a difficult operation when the inferior vena cava (IVC) is inadvertently injured. Massive hemorrhage begins and the surgeon's stress level rises significantly. The surgeon must use ability EI to recognize that the scrub nurse is also stressed and needs help activating the massive transfusion protocol. At the same time, the surgeon needs to use trait EI to maintain self-control while explaining to the anesthesia team members what is happening in the operative field and what is needed for successful repair. Trying to manage both aspects of EI while simultaneously managing the technical repair of the IVC is challenging and requires training.

Teaching Emotional Intelligence to Surgeons
EI training requires a combination of structured instructional sessions and helpful formative assessments. In terms of instruction, EI training is frequently simulation-based with carefully constructed learning goals and objectives with responses assessed by external predetermined criteria. These sessions could be based on hospital disciplinary reports or quality improvement data and will likely include an interprofessional communication or behavior issue. Given the expense and time commitment to create these scenarios, check the MedEdPortal site (*www.mededportal.org*) to see if a previously published scenario could be adapted for a particular need. These sessions should avoid role playing and allow participants to act in a manner appropriate to their level and occupation. Lastly, junior and senior surgery residents may have different EI needs because of their different service roles, so they may benefit from having separate sessions with different EI interventions.

Evaluating Emotional Intelligence

Ability EI may need to be evaluated separately using workplace performance instruments or patient satisfaction surveys as it is difficult to simulate occupational environments. Trait EI can be assessed using self-reported questionnaires such as the Trait Emotional Intelligence Questionnaire.[14] Trait EI interventions should be coupled with concrete suggestions for an individual to improve a particular facet of their EI. Because EI instruments lack the validity and reliability evidence for high-stakes assessment, these instruments should be used for formative feedback and individual growth rather than selection or advancement criteria.

Table 1. The five components of emotional intelligence at work

EIQ component	Definition	Hallmarks
Self-awareness	The ability to recognize and understand your moods, emotions, drives, as well as their effects on others	Self-confidence; realistic self-assessment; self-deprecating sense of humor
Self-regulation	The ability to control or redirect disruptive impulses or moods ... the propensity to suspend judgment, to think before acting	Trustworthiness and integrity; comfort with ambiguity; openness to change
Motivation	A passion to work for reasons that go beyond money or status ... a propensity to pursue goals with energy and persistence	Strong drive to achieve; optimism, even in the face of failure; organizational commitment
Empathy	The ability to understand the emotional makeup of other people ... skill in treating people according to their emotional reactions	Expertise in building and retaining talent; cross-cultural sensitivity; service to clients and customers
Social skills	Proficiency in handling relationships and building networks ... an ability to find common ground and build rapport	Effectiveness in leading change; persuasiveness; expertise in building and leading teams

Table 2. Proposed curricular elements for teaching professionalism using the emotional intelligence model

Quadrant 1: Enhancing your personal discovery	Quadrant 3: Enhancing your awareness of groups
• Meyers-Briggs Type Indicator • 360° feedback • Learning styles inventory • Identifying your ideal self	• Active listening • Empathy • Cultural competence • Systems thinking
Quadrant 2: Enhancing your ability to manage yourself	**Quadrant 4: Enhancing your ability to manage relationships**
• Time management • Communicating with patients • Communicating with groups • Coping strategies • Stress management • Developing a vision for yourself	• Team building • Conflict resolution • Creative problem solving • Change management

Professionalism

What Is Professionalism?

Professionalism is a set of values and behaviors through which physicians apply their scientific mastery to serve patients and the community. The word profession derives from Latin professus which means an "open declaration," and intimates that those in a discipline have specialized knowledge, shared standards of behavior with a way to implement them, and have the prime purpose of providing a public service. A medical "professional" implies a responsibility to maintain specialized knowledge and standardized behavior in service to patients. Medicine is a profession that includes:

- A vocation or calling associated with advanced knowledge, skills, and competence
- A code of conduct or ethics with a discipline system with enforcement capability to ensure compliance among members
- Commitment by every member to the greater public interest

Several important features are implicit in the definition:

- *The uneven nature of the physician-patient relationship.* In general, the medical community is in a position of power in relation to its patients. Physicians have the expertise whereas the ill or injured patient is inherently vulnerable. From this arises the fiduciary responsibility of a physician to act in the patient's best interest.
- *The physician's duty to be competent, skillful, ethical, altruistic, humanistic, and trustworthy regarding the health and well-being of an individual and the public.* Trust is essential to the physician-patient relationship and relies on the public's assurance that physicians can be expected to live up to defined standards for training, skills, methods, and continued study. The articulation and enforcement of these standards allows patients to identify physicians who fall short, and it allows physicians to refer to explicit and public policies for guidance about duties for training and practice.
- *The relative autonomy of the medical community to define its own standards of conduct.* Society expects physicians to be trustworthy and dedicated to the public's health and, in turn, grants them autonomy to admit, train, graduate, certify, monitor, and, if necessary, discipline its members. Society provides additional support through subsidies for training, funding for indigent care, and research programs. This relationship between society and the profession is called the "social contract" and is based on the requisite professionalism of the medical community.[15]

Why Is It Critical to Support Professionalism?
The legitimacy of a profession depends on how well it ensures its practitioners are trustworthy. Real and perceived assaults on professionalism may weaken the social contract between the profession and the public it serves. Surgeons, including trainees, should identify factors that dehumanize health care, undermine the physician-patient relationship, or weaken the public's confidence in the profession. To be a professional means believing that society is best served when health care is entrusted to medical professionals who establish, support, and enforce standards. Other proposed systems for organizing and delivering medical care show the dangers of what an erosion of professionalism that weakens public confidence and undermines medicine's position as a profession could lead to.[16]

Here is why physicians and trainees must focus on maintaining their professionalism:

- Patients are invited routinely to evaluate the quality of care and their satisfaction with their provider. High patient ratings for quality and satisfaction are associated with characteristics of professionalism. The ideal physician shows respect, courtesy, empathy, compassion, and communication skills when listening and providing information to patients. In some cases, patient assessments of professional behavior affect physician career opportunities and compensation. Additional information can be found at: *www.pressganey.com/resources/program-summary/workforce-engagement-solution-360-and-180-assessments.*
- In the competitive health care market, reputation and rankings are important to institutions. In addition to quality, safety, and efficiency, a positive professionalism rating for their medical staff helps institutions meet accreditation standards and attract patients.
- The American Board of Medical Specialties (ABMS) specialty boards address professionalism by requiring assessment, monitoring, and interventions as needed. They call for standards that define acceptable behavior, processes that identify and address unprofessional behavior, and directives to teach professionalism to physicians. To maintain board certification, surgeons must offer proof of professional standing as a component of the continuous certification process (*www.absurgery.org/default.jsp?policyethics*).
- The Accreditation Council for Graduate Medical Education (ACGME) lists professionalism as one of six core competencies to be embedded in graduate medical education and residency training. It is outlined by the ACGME Milestones and measured with annual reporting and periodic site visits.[17]
- The ACS is dedicated to the ethical practice of medicine, which establishes and ensures an environment in which all individuals are treated with respect and tolerance. Discrimination or harassment on the basis of age, sexual preference, gender, race, disease, disability, or religion, are inconsistent with the ideals and principles of the profession, as are unacceptable financial practices or other unethical behavior. As a result, the ACS has developed a Statement of Principles that includes a pledge and code of conduct for the surgical profession (*www.facs.org/about-acs/statements/stonprin*).
- Good patient outcomes are linked to professionalism and physician well-being. Data show that medical error is more frequent for a distressed physician with reduced empathy, poor communication, and disruptive behavior. Unprofessional behaviors result in more patient complaints, negative impact on associates, and increased risk for both adverse events and litigation.

Key Attributes and Responsibilities of the Professional
How a profession is defined varies with the conceptualization or framework used to discuss professionalism.[18] One approach is character-based and focuses on the values, virtues, and other internalized principles that lead to appropriate behavior. Sound ethical reasoning, caring, and compassion are component attributes, as are justice, honesty, altruism, and service. Another approach is behavior-based and considers the physician's role. It identifies and emphasizes competencies, such as responsibility, reliability, conflict negotiation, diplomacy, patient rapport, teamwork, and judgment dealing with specific situations. By focusing on doing rather than being, the latter approach is easier to examine and monitor because there is a set of behaviors for which specific outcomes can be observed.

This dichotomy in thinking about professionalism is why published lists of the key attributes and responsibilities of a professional vary so much. The character-based approach refers to virtues, aspirations, and the humanism embodied in the good physician who limits self-interest and demonstrates compassion as a humane person; the behavior-based approach refers to lists of expected behaviors such as accountability, confidentiality, collegiality, listening skills, acknowledging error, boundaries, fatigue management, social responsibility, and patient advocacy. While both approaches have merit and utility, the wide variation and differences among codes and guidelines can be confusing. Although they are different frameworks, they ultimately converge in the character and behavior of a good physician. The ACS Code of Professional Conduct illustrates this application of both character and behavior-based characteristics (*www.facs.org/about-acs/statements/stonprin#code*).

Professionalism is not a separate area of competence, distinct from a physician's other responsibilities. High-quality care requires a surgeon to acquire and maintain the necessary technical skills founded on a solid base of knowledge that go hand-in-hand with character traits and principled behavior required of the professional.

Ethical Foundations of Professionalism

The traditional view of medical professionalism relied on the physician to be a moral agent who, in ambiguous situations, applies ethical reasoning based on internalized values. Physicians were expected to make decisions and take action based on the application of ethical principles, such as autonomy, beneficence, nonmaleficence, and justice. So prevalent was this view that the terms "ethics" and "professionalism" were often used interchangeably. Used for generations, this virtues-based approach fell short when physicians had to make increasingly complex ethical decisions as new technologies and therapeutics were introduced. The physician remains a moral agent, but clinical ethics evolved into a separate area of competence.

There is a saying that a good doctor will make the right decisions, and ethics is just a matter of integrity. But ethics extends beyond moral behavior. Morality rests on values or beliefs that cannot be proven; they must simply be accepted. In addition, ordinary moral rules, which guide daily conduct, often fail to provide a clear direction in medical situations. Decisions are difficult when beliefs and values conflict and people of integrity and goodwill disagree about what to do. In these situations, common sense, experience, and integrity may be too little to guide decisions. In these situations, clinical ethics come into play.

Clinical ethics deals with situations in which there are dilemmas with strong reasons both for and against a course of action. Philosophers distinguish among actions that are obligatory, permissible, and wrong. It is obligatory to tell a patient when there are different options for care; it is wrong to bill fraudulently. But some actions are ethically permissible and optional because they are neutral, with arguments for and against them so evenly balanced that reasonable people would disagree. Or they might be optional in the sense that it would be praiseworthy to perform them, but failure to do so would not be blameworthy.

Clinical ethics provides guidelines, takes a systematic approach, requires making thinking explicit, helps to avoid overlooking important considerations, and supports achieving consistent resolutions. For the physician dealing with uneasy situations or difficult patients, underlying ethical issues often are at stake. For example, if caught in a family dispute over the care of an obtunded relative, it is beneficial to know that a surrogate can use certain standards to make decisions for the patient.

Familiarity with clinical ethics does not require a detailed understanding of philosophical theories or bioethics expertise. Instead, it supports professionalism by preparing a physician to identify the key issues in clinical cases, existing standards to deal with the issue, and the steps leading to good judgment: gather information, review the principles, articulate the options, and achieve resolution through agreement or negotiation. Clinical ethics in surgery is not catharsis or discussion, but a roadmap to an orderly approach for an informed professional to use. A review of relevant articles on basic medical ethics with specific applications to surgical practice can be found in *Selected Readings in General Surgery* Volume 45, No. 3. A comprehensive review of ethical issues in surgery can be found in *Ethical Issues in Surgical Care*, which the ACS Committee on Ethics prepared and includes sections on General Considerations in Ethics, Surgeon-Patient Relationship, Surgeon and Surgical Profession, and the Surgical Society.[19]

Principles for Teaching Professionalism

Traditionally, professionalism was not taught didactically but through exposure to respected role models. The success of this method presumes shared values within a homogenous group of practitioners with a primary focus on the physician-patient relationship. Today, physicians come from more diverse backgrounds, work in less autonomous niches within large institutions, and are employees expected to work with the greater efficiency and productivity that corporate health care demands. With increasing challenges to the role of physicians, by the late 1990s, organized medicine understood the need for thorough descriptions and formal teaching of professionalism. Although no unifying theoretical or practical model has been developed for teaching it, some best practices have emerged.[20]

Environmental and institutional modeling of values. Physicians learn and retain from the "hidden curriculum"—the day-to-day experiences of working in the clinical environment while observing peer and leadership behaviors—positive examples to emulate and negative examples, such as rudeness, cynicism, or misbehavior, to avoid. Many institutions and teaching hospitals have allocated resources and implemented programs to teach medical professionalism, and some have tried to develop methods of evaluating how well that goal has been achieved. When done effectively, the entire culture and environment respects and rewards professional behavior while rejecting unprofessional behaviors. Within the university, academic leadership must ensure this climate exists and is sustained with authentic and public support.

An explicit cognitive curriculum for teaching and sustaining professionalism is needed. The core professional values in medicine are not always intuitively apparent in today's health care environment. New expectations emerge with societal change and technical innovation, and responsibility falls to medical organizations and institutions to update codes of professional conduct and to lay out an explicit curriculum as a "cognitive base" for teaching professionalism. A standard curriculum would provide information and improve knowledge about historical background, definitions, obligations necessary to sustain professional status, and medicine's social contract with society that includes values, attitudes, duties, responsibilities, and behaviors. Specific topics would include honor codes, clinical ethics, moral development, humanism, competencies, patient communication, diplomacy, crisis communication, setting boundaries, conflicts of interest, and systems thinking.

Integration of moral development with biomedical and clinical areas of education. Although professionalism has a cognitive base, didactic teaching isolated from the workplace experience is insufficient. Issues can be identified and discussed in the abstract, but more nuanced circumstances that call for professionalism occur with real-life clinical encounters. It is in everyday situations that routine diagnostic and treatment decisions are overlaid by the opinion of the patient, pressures of time, health system requirements, and the intrusion of personal problems that may cloud vision and distract focus. Didactic sessions are insufficient for teaching attitudes; the physician's attitude and behavior reside in the physician's milieu of patients, hospital, and practice.[21]

Continuity and a longitudinal course of learning. Professionalism is learned through long-term continuity of experience coupled with role models in real practice settings. One key to success is the longitudinal nature of the learning in which the physician has increasing clinical responsibility or exposure to a widening variety and intensity of clinical situations. There is evidence that didactic information and even moral reasoning can be learned in a limited number of sessions or interactions. However, professional behavior is an adaptive process that evolves through repeated participation and interactions with others.

Teaching that is experiential, not theoretical. Physicians learn to practice as health care professionals in workplaces that are simultaneously involved in education and delivering real-life services. In this setting, the core condition of learning is participation. Merely being present is insufficient; the workplace must offer structured opportunities for learning through involvement. To teach professionalism requires stage-appropriate opportunities for learners to encounter professional issues, discuss them with trusted mentors, personalize them, and ultimately internalize them. This situational or experiential learning is built on involvement in clinical encounters, associated explicit teaching, reflection and reinforcement, and progressive incorporation of professional values and aspirations into the learner's identity. Rather than relying on the random interactions of an informal curriculum, experiential learning guides and supports a transition to the values, aspirations, and behaviors of professional practice.[22]

Experiential learning is enhanced when the topic is relevant. Learners are more engaged in learning professionalism when it is considered in the context of their specialty; that is, vascular or endocrine surgeons best appreciate a professionalism consideration if it relates to the individual's practice. To strengthen situated learning, the curriculum should be practical and organized by identifying and addressing professionalism challenges the learner is likely to encounter.

Teacher and role model engagement. Because the clinical environment shapes the attitudes of physicians, physicians must recognize how they themselves model positive or negative aspects of professionalism. "Faculty development" is essential to enhance the teacher's ability to foster caring attitudes and to develop the resources necessary to educate residents and medical students. Some institutions offer resources for learning communication and interpersonal skills, but it is unusual to find programs that offer faculty-development activities focused on the cognitive base of professionalism, methods of expressing and teaching professionalism in their setting, and how to assess and discuss it with others. Time pressures and productivity requirements may undermine humanist values, including support for faculty development programs about caring attitudes and role modeling. In general, faculty need further development to successfully incorporate teaching professionalism into everyday clinical activities.[23]

Methods for Teaching and Learning Professionalism

The educational theory of "situated learning" is most successful when used to design programs aimed at teaching professionalism. Values are implanted through authentic activities that require both abstract knowledge and the application or use of principles. Thus, a balance between the explicit teaching of a subject and the supporting involvement in activities must be struck to ensure the information is relevant, required, useable, and useful. The former is easier and more commonly done; the latter is harder to develop and sustain.[24] Following are several methods for teaching professionalism:

Didactic sessions. Didactic lectures summarize information. They are essential groundwork because physicians must be aware of obligations before they can meet them in everyday life. Physicians need to know, articulate, and explain values, as well as the personal and societal consequences of failure. A curriculum with a formal list of topics ensures that necessary information is covered. Didactic approaches include lectures, panels, videos, and specialty-specific venues, such as grand rounds. To engage the listener, many lecturers use an audience-response system in which audience members are asked to select an answer from a list. Exposure to multidisciplinary experts, including ethicists, attorneys, or hospital-based chaplains, can enrich the didactic program.

Online curriculum/self-study. Web-based teaching modules are increasingly used because they offer several advantages over didactic lectures. A well-designed module covers a range of topics, is available and accessible to many users, and offers the same learning opportunities for all. They can be enhanced with video and interactive features to engage the user and can embed questions in web-based modules to enable feedback on the learner's comprehension. Additional information is available at: *www.surgicalcore.org/* (American Board of Surgery SCORE Curriculum: Surgical Professionalism and Interpersonal Communication Education [SPICE]).

Small group/case-based discussion. According to a recent survey, the most used method for teaching professionalism is the guided discussion of challenging cases in a structured environment facilitated by a group leader.[25] Vignettes or case studies may be used to trigger discussion, encourage questions, and present potential solutions and skills to address the dilemmas that arise from the case. The type and number of topics can be customized for learners based on material drawn from clinical cases or vignettes supplied by professional organizations, such as the ACS (see "Professionalism in Surgery: 2nd Edition DVD" at *https://web4.facs.org/ebusiness/ProductCatalog/product.aspx?ID=169*). Using cases drawn from the lived experiences of a practicing professional, the educational content can teach skills required for professional regulation at the individual, social, and system level. Although case-based discussions stimulate participation, they are limited by the availability and skills of a faculty facilitator and their relevance to the learner's personal experience.

Role playing/simulation. Courses that use role play with standardized patients effectively provide practical experience in a safe environment. When used to explore topics in professionalism, role play can also be done by peers, which is less expensive, less time-consuming, and possibly more likely to stimulate empathy when their colleagues are their "patients." Topics, such as communication theory and professional behavior, are well suited to role play and could include breaking bad news, speaking up regarding an impaired colleague, or a difficult interaction with a patient. To formalize the course content, the theoretical framework behind a situation can be presented in a lecture format before the assigning role scripts.

Role modeling/mentorship. The most effective means of teaching professionalism is the physician role model. The ideal role model demonstrates good clinical skills, desirable personal qualities, and positive interactions with patients and other health care professionals. The good role model spends time with the learner, stresses the importance of the physician–patient relationship, emphasizes the psychosocial aspects of patient care, and gives in-depth, specific feedback to learners. In Figure 1, Cruess and colleagues offer strategies for physicians to consciously improve their effectiveness as role models, starting with being aware that they are role models.[26] Other measures include showing a positive attitude, using clinical interactions as opportunities to teach, discussing a clinical experience, and calling out what is being modeled. Termed "reflection in action," this interactive teaching method draws learning points from what learners may observe but not fully appreciate until brought to their attention.

Figure 1. Characteristics of role models[26]

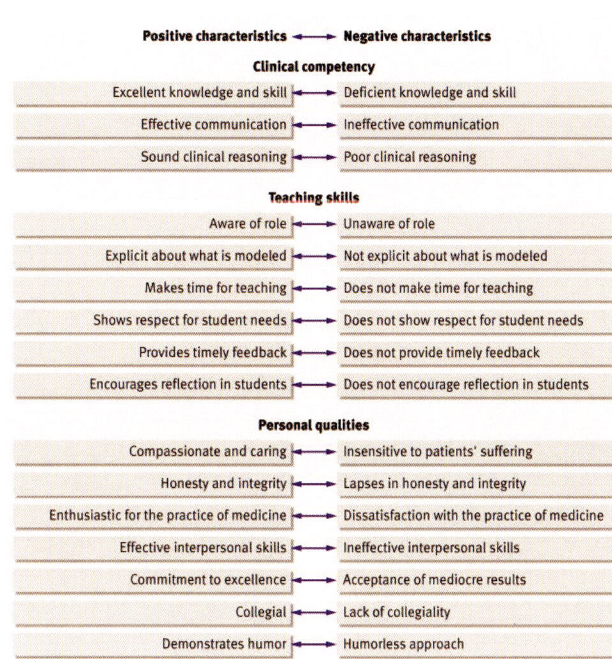

Reflective exercise. Reflection is an essential part of experiential or situated learning that shapes professional identity. Trainees gather impressions as they move through a clinical experience. Active reflection converts these into conscious insights that can be used to build a set of principles and a plan for future action. With increased self-awareness and understanding of their attitudes and beliefs, physicians can more effectively control and direct their behavior. Medical educators have introduced formal, guided reflection by asking learners to write a reflective essay, or "critical incident report" describing a meaningful patient care encounter. This reflective exercise is most useful in conflict-prone settings. This educational approach brings the learner and the mentor together in a deeper, more meaningful way. A challenge, however, is to train the facilitators to help manage and resolve the tensions and emotions expressed in written or verbal reflective exercises.[27]

A recent systematic review of published curricular designs failed to identify best practices for teaching professionalism.[25] The study showed that the heterogeneity of curricular designs made it difficult to compare quality and validity. While work is ongoing to develop and refine teaching tools for professionalism, many different techniques appear suitable, depending on the curricular content (pure information, experiential activity), the setting (computer-based, OR), the topic (teamwork, conflict of interest), and the status of the learner (student/resident, senior faculty). Given the overriding influence of the physician role model on the positive and negative attributes of professionalism, more faculty development and institutional support is needed to promote professionalism.

Methods for Assessing Professionalism

Educational assessment documents a learner's mastery of a subject or acquisition of a skill and evaluates the educational program's efficacy. Formative assessments with feedback assist the learner's progress along the educational pathway. In professionalism, another purpose for evaluation arises from the social contract that grants the profession autonomy for self-regulation. With professional autonomy comes the obligation for the profession to show that it sets and maintains standards and can assess the competence and character of its practitioners at all levels. To demonstrate the professionalism of its members and its own accountability, a profession must develop, refine, and use rigorous assessment tools to gauge professionalism. At present, many different evaluations are used to capture the many dimensions of professional conduct.[28] These professionalism assessments are often adopted before their scoring systems are validated. Further work needs to be done to test the validity of the tools and their ability to affect a physician's actual performance.[15]

Professional assessment can be categorized into cognitive testing, performance-based evaluations, self-assessment, and multisource ratings and reviews (Table 3).

Table 3. Tools for assessing professionalism

- Cognitive testing
- Observations and feedback
  - Clinical setting
  - Simulated (OSCE) setting
- Reflective writing exercises/Self-administered rating scales
- Multisource reviews
  - Patient surveys
  - 360-degree reviews
- Rating forms
- Critical incident reports on lapses

Assessment results and feedback can help physician learners advance as part of a career-long process. Knowledge can be tested through written, oral, and online programs, while observations with ratings and feedback are made in both the clinical setting and through objective structured clinical examinations (OSCEs). Patient surveys are used widely to measure physician performance, whereas multisource evaluations using 360-degree reviews take a deeper look at physicians in their work settings. Incident reports and patient complaints may identify professional lapses and be used to initiate feedback and performance improvement.

Assessment of professionalism is an evolving field with instruments that will need more work to ensure their reliability. For many of them, accuracy and legitimacy depend on adequate sampling and the expertise of those making judgments. Goldie suggested that assessment should include monitoring the practice environment because situational and contextual phenomena can influence a physician's behavior; in fact, observers who ignore contextual circumstances may unfairly label physicians as "unprofessional."[28] In summary, further research and improvements in the professional assessment process will ease some of its associated tensions, engage the physician in an authentic way, and assure the public that the profession tries to ensure the competence and character of its member physicians.

Interprofessional Education

Interprofessional Education

To enable effective collaboration, interprofessional education (IPE) brings together learners from two or more professions to exchange information and perspectives. The goal of IPE is "to improve health outcomes through the education of a practice-ready health care team that is prepared to respond to local health needs," according to the World Health Organization. The skills necessary for teamwork, as described earlier in this chapter, are an essential element of IPE. Communication, mutual support, and situation awareness are modified and reinforced as health care workers learn to collaborate to solve complex problems.

Why Interprofessional Education Is Important

A team's safe practice of medicine requires effective and constant communication with colleagues and patients as well as intentional listening, assertiveness, and timeliness. In contrast, most health professions today are taught in relatively siloed institutions. In fact, very limited dialogue takes place between the schools of nursing, medicine, and social work, even in universities that house all three, and the same is true for pharmacy, nutrition, physician assistant, and other programs. Training emphasizes that each member of the profession is responsible for the care of the patient; yet as medicine has become more complex, requiring many individuals with specialized expertise to care for a patient, there is a heightened need to coordinate and appropriately distribute tasks and responsibilities among those individuals. Thus, there is the need to create teams composed of individuals with different fields of expertise capable of efficiently working together toward a common goal. Team-based care has been proven to improve patient satisfaction, health outcomes, and resource utilization. In response, the Institute of Medicine (now the National Academy of Medicine), followed by The Macy Foundation and other organizations, have developed the concept of interprofessional education.

This concept is based on the notion that, if students from different medical professions (medicine, pharmacy, nursing, social work, dentistry, and so on) learn how to work together during the early stages of their training, they will be better prepared to work as teams in providing patient care. This approach is supported by the evidence that improved communication and collaboration in interprofessional teams leads to better patient care.

In contrast, failures in the provision of care by a team are often related to failures of communication. In fact, The Joint Commission identified the failure of interprofessional teamwork—usually the result of communication failure—as the most common cause of sentinel events. Sometimes turf battles lead to adversarial relationships between professionals; at other times, roles are not clearly defined or the use of different terminology by different professionals leads to a communication failure. Interprofessional education addresses these failures and builds a foundation of communication and coordination by establishing an exchange between students of various health professions.

Barriers to Interprofessional Education

Despite the relative simplicity of the concept, substantial barriers inhibit implementation of IPE. Most relate to the reluctance to move away from traditional curricula or the perception of a hierarchy among the professions. Moreover, bringing together students and residents from different professions from different geographic areas requires travel and time, which some health professionals believe increases cost and decreases efficiency. In addition, scheduling can be complicated by differing work schedules and requirements from school to school and the lack of an identifiable owner responsible for implementing IPE.

This lack of a specific "owner" of IPE has been overcome with support from foundations such as The Macy Foundation and has found a place in some of the ACS-accredited Educational Institutes (ACS-AEIs). In other instances, health science-related colleges have created specific IPE centers to implement appropriate curricula. An example is presented at *https://collaborate.uw.edu/online-training-and-resources/simulation-team-training-toolkit/*.

Teaching IPE

IPE can be taught in four steps: Identify a program owner, develop a curriculum, use simulation modules, and consider alternative teaching methods.

Determine who is in charge. The first step in teaching IPE is to identify an "owner" of the program. This process is often challenging because most institutions are organized and operate in relative silos (medicine, nursing, public health, and so on) whereas this new unit needs to be part of every college or school as well as serve as an "umbrella" capable of developing curricula and authorized to direct students and residents from the different institutions to the program. This new unit must be clearly identified with defined resources and relationships with participating schools and colleges.

Develop the curriculum. A curriculum must be developed to expose trainees in advanced health professions to how teams can effectively collaborate in the care of a patient with a complex condition. The goals of the curriculum should be as follows: instill a culture that respects the dignity, privacy, and values of patients; define roles and responsibilities of the interprofessional team and how its members work together and care for their patients; and define how each member contributes to the effectiveness of teamwork. Implementation of this curriculum may be facilitated by existing programs on team training. For example, the TeamSTEPPS training model, widely used to train health care teams, is a great resource for training interprofessional teams. This training model has been shown to improve students' attitudes, knowledge, and skills in interprofessional work.

One unique aspect of IPE curriculum development is the development of a curriculum for trainers. Trainers are usually members of a specific profession and, as such, act within the silo of their profession. They will need to develop all aspects of team training and a deep understanding of the unique contributions that the students from other professions bring to the team. They also will need to develop expertise on assessment and evaluation in this relatively new field.

Use simulation to teach IPE. The ACS-AEIs offer a unique site for IPE that allows the creation of interprofessional training modules to teach the key elements of effective teamwork in simulated settings in a controlled environment. Trainees from various professions can be paired together.[29] For example, videos of scenarios in which a case progressively unfolds helps facilitators to establish collaborative dialogue among advanced learners. One of the leading institutions in the development and use of IPE uses a series of web-based cases, lectures, and simulated scenarios with human patient simulators or standardized patients. These scenarios are part of the existing curriculum of each school involved. This project provides integrated training to medical, nursing, pharmacy, and physician assistant students in four error-prone areas: acute care events, chronic care coordination, error disclosure, and conflict resolution (*https://collaborate.uw.edu/*). The aim is to help these health care professionals provide safe, high-quality care during challenging clinical situations.

One program that trained faculty from the schools of medicine, nursing, pharmacy, and the physician assistant program resulted in the appropriate training of the trainers and enriched the culture of those schools as well. A toolkit was developed that can be accessed at Developing a Program for Interprofessional Education, *https://collaborate.uw.edu/online-training-and-resources/simulation-team-training-toolkit/*.

Consider other teaching methods, such as online training. The Coronavirus Disease 2019 (COVID-19) pandemic forced education and training programs to find alternatives to traditional teaching methods. The program described above made a shift to online delivery of content for students affected by stay-at-home orders across the five-state WWAMI Region (Washington, Wyoming, Alaska, Montana, and Idaho). They achieved their goal of focusing on communication, leadership, and team functioning by breaking the larger group into smaller discussion groups for scenario vignettes. Overall, in two weeks, they were able to fully offer an IPE program online to hundreds of students from medicine, nursing, and pharmacy schools.

Assessing IPE

There are several ways to assess competence in the field of IPE. First, is direct observation by the faculty of the student's interactions during role playing. This assessment should evaluate teamwork and communications and is a good way to determine overall effectiveness of training.

Another way is through a comprehensive pre-/post-assessment. These assessments include individual questions using the Likert scale that allows for a quantitative measurement and open-ended questions that allow students to reflect on their observations and the actual experience regarding attitudes, mutual respect, privacy, patient values, and so on.

Specific areas such as communication, leadership, and mutual support can be measured using the TeamSTEPPS methodology. Additionally, measurement can be supported with self, team, and peer assessments that students complete for evaluation, reflection, and debriefing after the simulation exercise.

Lastly, the organization, utility, and facilitation effectiveness of IPE programs should be evaluated and its effects on the different professions compared.

Evaluations show that both students and faculty who participate in IPE benefit significantly as reflected in improved attitudes toward the members of other professions, a better mutual understanding of values and beliefs, and increased motivation to participate in future trainings. IPE participants recognize the utility of TeamSTEPPS communication training and develop an increased sense of self-efficacy in their ability to translate the skills learned in training into the practice of team medicine.

Leading a Diverse Team

Leading a Diverse Team

Leadership is a key quality of a surgeon. Most surgical programs try to identify leadership qualities among applicants for internships and consider the development of leadership skills during surgical residency to be a critical component of the training process.

There are at least three important clinical scenarios in which surgical leadership is key, including leading the team on surgical ward rounds, leading in the trauma bay, and leading the OR. Each of these situations requires surgical leaders to have some of the same skills, such as situation awareness, but also requires distinct ones unique to the scenario.

Leading Surgical Rounds

Leading a surgical team on surgical rounds is often the surgical resident's first leadership responsibility. This skill is seldom taught in a "traditional manner." Most residents begin the learning process by observing their senior or chief residents when rounding as a medical student, intern, or junior resident. Occasionally, they observe attending surgeons during "teaching rounds." Surgical residents may begin leading surgical rounds as early as their second postgraduate year on some services or perhaps on "morning work rounds," maintaining this responsibility throughout residency and even into fellowship.

Leading ward rounds requires: gathering data, such as vital signs, inputs and outputs, physical examination, and lab data; assessing the patient with some level of communication to the patient and family; and, finally, developing a tentative plan for the day or the remainder of the hospitalization. All of this, plus creating teaching moments, must be accomplished in a timely and efficient manner to allow the team to get to the OR in the morning and to respect their need for work-life balance and personal autonomy. The necessary skillsets include listening, careful observation of the patient, decision-making, prioritization, 360-degree communication, and efficiency. Specific challenges include unexpected findings, the variable learning curves of students and junior residents, and balancing the team's "service versus education" at both ends of a busy day. Providing leadership on surgical rounds often allows the team to work together throughout the rotation. Thus, leadership improves as surgeons or residents get to know team members and can better anticipate what to expect in most situations.

To successfully develop junior surgical resident leaders, the observations of experienced team leaders are needed to reinforce good traits and avoid the undesirable traits. Textbooks, lectures, videos, or even simulation cannot replace experience gained by repeating this process over the years of training, which is why rounding responsibilities typically continue throughout the five-plus years of clinical training. Finally, it is important that the "leader of rounds" have the opportunity to express the knowledge gained on rounds with the attending by reporting the key findings and sharing the plan that the resident has developed. Attending surgeon feedback is important but must avoid simply dictating to the learner "what to do." A good attending surgeon listens and allows the resident to learn by trial and error in development of their plan.

Leading the Trauma Bay

Gaining leadership experience in the trauma bay is usually reserved for more senior residents. Although all the qualities of leading ward rounds are necessary in the trauma bay, there are distinct differences.

The most obvious is urgency, particularly given the needs of the critically ill, unstable trauma patient. Quickly making life-or-death decisions with limited information requires the leader to remain composed and in control so they can function at the "top of their game" and maintain the team's confidence.

Another major difference is delegating aspects of patient care and responsibility for completing specific tasks to caregivers outside the core surgical team, such as emergency room nurses, emergency medicine residents, and attendings. Those relationships can often create issues related to "who is really in charge." The surgical senior resident or fellow (or even the attending) must set aside his or her ego and defer to others as appropriate while avoiding conflict, especially in the heat of the moment. There is little room for argument in the trauma setting; ultimately the decision falls on the responsible trauma surgeon, with any differences that arise during the case to be discussed and settled in a post-event performance analysis. Simulation with "team training" can play an important role in this process and should be part of all surgical training programs. The ACS Advanced Trauma Life Support® (ATLS®) course offers valuable educational resources for teaching interprofessional cooperation and teamwork.

Leading the OR

The final and most important opportunity for surgical leadership is in the OR, where the surgeon needs to orchestrate every aspect of the operation, including the role of assistants and learners, regardless of case complexity. This leadership is particularly necessary in times of stress, such as bleeding, intraoperative difficulty, or complications. The tone of the case changes with the setting, such as an elective procedure versus an emergency case including the unstable trauma patient. The OR environment, perhaps more than any other setting, requires leadership, decision-making, and addressing all technical aspects of a case; it also requires professional behavior, including respect for all team members, protocols or policies, and the "team culture." The leadership and composure of the surgeon in the OR determines the quality of the contributions and the overall experience of all team members and, in many cases, the outcome of the procedure. Patient outcomes are enhanced if the surgeon leader has previously worked with team members, including anesthesiologists and nurses, and knows their familiarity with the type of operation being performed.

At various stages of the residents' training, it's essential to provide them autonomy in the OR. This process begins with case components but progresses to full autonomy with supervision. Such autonomy must be balanced with OR efficiency and the clinical setting of the case. In some settings, years of interaction between an attending surgeon and scrub nurse or circulator may enable the resident to learn as much from the scrub nurse as from the attending. A good resident never turns down the opportunity to learn from more experienced professionals, regardless of whether the attending is in the room or not. The classic example of "give me what I need, not what I asked for" requires the resident to have the situation awareness to recognize the importance of the experience of all members of the team. Conducting the case autonomously requires humility and willingness to obtain feedback, both of which allow a junior surgeon to learn and still achieve quality outcomes. In the OR, leadership can be taught not just through close observation and graduated experience, but also with team training simulation.

Issues of Gender Equity, Diversity, and Inclusion
Over the last few decades, more women have joined the surgical workforce to the point where women are now the majority of trainees in many U.S. surgical residency programs. (How these changes promote the best of surgical care and create a strong pipeline for future leaders is a discussion beyond the scope of this chapter.)

Nonetheless, this change creates distinct challenges in leadership at all levels. Unfortunately, the biggest challenge associated with gender diversity in daily surgical practice is the unwillingness of some patients, nurses, and others to acknowledge a woman surgeon as a leader because of gender bias or stereotyping. Female chief residents have been treated in a demeaning, gender-biased manner on rounds or in clinic by patients and on the wards or in the OR by nurses and even attendings. Most women residents and attendings have at some point had patients refer to them as nurses or ignore their leadership position. Some female surgeons have even been sexually harassed by patients, patient family members, or colleagues.

All team leaders must work to ensure that female team members receive appropriate respect in every setting, including being referred to as "doctor." This practice establishes respect for the medical degree and additional training achieved by the surgeon or resident. Women leaders need to develop and practice how to react in situations where they face bias or harassment. Whatever the setting, they should exhibit professionalism and leadership by correcting any misconceptions of the patient or members of the patient care team, in clinic settings, in inpatient units, or in the OR. They should be appropriately assertive when reacting to episodes of gender bias without creating dysfunction in their relationship with the patient or in the workplace. In this way, women leaders can gain the respect of individuals who question their role as a leader. Finally, institutional leaders, particularly division chiefs or surgical chairs, should be sure that bias is appropriately managed and corrected. This may require dealing with nursing leadership, patient care services, or even hospital security.

Nowhere in the U.S. is immune from bias, prejudice, or even systemic racism. The same challenges that women leaders face are matched or magnified for leaders who are underrepresented minorities. Combatting these issues requires emphasis on the professional qualities of the individual and the support of surgical and institutional leadership. Similarly, team leaders must immediately respond to any example, no matter how subtle, of prejudice, bias, or racism, particularly during one-on-one interactions with a patient (or family). Team leaders must also respond to similar behavior demonstrated by any team member, be it a physician, nurse, or other health care provider, in the wards, trauma bay, or the OR.

Efforts to improve inclusion of a diverse population of residents is important for the present success of surgical training programs and will help pave the way for a more diverse set of leaders in the future. To ensure this transition, all surgeons, including senior or junior residents, must help enable residents of any gender or race to lead without bias or prejudice in every clinical setting.

Psychological Safety in Surgical Leadership
The final component of this discussion, psychological safety in leadership, is the ability to lead without fear of negative consequences on self-image, status, or one's career. Psychological safety requires a shared belief that the team is safe for interpersonal risk taking and allows team members to feel accepted and respected. The four stages of psychological safety include a condition where an individual feels included, safe to learn, safe to contribute, and safe to challenge the status quo – all without fear of being embarrassed, marginalized, or punished. Psychological safety will enable teams to learn and perform at the highest level and to be effective in every setting. The process allows team members to share ideas for improving performance, even in settings where they frequently remain silent for fear of being judged harshly. Thus, an important part of teaching surgical leadership is to ensure all learners understand the value and presence of psychological safety. This shared understanding across all levels of an institution will improve process innovation, promote learning from mistakes, foster engagement, and motivate teams.

This culture must be encouraged from the top, including chairs, division chiefs, and program directors to allow surgical trainees to become the most effective team leaders.

Conclusion

This chapter focuses on the skills a surgeon must acquire beyond those purely related to technique. Most training programs in general surgery traditionally focused on the acquisition and mastery of technical skills. During the last two decades, with the substantial increase in the complexity of surgical procedures which require the combined and coordinated work of a larger group of people, the handling of different devices and the integration of systems within the OR, it has been recognized that a number of other skills, grouped under "non-technical skills" such as situation awareness, communication, shared mental models, emotional intelligence and professionalism are essential to achieve excellence in the performance of surgery.

In this chapter we describe the importance of these "non-technical skills" in surgery and define ways in which each skill can be taught, learned, and measured. Furthermore, the chapter includes a section on interprofessional education, describing this novel way of integrating–at the student level–members of different professions that will eventually come together to provide clinical care. It spells out the methodology for developing interprofessional education programs, delivering it, and for the evaluation of results. In addition, the chapter defines leadership with emphasis on aspects pertinent to surgeons, providing examples on leading on rounds, in the trauma bay, and in the operating room itself. Lastly, we discuss how diversity and inclusion relate to leadership, and how we all must effectively address bias, racism, and other notions that profoundly affect our ability to work together. The chapter ends with a discussion on psychological safety and how, when appropriately exercised, it positively impacts the delivery of care.

Suggested Readings

Agency for Healthcare Research and Quality. TeamSTEPPS. Available at: https://www.ahrq.gov/ teamstepps/index.html. Accessed October 12, 2020.

American College of Surgeons. Residents as Teachers and Leaders Course. Available at: https://www.facs.org/education/division-of-education/courses/residents-as-teachers. Accessed October 8, 2021.

Arriaga AF, Gawande AA, Raemer DB, et al. Pilot testing of a model for insurer-driven, large-scale multicenter simulation training for operating room teams. *Ann Surg.* 2014;259(3):403-410.

Brock D, Abu-Rish E, Chiu C, Hammer D, Wilson S, Vorvick L, Zierler B. (2013). Interprofessional education in team communication: working together to improve patient safety. *BJM Quality & Safety.* 2013;22(5):414-423.

Clark TR. *The 4 Stages of Psychological Safety: Defining the Path to Inclusion and Innovation*. Oakland, CA. Berrett-Koehler Publications, Inc.;2020.

Ericsson KA. Deliberate practice and acquisition of expert performance: a general overview. *Acad Emerg Med.* 2008;15(11):988-994.

Flin R, Youngson G, Yule S. How do surgeons make intra-operative decisions? *BMJ Quality & Safety* 2007;16:162.

Greenberg CC. Association for Academic Surgery presidential address: sticky floors and glass ceilings. *J Surg Res.* 2017;219:ix-xviii.

Greenberg CC, Ghousseini HN, Pavuluri Quamme SR, et al. A statewide surgical coaching program provides opportunity for continuous professional development. *Ann Surg.* 2018;267(5):868-873.

Gutierrez D, Mullen PR. Emotional intelligence and the counselor: examining the relationship of trait emotional intelligence to counselor burnout. *J Mental Health Couns.* 2016;38(3):187–200.

Pradarelli JC, Gupta A, Lipsitz S, Blair PG, Sachdeva AK, Smink DS, Yule S. Assessment of the Non-Technical Skills for Surgeons (NOTSS) framework in the USA. *Br J Surg.* 2020;107(9):1137-1144.

Sevdalis N, Davis R, Koutantji M, Undre S, Darzi A, Vincent C. Reliability of a revised NOTECHS scale for use in surgical teams. *Am J Surg.* 2008 Aug;196(2):184-190.

Willgerodt M, Sonney J, Liner D, Barchet L. (2018). The power of a team: using unfolding video cases in interprofessional education for advanced health trainees. MedEdPORTAL. 2018;14:10707.

Wilson S, Vorvick L. (2016). Dyspnea in a hospitalized patient: using simulation to introduce interprofessional collaborative practice concepts. MedEdPORTAL Publications. 2016;12:10488.

Yule S, Flin R, Paterson-Brown S, Maran N, Rowley D. Development of a rating system for surgeons' non-technical skills. *Med Edu.* 2006 Nov;40(11):1098-1104.

Yule S, Gupta A, Gabler Blair P, Sachdeva AK, Smink DS on behalf of the American College of Surgeons Committee on Non-Technical Skills. Gathering validity evidence to adapt the Non-technical Skills for Surgeons (NOTSS) Assessment Tool to the United States context. *J Surg Edu.* 2021;78(3):955-966.

References

1. Salovey P, Mayer J. Emotional intelligence. *Imag Cogn Person.* 1990; 9:185–211.
2. Hogeveen J, Salvi C, Grafman J. 'Emotional Intelligence': Lessons from lesions. *Trends Neurosci.* 2016;39(10):694-705.
3. Daffey-Moore EK. Is emotional intelligence relevant to a fighting force? *J R Army Med Corps.* 2015;161 Suppl 1:i14-i16.
4. Shouhed D, Beni C, Manguso N, et al. Association of emotional intelligence with malpractice claims: a review. *JAMA Surg.* 2019;154:250-256.

5. Ranjha AY, Shujja S. Emotional intelligence and psychological adjustment of nurses serving in emergency and non-emergency wards. *J Behav Sci*. 2010;20(2):36–48.
6. Şenyuva E, Kaya H, Işik B, Bodur G. Relationship between self-compassion and emotional intelligence in nursing students. Int. *J Nurs Pract*. 2014;20(6):588–596.
7. Ezzatabadi M, Bahrami MA, Hadizadeh F, Arab M, Nasiri S, Amiresmaili M, Tehrani GA. Nurses' emotional intelligence impact on the quality of hospital services. Iran. *Red Crescent Med J*. 2012;14(12):758–763.
8. Schneider TR, Lyons JB, Khazon S. Emotional intelligence and resilience. *Pers Individ Diff*. 2013;55(8):909–914.
9. Montes-Berges B, Augusto JM. Exploring the relationship between perceived emotional intelligence, coping, social support and mental health in nursing students. *J Psychiatr Ment Health Nurs*. 2007;14(2):163–171.
10. Gutierrez D, Mullen PR. Emotional intelligence and the counselor: examining the relationship of trait emotional intelligence to counselor burnout. *J Ment Health Couns*. 2016;38(3):187-200.
11. Caruso DR. Emotions and the ability model of emotional intelligence. In: Emmerling RJ, Shanwell VK, Mandal MK eds. *Emotional Intelligence: Theoretical and Cultural Perspectives*. New York, NY: Nova Science Publishers; 2008:1–16.
12. Petrides KV, Pita R, Kokkinaki F. The location of trait emotional intelligence in personality factor space. *Br J Psychol*. 2007;98(2):273–289.
13. Mayer JD, Salovey P. What is emotional intelligence? In: Salovey P, Sluyter D, eds. *Emotional Development and Emotional Intelligence: Educational Implications*, 2nd ed. New York, NY: Basic Books; 1997:3–31.
14. Petrides KV. Psychometric properties of the trait emotional intelligence questionnaire (TEIQue). In: Stough C, Saklofske DH, Parker JDA, eds. *Assessing Emotional Intelligence*. New York, NY. Springer;2009:85–101.
15. Mueller PS. Teaching and assessing professionalism in medical learners and practicing physicians. *Rambam Maimonides Med J*. 2015;6(2):e0011.
16. Wynia MK, Papadakis MA, Sullivan WM, Hafferty FW. More than a list of values and desired behaviors: a foundational understanding of medical professionalism. *Acad Med*. 2014;89(5):712-714.
17. Wagner R, Koh N, Bagian JP, Weiss KB, on behalf of the CLER Program. *CLER 2016 National Report of Findings. Issue Brief #8: Professionalism*. Chicago, IL: Accreditation Council for Graduate Medical Education; 2016.
18. Irby DM, Hamstra SJ. Parting the clouds: three professionalism frameworks in medical education. *Acad Med*. 2016;91(12):1606-1611.
19. Ferreres AR, Angelos P, Singer EA. *Ethical Issues in Surgical Care*. Chicago, IL: American College of Surgeons; 2017.
20. Glass N, Wilson I, Harrison M, Usherwood T, Nass D. (2013). Teaching professionalism in medical education: a Best Evidence Medical Education (BEME) systematic review. BEME Guide No. 25. *Med Teach*. 2013;35:e1252-e1266.
21. Huddle TS. Viewpoint: Teaching professionalism: is medical morality a competency? *Acad Med*. 2005;80(10):885–891.
22. Yardley S, Teunissen PW, Dornan T. Experiential learning: transforming theory into practice. *Med Teach*. 2012;34(2):161-164.
23. Lown BA, Chou CL, Clark WD, et al. Caring attitudes in medical education: perceptions of deans and curriculum leaders. *J Gen Intern Med*. 2007;22(11):1514-1522.
24. Cruess RL, Cruess SR. Teaching professionalism: general principles. *Med Teach*. 2006;28(3):205-208.
25. Berger AS, Niedra E, Brooks SG, Ahmed WS, Ginsburg S. Teaching professionalism in postgraduate medical education: a systematic review. *Acad Med*. 2020;95(6):938-946.
26. Cruess SR, Cruess RL, Steinert Y. Role modelling--making the most of a powerful teaching strategy. *BMJ*. 2008;336(7646):718-721.
27. Cruess RL, Cruess SR, Boudreau JD, Snell L, Steinert Y. A schematic representation of the professional identity formation and socialization of medical students and residents: a guide for medical educators. *Acad Med*. 2015;90(6):718-725.
28. Goldie J. Assessment of professionalism: a consolidation of current thinking. *Med Teach*. 2013;35(2):e952-e956.
29. Zierler B, Ross B, Liner D. (2010). A WHO report: the Macy Interprofessional Collaborative Project, the University of Washington. *J Allied Health*. 2010;39 Suppl 1. e131-e132.

AMERICAN C
SURGEONS A
OF SURGEON
COLLEGE OF
AMERICAN CO
SURGEONS A
OF SURGEON
COLLEGE OF
AMERICAN C
SURGEONS

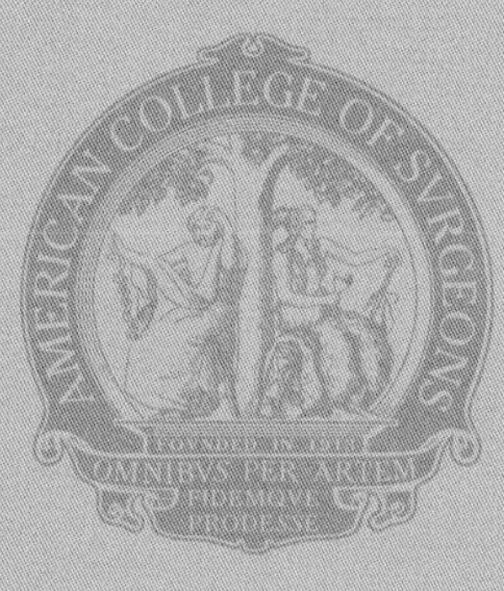

CHAPTER 8
Resident Training in Scholarship and Research

Lead Author

Kelly M. McMasters, MD, PhD, FACS

Co-Authors

Timothy J. Eberlein, MD, FACS, MAMSE

James S. Economou, MD, PhD, FACS

Mary T. Hawn, MD, MPH, FACS

Allan D. Kirk, MD, PhD, FACS, MAMSE

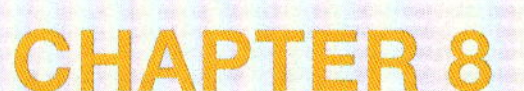

Resident Training in Scholarship and Research

Executive Summary

This chapter focuses on the importance of engaging residents in scientific inquiry. Training programs should provide opportunities for residents and fellows to investigate surgical diseases, solve scientific questions, and publish or present their findings. The research process is relevant to all surgeons, regardless of whether they aspire to be academicians, scientists, or clinicians.

In this chapter, we answer the following questions:

- Why should surgical trainees participate in research?
- What are the common scholarship elements/requirements for all surgical trainees?
- How do we train surgeon-scientists to become independently funded principal investigators?
- What are the research and scholarship requirements for most academic surgeons?
- What resources are needed to support resident research, scholarship, and career development?

The Value of Surgical Trainee Participation in Research

Research and Scholarship in Surgical Disciplines

The 1910 Flexner Report established that it is important for physicians to engage in scientific research. Ever since, the disciplines of surgery have embraced these recommendations, with some residency programs requiring additional biomedical research training. A critical component of the philosophy of surgeon education is that scientific inquiry is part of a physician's professional responsibility. Ample evidence shows that the use of the scientific method in clinical practice and discovery-based medical research has improved the care of surgical patients over the last century.

However, learning to conduct structured, scientific research and write scholarly articles requires training. And although all residents should be exposed to research, many residents will not have an interest in pursuing formal research training. For residents who are driven by a strong sense of inquiry, however, preparing for a career in surgical research needs to be deliberate and strategic.

There are many opportunities for surgical research to impact patient care today, but they require deliberate strategies and training paradigms. For example, genetic medicine has strengthened our understanding of disease biology through large scale DNA/RNA sequencing, bioinformatics, cell and gene therapy, molecular diagnostics, and biomarker-driven clinical trials. To become authentic participants in disease-altering discoveries for patients who present with traditional surgical diseases, surgical investigators will need to train and adapt to a new model of biomedical research called "team science," which is a collaborative effort to address a scientific challenge by leveraging the expertise of professionals from different fields. In addition to biomedical research, fields such as outcomes science, implementation science, and educational research have grown in sophistication and also require specific training.

A Culture Change

Our current organization of academic medical disciplines—surgery, internal medicine, pathology—inherited from the 19th-century German schools, once made good sense. But since the 1950s, it has become clear that addressing the biology of most diseases benefits from research teams with diverse education and training backgrounds. The most successful of these multidisciplinary team science enterprises generally are dedicated to producing solid discovery science that improves patient care. These teams recognize that each member has a role that should be valued and rewarded, including junior members.

Research Training for Surgeons

Clinical training in surgery often lasts more than five years after medical school and includes specialty training. Scientists on a traditional PhD track may require up to a decade of graduate school and postdoctoral fellowship(s) before employment in academia or industry. Although both disciplines employ the scientific method, there is often inadequate overlap between the scholarly activities of clinical surgery and discovery-based biological research.

Medical scientist training programs (MSTPs) produce a small number of MD/PhD-trained physician-scientists who make substantial contributions through their own scientific research, the trainees they mentor, and their leadership of academic institutions and scholarly societies. However, one does not need to be a dual-trained physician-scientist to become a leader in scientific discovery and innovation. In fact, in every medical subspecialty the scientific contributions and accomplishments of MD-trained investigators greatly exceed those of MSTP-trained physicians. Surgeons with a variety of backgrounds can contribute to important research endeavors if research programs are properly structured. By participating in a one- to two-year research experience, surgical residents often develop an appreciation for scientific discovery and the curiosity to ask the questions required for research efforts to improve patient care. Some residents spend additional time in research programs to learn specific techniques, even though it may not lead to a formal degree.

Many surgical residents who interrupt their clinical training for a one- or two-year research experience often are surprised at its rewards. If they join a rigorous and productive research environment with experienced investigators and trainees and are mentored well, they will learn which types of scientific discovery environments they would prefer to join later in their careers. Trainees engaged in research also will learn scientifically rigorous thinking and how to appropriately ask and answer scientific and clinical questions. The laboratory hones investigative skills that will improve the quality of clinical work. Both contribute to better science and advancements in patient care.

Frequently, the best training experiences come from being part of a diverse, multidisciplinary team of investigators who are tackling an important problem in human disease biology. The simultaneous acquisition of technical expertise and intellectual skills will improve the resident's research training experience. Aside from learning how to design and critically interpret research experiments, residents will learn the interpersonal skills required to work with research colleagues to achieve a common objective. Also, they will learn that good scientists are driven by intense curiosity and always try to disprove their favorite hypotheses.

Surgeons entering academic and community practice may engage in a range of scholarly activities as well. They do not need to work in a wet laboratory to make important scholarly contributions. For example, participation in quality outcomes research or well-designed clinical trials may significantly benefit surgical patients.

Career development of junior faculty is dependent on the quality of mentorship and the supportive multidisciplinary team structure to ensure trainees achieve necessary training. Academic surgeon leaders who recruit and support junior surgical investigators adhere to the triad of resources, space, and protected time. More important to the resident's success, however, is a supportive scientific team and community, as well as quality mentorship. Ideally, well-trained surgical investigators are immersed in a scientific team in which members teach each other and help junior members grow. The National Institutes of Health has long recognized the value of mentored training platforms for junior faculty through its support of K-Award programs.

Traditionally, physician-scientists achieved academic success once they became independent investigators who supervised a research team, such as the principal investigator on a federally funded grant. This paradigm is increasingly regarded as unrealistic because of the demands of apportioning effort between clinical practice and research and the recognition that human disease biology research requires tools that most "independent" investigators, even those who are devoted fully to research, cannot realistically master. Although surgeons remain important as principal investigators and leaders in scientific discovery and innovation, high-functioning scientific teams have become the best model to develop faculty careers and achieve meaningful scientific progress.

A 21st century model of *team science* focuses relentlessly on a challenging scientific problem, takes full advantage of diversity in training and expertise, and values and supports all team members. To prepare for this challenge, residents must acquire basic skills, supervise a research program, and manage their time so they can simultaneously develop their clinical career and maintain a research program.

Common Scholarship Elements/ Requirements for All Surgical Trainees

Scholarship

Scholarship in surgical training provides surgeons with a structure to acquire and assess information relevant to their practice. Sound surgery requires a working understanding of normal human biology, the mechanisms underlying surgical diseases, and the biophysical principles of surgical practice.

Scholarly activity, such as research (hypothesis generation and testing) and publication (peer review and dissemination of validated insights), is critical to understanding these cornerstones. State-of-the-art information for all specialties is always evolving; as a result, surgeons are distinguished from technicians by their capacity to assimilate new knowledge and apply it in evolving situations. For surgeons to develop and maintain the knowledge base needed to conduct a safe and effective practice, they must understand scholarly conduct and be able to acquire, assess, and reformulate the necessary information.

To instill and satisfy trainees' desire to acquire and maintain a robust fund of knowledge, training programs offer independent reading, didactic coursework, apprenticeship and experience-based training, and other means of cultivating information. However, for a surgeon to stay competent throughout practice, training programs must also teach residents how to stay current throughout their careers while amassing the experience needed to handle various situations faced in practice. For example, a training program might incorporate the use of academic practice tools, including a framework to approach research and publication, to improve trainees' clinical approach.

Establishing a Knowledge Base

All trainees should have access to a reliable source of contemporary literature pertinent to surgical practice overall as well as to the specifics of their specialty. This should include access to the primary literature, ideally through subscription access to relevant content of the National Library of Medicine through PubMed.gov (*https://pubmed.ncbi.nlm.nih.gov*). For practical purposes, access to reputable derivative works, such as textbooks and peer-reviewed summaries, is helpful but not a substitute for primary literature. Trainees should not, for their foundational learning, rely on commercially biased or non-validated sources of information, such as non-peer-reviewed writings, social media, lay accounts, online videos, materials provided by the biomedical device and pharmaceutical industry, and so on.

If access is important, so is time to read. Programs should identify time for staying current on the scientific and clinical literature and faculty should model effective study habits. Residents' use of curated curricula of the current literature, such as *Selected Readings in General Surgery*® (*www.facs.org/publications/srgs*), should give way over time to keeping up with relevant specialty journals. Experiential and didactic sessions should be integrated into, but not replace, a formal reading curriculum.

The Value of Primary Literature

All programs should have a structured approach toward the primary literature that includes teaching a basic understanding of the peer-review process, the various classifications of strength of evidence, the concepts of bias and conflict, and the general approach to a peer-reviewed article. Journal clubs or other group conferences can help structure readings. Ideally, these reading groups should be proctored by mentors experienced in peer review and capable of dissecting an article's strengths and weaknesses. When possible, assign articles with a variety of evidence levels from foundational preclinical science, through case reports and descriptive series, to randomized controlled trials, and, when available, meta-analyses and structured consensus reviews. Standardized tests should periodically assess trainee knowledge, and trainees should be required to present new topics at journal clubs or other peer conferences.

Trainees learn best through experience. Just as trainees learn best how to perform an operation through operative experience, their understanding of the primary literature and how articles are composed is enhanced through writing and submitting articles for publication. In fact, writing an article helps residents learn how the primary literature emerges; this is especially true for trainees who participate in discovery-based investigation, but it is also true for those who compose descriptive works, case reports, or review articles. Likewise, just as operative feedback from a senior clinician helps trainees learn a procedure, feedback from an experienced senior author can help residents learn how to contribute to the scientific literature. Programs should enable every trainee to participate in the publication of some scholarly work.

Discovery

Essentially all innovations shaping surgical practice derive from creative research that begins with a problem; formulates and tests a hypothesis; and then defends, validates, and publishes results. Understanding this process is valuable to all surgeons who seek to improve their practice by adopting their own innovations or those that other surgeons have developed; it also prevents surgeons from adopting unvalidated practices. Thus, all programs should have a formal mechanism to teach trainees the process of discovery. Trainees who participate in a formal research project will benefit from the experience regardless of whether they go into academic or clinical practice. Though it may be impractical to require a formal research experience for all surgical trainees, these opportunities indicate a broad commitment to scholarly development and should be encouraged. Regardless of a program's ability to offer a research experience, all programs should encourage trainees to ask questions, formulate potential solutions, seek evidence to support or refute an idea, and disseminate the conclusions.

Facilitated Critical Thinking and Inquiry

There are many opportunities, besides formal research projects, to help trainees understand the discovery process. Morbidity and mortality conferences, grand rounds, and other gatherings should be used to discuss challenges and solutions. Speculation about potential solutions should lead to generating and testing a formal hypothesis or appraising the existing evidence to validate emerging options. Trainees can also learn to understand the process of evidence creation by serving on hospital committees, such as those that evaluate new technology. Every sound curriculum exposes trainees to the principles of statistical analysis and bias. All programs should develop a formal initiative that requires residents to periodically present their own investigative work or interpret the scholarly work of others. In fact, every trainee should make a public presentation to their peers during their training that demonstrates a logical thought process, improves communication skills, and exposes flaws that interfere with evidence-based practice.

Training Surgeon-Scientists to Become Independently Funded Principal Investigators

Developing Successful Mentoring Programs

Development of a resident into a successful surgeon-scientist in basic science or health services research requires a major commitment from the individual, the department/interdepartmental and institutional leadership, and appropriate mentoring faculty, as well as the necessary laboratory resources. In other words, success requires appropriate strategic planning, leadership commitment, and sufficient investment of time and resources.

Departmental or institutional SEED (supporting effective educator development) grants or philanthropic support, small foundation grants, formal government training grants (T32, K08, and so on), and professional society research grants (American College of Surgeons, American Surgical Association, American Association for the Surgery of Trauma, Society of Thoracic Surgeons, and so on) can provide a young investigator with the technical support, equipment, and supplies to get started.

Frequently, after completing residency and related research training, young faculty surgeons request "protected time." Unfortunately, young surgeons must recognize that the nature of surgical disease makes it difficult to protect large blocks of time. Medicine, pediatrics, and other similar specialties can frequently guarantee a young physician's minimal clinical involvement for a substantial portion of the year; however, it is harder for young surgeons to obtain and requires a combination of departmental commitment, senior partner support, and self-discipline. The available research time should be tailored to the needs of the academic surgeon; different surgical subspecialties will require different solutions.

Mentors are critical to academic career advancement during and after residency. The ideal mentor is a successful surgeon-scientist or surgeon-health services researcher. Mentors can serve as role models and advisors for young surgeons; more than one mentor is usually required. For example, a division chief or section chief can help identify local funding, supporting contacts, and collaborations, and assure protected time. Meanwhile, a successful senior basic scientist with the expertise and the interest to help develop the young surgeon may be needed to provide the scientific expertise needed for a young surgeon's research that is often outside the surgical discipline, such as genomics, immunology, and other basic science disciplines. Although working in a well-known investigator's laboratory can be attractive, for the young surgeon to have an authentic, successful experience, it is important to find an investigator willing to develop a genuine mentor-mentee relationship that includes frequent meetings and involvement in all aspects of scientific progress. The young surgeon may start in an organized wet lab and then, once experienced and self-sufficient, move to an independent space.

The young surgeon should be embedded in an environment with a critical mass of expertise that can ensure day-to-day oversight, problem solving, and advice to technical staff, residents, or fellows when the young surgeon is unavailable because of duties in the clinic, hospital, or operating room.

Finally, learning how to collaborate is an important part of a resident's research experience. Young surgeons who develop technical skills and publish with collaborators can show that a grant application's methodology works; it also is a way to enhance criteria for their academic advancement.

Surgeons who aspire to a successful science career will need to decide where to publish their best research. While publishing in field-specific journals gains recognition from the basic science or health services research communities, it is also important that the surgeon-investigator publish in prestigious surgical journals. Balancing the two types of publications helps surgeons establish a reputation in their scientific discipline and documents success in their surgical profession. Mentors should advise the surgeon-investigator on how to achieve this balance.

Alternative Areas for the Surgeon-Investigator

The traditional surgeon-scientist investigates basic science concepts related to surgery, but other opportunities also can enhance an academic career in surgery. For example, in addition to health services research, surgeons can become clinical trialists; although initiating novel, prospective clinical trials may require writing a grant proposal, it may also meet the needs of surgeons focused on clinical outcomes, new technologies, and innovative therapeutic interventions.

Similarly, surgeons can advance their careers by emphasizing quality, safety, and standardization; surgeon-investigators may apply for grants to prospectively demonstrate how interventions can reduce morbidity, costs, length of stay or readmission, or improve outcomes and patient satisfaction. Finally, surgeons focused on education may study education methodologies and interventions in a prospective, controlled fashion that can lead to novel education pathways and career advancement.

Keys to Writing a Successful Grant Application

General Principles

To write a successful grant proposal, resident researchers should start by reading through other successful grant applications to note style and technique. To learn to write grant applications, they will need time to review literature, practice writing an application, and most importantly, receive dedicated mentoring from an experienced scientist.

The grant writing process begins with creating a hypothesis related to a clinical or scientific problem, developing specific aims with mentors and advisors, and composing questions related to the hypothesis that the research project will answer.

The writing process should start early to avoid errors and ensure important details are included. The best grants are simple, logical, and straightforward. Introducing too much complexity and too many contingencies may confuse a reviewer and lead to criticisms. Aims should be specific and hypothesis-driven. A frequent fatal flaw in grant writing is to make the first specific aim a discovery on which all the subsequent aims depend.

The scientific team should have experience in all the techniques cited in the grant application. The application should include preliminary data to demonstrate the capability of the proposal's investigators. It also is wise to reassure the grant reviewer by attaching previous publications to demonstrate familiarity and success with the technology.

A grant application must have the appropriate statistical methodology and expertise needed to analyze the results of each of the specific aims. The use of improper statistical analysis will undermine a successful grant application because it can lead to erroneous results.

When complete, the draft of the grant application should be shared with other mentors and advisors who know the proposed science and techniques. These advisors must have time to critically review the grant application; for the first few applications, the surgeon should review the application with the advisors in-person. This is why grant writers need to start well ahead of the grant deadline. Resident researchers greatly benefit from a departmental resource for grant development.

Grant applications must be written in clear, concise, focused language so that the proposal's goals and significance are easily understood by someone who is not an expert in the field. The styles and areas of emphasis of health services research grant applications can differ from basic science research grants. In general, the grant should be prospective and hypothesis-driven, and with proper powering of the sample size and emphasis on appropriate statistical methodology. Descriptive, retrospective database queries are important to help define and identify potential hypotheses but are rarely funded by peer-reviewed organizations. The above principles, such as early preparation and appropriate mentors or advisors, also help generate successful health services research grants.

Specific Suggestions

The first and most important aspect of a successful grant is idea development, which may be driven by a federal institution, focus of a foundation, or a current urgent health need. Research-funding organizations vet their interests through advisory councils that determine their research focus and issues requests for proposals. Opportunities can be found by scanning the websites or subscribing to services that publish these offerings. Depending on the agency offering funding, potential interest can be assessed through a short query letter or may require a full proposal. Most organized research funders have program officers who welcome phone calls or other communications to see if the interests of the organization and the investigator are aligned. Finding the right source of funding can be as important as crafting a well-written proposal.

Generating a good idea that matches a funding agency's interests may require the input of critical peers who can objectively assess the importance of the young surgeon-investigator's question. Investigators should outline their approach to solving the problem and develop a hypothesis that can be reviewed by advisors and mentors. The title should be broad enough for further development yet specific enough so that the application is directed to the proper study section. Talking to a grant officer can help to triage the process to an appropriate study section or give the investigator insights into a particular study section's interests. The title should not be too clever. Keywords should be used and clinical importance emphasized. Specific aims should be precise and feasible. There should not be too many specific aims proposed and the young surgeon-investigator must be able to perform each of them.

The abstract is another important part of the grant application. It should tell a story. It should bring perspective to observations, identify unresolved issues, and be comprehensive but not exhaustive.

The background and significance section should answer: "What is the state of the art?" A concise and relevant literature review should be provided. Like the abstract, it should put observations into perspective and identify the most important unresolved issues. Finally, it should state the goals of the research.

Preliminary data should show proficiency in using all proposed grant methods and that all collaborations are in place and functional. Original data should be shown and put into context. Preliminary data that show promise are useful and demonstrate the importance of a proposal. There shouldn't be an attempt to perform all the work of the specific aims; rather, familiarity should be demonstrated with every technique needed to execute the grant.

The experimental design and method should relate to the specific aims. References to prior work must be minimized. Investigators should be specific and also include all controls and assure that statistical methods are appropriate to the question asked. Potential problems and alternative approaches should be briefly described.

In the summary, the story is briefly retold. The objectives and logical next steps are stated and investigators should be realistic. Successful grants have good ideas, good science, good application, good data quality, appropriate statistical design, properly powered patient populations, and investigators who have demonstrated their ability to complete the work.

Research and Scholarship Requirements for Most Academic Surgeons

Only a small fraction of surgical trainees will aspire to become independently funded surgeon-scientists. Most will spend their careers in "community" practice; however, the lines have blurred between traditional academic practice and community practice. Many community practice surgeons may conduct clinical trials or participate in other types of research and scholarship opportunities. Meanwhile, most academic surgeons devote much of their careers to patient care and surgical education while also conducting clinical, outcomes, or educational research and/or collaborating in translational laboratory research. Whether in traditional or nontraditional academic environments, surgeons have ample opportunity to participate in research and discovery, most often as part of a research team. Therefore, it is important that all surgical trainees learn the scientific process by participating in research or scholarly activity.

There are some common fundamental steps to surgical career development, whether along the academic surgery pathway or evidence-based community surgeon pathway (Table 1).

Table 1. Stepping stones in academic surgeon development

- Learn to critically evaluate the literature
  - Journal clubs and conferences that emphasize evidence-based medicine
  - Perform literature searches and evaluate levels of evidence
  - Write a review article or book chapter
- Learn to communicate your research
  - Write an abstract—succinct, precise, and compelling
  - Poster presentations
  - Case reports/Small case series
  - Oral presentations
    - Local/Regional meetings
    - Resident forums at national meetings
    - National/International meetings
  - Manuscript preparation, submission, and response to peer review
- Understand the basics of clinical research
  - Education in the basic tenets of ethical human subject research
  - Learn the fundamentals of statistical analysis
  - Perform retrospective clinical studies
  - Health services/outcomes research (large databases)
  - Write a clinical trial
- Learn to think in a scientifically rigorous manner
  - High-quality scientific team and dedicated mentorship
  - Learn to state a hypothesis appropriately, explicitly, and precisely
  - Learn to use the existing literature and evidence to develop specific aims and an experimental plan
  - Learn how to evaluate and understand bias, limitations, and pitfalls
  - Critically evaluate results and understand how to design complementary and confirmatory experiments/studies
  - Write a grant
    - Local and intramural grants
    - Foundation or professional society grants
    - Career development awards
    - Mentored grants (such as K-awards)

To appropriately engage in the surgical and scientific literature, it is first necessary to learn to read and critically evaluate it. Doing so requires understanding the levels of scientific evidence, as well as how to perform a literature search and prioritize the most important and authoritative articles. These basic tenets of academic success can be taught through reading assignments, journal clubs, and conferences that emphasize evidence-based medicine. Since research training is best accomplished through experiential learning, in addition to searching, evaluating, and comprehending the medical literature, programs should assign trainees to write review articles or book chapters and to learn how to write in the style appropriate for biomedical publications. They should be mentored through the process of writing a grant application or a clinical trial study.

Residents should learn how to properly present at a medical or scientific meeting, including the basic principles of how to create an effective poster presentation. Although case reports or small case series may not be accepted by high-impact factor journals or as a podium presentation at major national meetings, they are valuable entry-level research and scholarship-training tools for residents. There may be opportunities for such presentations at the institutional level or at larger gatherings, such as state chapter meetings of the American College of Surgeons (ACS), regional surgical societies, or at residents' forums of other general surgery and subspecialty societies. These types of studies teach the skills of asking a basic clinical or scientific question, searching and assimilating the literature, presenting the findings in a public forum, learning to answer questions about the study in a clear and succinct fashion, and preparing a basic manuscript.

Trainees should understand how to obtain and maintain institutional review board (IRB) approval for clinical studies. They must be trained in human subjects' protection and the basic tenets of ethical clinical research. The IRB presentation should describe the research, the roles of the principal investigator and other team members, and the characteristics of participating patients, with a strategy for increasing participation of traditionally underrepresented minorities. The measures to protect patients should be clearly described, particularly vulnerable populations. Residents preparing to lead clinical trial research efforts should practice creating these presentations.

To learn the principles of performing retrospective clinical studies, residents should start by performing chart reviews or using available databases. The best retrospective studies often are driven by a fundamental question properly stated as a hypothesis. Initially, faculty mentors may need to help trainees develop these questions. As trainees gain confidence in their ability to ask relevant questions, think critically, evaluate the literature, and identify the proper source of data to test the hypothesis, their intellectual curiosity will be stimulated, and trainees will learn what it takes to become an investigator.

Retrospective studies often are clinically meaningful and may lead to new hypotheses and investigations; they also teach the limitations and biases inherent in such studies. Retrospective studies require proper statistical analysis, which increases the trainee's level of education and experience. The basics of statistical analysis and the pitfalls of improper statistical methodology should be part of every program's curriculum. Training programs should foster an environment in which faculty show trainees how to properly perform retrospective clinical studies; in fact, learning this technique should be a basic milestone for trainees who aspire to be involved in clinical and outcomes research.

Another step on the academic surgeon training ladder is performing outcomes or health services research using large databases, surveys, and other tools to evaluate a variety of patient care and economic endpoints. Such studies require experience and statistical expertise to avoid the common mistakes of failing to account for incomplete or biased data or failing to recognize statistically significant but clinically unimportant distinctions; therefore, an experienced statistician should participate in the study. Effective collaboration with other scientists and experts from other disciplines is best learned from mentors or by experience.

Because most academic surgeons devote their research efforts to clinical, outcomes, or health services investigation, residents on this track should learn how to perform these types of studies. Thus, residents should be afforded dedicated time for research. Not all general surgery residents will take time off during residency to perform research (typically one to three years); those who do have an opportunity to obtain an advanced degree during their research time (for example, Master of Science, Master of Public Health, PhD, and so on). Many university programs offer tuition remission or assistance to help trainees participate in these graduate programs. Although it is not possible to mandate that institutions provide graduate assistance for trainees, the institutions that do make an invaluable contribution to developing academic surgeons.

Surgical education is an underestimated area of research opportunity. Rapid advances in science and technology, along with the evolution of the needs of learners in the digital era, require creative, effective new ways to educate students, residents, fellows, and practicing surgeons.

Once the trainee has been mentored through the process of performing a research project, the next step is to submit an abstract of the work for presentation at a scientific meeting. Abstracts must be clear, succinct, and compelling. If the abstract is accepted, the trainee should expect to prepare a presentation and/or a full manuscript. Firm target dates for abstract submission, presentation at a meeting, and timely submission of a manuscript help residents learn how to plan and avoid the stress and anxiety of deadlines. The discipline it takes to go through this process motivates the resident to see a research project through to completion. In addition to learning how to plan for and manage deadlines, trainees also learn how to respond to questions and critiques during a presentation or the manuscript-review process—another important step in their development as academic surgeons.

Trainees who present at a national meeting of their peers are rewarded with a sense of accomplishment and confidence. At the least, they get a trip out of town and the opportunity to meet new people with similar interests. These conferences offer trainees a chance to network with colleagues from around the world and discuss new ideas and the latest research findings with them. They also offer trainees the opportunity to meet some of the most prominent surgeons and scientists in their field, including some whose articles they have read and studied. They also may see their mentors engaged in conversations about their areas of expertise with national or international experts. These meetings can result in meaningful scientific collaborations, new scientific investigation and clinical trials, and lifelong friendships. Because surgical trainees who share in the full range of these national meeting experiences are more likely to seek out academic careers, training programs should support their attendance, including reimbursement for travel expenses. As a guideline, every trainee should attend at least one professional meeting during residency.

Finally, surgeons need not be a principal investigator to make meaningful contributions to translational research. They can often participate as collaborators or co-investigators and contribute patients and clinical specimens while giving their patients access to new treatments. An interested surgeon may participate as a member of a multidisciplinary research team and participate in hypothesis generation, study design and execution, grant writing, data analysis, and publication.

Resources Needed to Support Resident Research, Scholarship, and Career Development

Resident Participation in Research and Scholarship

The extent of surgical trainee participation in research and scholarship varies significantly across surgical training programs. For example, at the University of Minnesota, Minneapolis, the general surgery training program once required every trainee to obtain a PhD during their residency, whereas many other programs required little or no dedicated research time of their trainees. Today, the variation in research requirements is one of the most significant difference across training programs. Some have a mandatory research time requirement, whereas for others, research time is optional or not expected. This variability is due, in part, to the fact that more than 70 percent of general surgery residents prolong their training time by going on to clinical fellowships; for them, devoting an extra year or more to research may be of questionable value.

For residents choosing an academic career path, one year of research is seldom enough to assure research training and success. As a result, various research models have evolved. The Accreditation Council For Graduate Medical Education (ACGME) Common Program Requirements (CPR) for scholarship are found under Section IV.D in the CPR for Residency and state the following (as of July 1, 2020):

> *Medicine is both an art and a science. The physician is a humanistic scientist who cares for patients. This requires the ability to think critically, evaluate the literature, appropriately assimilate new knowledge, and practice lifelong learning. The program and faculty must create an environment that fosters the acquisition of such skills through resident participation in scholarly activities. Scholarly activities may include discovery, integration, application, and teaching.*

ACGME and RC Research Requirements for Programs

As specified by ACGME, programs are responsible for the following:

- Demonstrate evidence of scholarly activities consistent with its mission(s) and aims.
- In partnership with its sponsoring institution, allocate adequate resources to facilitate resident and faculty involvement in scholarly activities. [The review committee (RC) may further specify.]
- Advance residents' knowledge and practice of the scholarly approach to evidence-based patient care.

The RC for Surgery stipulates the following:

- IV.B.1. Program curriculum must advance residents' knowledge of the basic principles of research, including how research is conducted, evaluated, explained to patients, and applied to patient care.
- IV.B.2. Residents should participate in scholarly activity.
- IV.B.2.a) The participation of residents in clinical and/or laboratory research is encouraged.
- IV.B.3. The sponsoring institution and program should allocate adequate educational resources to facilitate resident involvement in scholarly activities.

Other surgical RCs have explicit expectations for scholarship among trainees. For example, Complex General Surgical Oncology requires that the fellow complete a course on protecting human subjects as well as conduct clinical research. The RC for Thoracic Surgery specifies that the residents must produce at least one scholarly product per year (for instance, a paper, book chapter, presentation, and so forth) and that the institution should provide support for attendance at a national professional meeting. In addition to resident requirements, the ACGME annual faculty survey collects information on faculty scholarship activity, including peer-reviewed publications and presentations.

Resources for Surgical Trainee Research

In principle, program resources should match its trainee requirements. For example, community-based programs resources are quite different from those of an academic program with a mandatory research requirement.

Mentorship

We have seen that to foster trainee research, faculty must not only teach the trainee the fundamentals of research, but must also serve as mentors who provide guidance on critical writing, where to present or publish, and authorship ethics. Often with team-based science, a resident may have research mentors across several disciplines, which may introduce conflict for the trainee regarding research prioritization, authorship, and intellectual property. Hence, it is important that the primary mentor anticipate potential conflicts, develop clear expectations, and hold frequent mentor meetings. Departments should provide adequate resources and recognition for faculty who serve as research mentors.

Financial Resources for Trainee Research

Surgical departments leverage several sources of revenue to support and foster trainee research. Expenses include, but are not limited to, trainee salary, benefits, travel expenses, and professional support including statisticians, consumable supplies, and faculty mentorship time. For programs that require or offer dedicated trainee research time, trainee salary and benefits are typically the biggest expense. Training grants, such as the T-32 program, can support trainee research by helping to pay for salary expenses, trainee education (including advanced degrees in some cases), and supplies, such as a computer. These federally funded institutional training grants often are available through surgical departments and other departments at the institution. Trainees typically compete for a spot, and their research interest must align with the focus of the grant. Many academic research universities have other internal grants that provide trainee support. In addition, resources may be available at an affiliated Veterans Affairs Medical Center; financial research support is also available from professional organizations, such as the American Surgical Association (ASA), Society of Surgery of the Alimentary Tract (SSAT), the American Association for the Surgery of Trauma (AAST), Society of Surgical Oncology (SSO), and many from the American College of Surgeons as well as other organizations.

Trainees who pursue dedicated research time should compete for external funding, which brings many advantages. By applying for competitive research funding, residents learn through real-life experience how research is funded. They also have the experience of working closely with their research mentor to develop the project and write a compelling proposal for the research project. Regardless of funding success, these efforts help trainees be more productive and successful researchers. Those who write top proposals may win a prestigious award or be invited for an in-person interview by a surgical society, which introduces the trainee to leaders in academic surgery and may set up future mentoring opportunities.

Departments without grant support for research time must instead rely on discretionary funds and philanthropy. As academic medical center financial margins tighten, department leaders must make difficult choices about how they support research compared with other missions. In any case, departments can help trainees seek outside training opportunities at institutions that support intramural research programs. Some examples are the National Institutes of Health-sponsored intramural research fellowships and the ACS Research Fellowships, as previously mentioned. Although research fellowships outside the trainee's institution are a great resource, not all trainees can relocate for their research experience; in fact, many programs rely on these residents for clinical call coverage support to ease the burden of full-time clinical trainees. Again, programs must balance these competing priorities to meet their vision and the needs of the trainees.

Additional Resources for Research Conduct

Research Compliance

Minimal program support for trainee research includes mentorship, basic training in research ethics, and assistance with disseminating the research. The IRB requires research ethics training for any individual conducting research. Further training for animal use, proper handling of hazardous materials, and other special areas are required depending on the type of research methods. This training can be provided by the university, an online module, or both. The supervising investigator is responsible for ensuring that the trainee is compliant and proficient in these important and highly regulated areas.

Research Methods

Any research project requires an understanding of the scientific method, yet surgical trainees have varied backgrounds and research experience. Trainees who lack prior research experience should be considered candidates for formal training. Many research universities offer these types of introductory or 'boot camp' courses; some offer these through their Institutional Clinical and Translational Science Award (CTSA) or other similar initiatives.

For basic science research, partnering with nonsurgical laboratories for training of specific methodologies is often used. Another common model is for core laboratory services to be offered that supports many smaller labs. Training in specific methodologies and techniques can be taught here, as well.

Although trainees who pursue data science research projects may be able to teach themselves statistical programming skills, they also should be allowed, at a minimum, to consult a statistical expert. Trainees dedicated to this area should consider an advanced degree, or at least coursework, in statistics. At some institutions, the trainee may be able to audit these courses for free or a reduced fee.

Unique Considerations for Conducting Surgery Research in Low- and Middle-Income Countries

Some departments support residents who pursue surgery research in low- and middle-income countries, including several that offer fellowships to trainees outside their institution. Programs should ensure the trainee is entering a safe environment and work with their institutional officials to monitor the political stability and health of the environment while the trainee is there. Additionally, the conduct of research needs to follow the same guidelines that would be expected in the United States.

This type of research requires knowledge of available databases, including the strengths and weaknesses of the data, elements of statistical analysis, and clinical trials design. Research in low- and middle-income countries frequently includes analyses of educational activities and socioeconomic factors, which will require the trainee to learn appropriate and relevant analytic and statistical techniques.

Conclusion

As more surgical trainees aspire to a career in academic surgery, it is increasingly important that residents and fellows be prepared to engage in scientific inquiry, investigation, and publication or presentation of their findings. The process of defining a problem, studying the current and critical literature, working in a lab to investigate possible solutions, applying for grants, and offering an analysis of research findings is a rigorous process, but one with far-reaching benefits. It trains surgeons to think critically, to seek out mentors and mentees who share similar clinical and scientific interests, to work shoulder-to-shoulder with other team members, and to see a project through to completion. These skills will benefit all surgeons—surgeon-scientists, academicians, and clinicians—who are dedicated to lifelong learning.

AMERICAN C
SURGEONS A
OF SURGEON
COLLEGE OF
AMERICAN C
SURGEONS A
OF SURGEON
COLLEGE OF
AMERICAN C
SURGEONS A

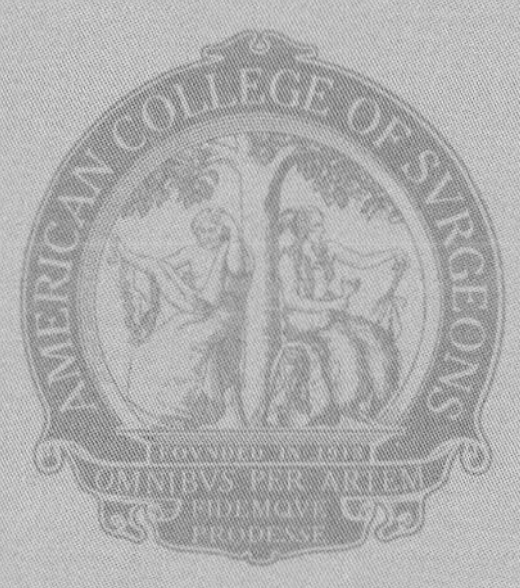

CHAPTER 9
Curriculum: Quality and Safety: Evaluation, Management, and Improvement

Lead Author
John F. Sweeney, MD, FACS

Co-Authors
Justin B. Dimick, MD, MPH, FACS
Clifford Y. Ko, MD, MS, MSHS, FACS, FASCRS
Susan Moffatt-Bruce, MD, PhD, FRCSC, MBA, FACS, MAMSE
Brigitte K. Smith, MD, MHPE, FACS, FSVS

CHAPTER 9

Curriculum: Quality and Safety: Evaluation, Management, and Improvement

Executive Summary

This chapter emphasizes the importance of introducing surgery residents to the concept of quality improvement (QI) and patient safety—why it is important in today's health care environment to continuously evaluate, manage, and improve the quality and safety of surgical patient care. This chapter addresses the following questions:

- Why is QI training important?
- How do you teach QI to trainees?
- What sources of information are available at the institutional level that trainees can use to identify a quality problem?
- Once the trainee has identified a quality problem, what are the next steps?
- How do we identify key stakeholders and develop consensus to ensure success?
- How do we measure the impact of QI interventions?

The Value of QI Training

In our ever-changing health care environment, with emerging and persistent systems issues and increasing patient acuity and complexity, providing high-quality care is both challenging and rewarding. To ensure delivery of high-quality surgical care, essential training is needed to support and promote clinical judgment, technical skills, professional resilience, and better teamwork. Surgery is uniquely positioned to treat the ill, improve outcomes, and support patients and their families. Surgical outcomes can be measured, and analyzed; as such, they can be improved.[1] That's why surgeons need to understand QI principles and closely integrate them into surgical training and practice.

From its very beginning, the American College of Surgeons (ACS) has focused on developing efforts to improve the quality of care. Starting with its hospital verification program (1918), which became the foundation of The Joint Commission, these efforts have continued over the last 30 years with QI programs for specific surgical diseases (Cancer, Trauma, Bariatrics, and more). All of these programs include the necessary educational frameworks to prepare surgeons and trainees to participate in the programs. The expectations set out in ACS training standards, now on an international basis, require that residency education occur in an environment that not only emphasizes excellence in safety and quality, but expects it. The expectation is that residents, in all specialties, constantly evaluate and analyze the care they provide and adopt the principles of continuous improvement. This requires that residents "work in a well-coordinated manner with other health care professionals to achieve organizational patient safety goals," according to the Accreditation Council for Graduate Medical Education (ACGME).[2] Graduate surgical education leaders and teaching faculty need to actively support quality and patient safety education; equally important, they must educate themselves and adopt these principles in their clinical activities.

More than two decades ago, the Institute of Medicine (now the National Academy of Medicine) released *To Err Is Human*, a report that alerted the world to the high number of patients harmed by medical errors and preventable adverse events and set an ambitious global goal to reduce harm by improving the quality and safety of patient care.[3] Calls to action included programming for integrated electronic health records (EHR), limiting resident work hours, quality-based reimbursement, and QI training for all physicians and trainees.[2] This initiative and subsequent public reporting have promoted the creation and enhancement of a culture of safety and accountability in our residency training programs.[2]

The ACGME has embraced these approaches and has worked to help ensure that residents are engaged in QI during their training years.[2] Similarly, the Royal College of Physicians and Surgeons, through the Canadian Medical Education Directives for Specialists (CanMEDS) program, provides a framework for improving patient care through enhanced resident training along seven key integrated competencies. In many cases, these programs built on the foundation of QI efforts already established by ACS.

Therefore, in training residents, QI should be integrated into the curriculum as well as the evaluation process. Integrating this training into curricula can prove to be challenging, especially considering the typically heavy schedules of residents and faculty. Creating a culture of QI means ensuring that striving to achieve the highest quality of care is not just a resident project or a trendy program but is instead the core of resident education. Furthermore, as part of the Next Accreditation System (NAS), the ACGME has helped develop a required program called the Clinical Learning Environment Review (CLER) program[4] to ensure the successful implementation and development of safety and QI training in all U.S. residency programs. CLER focuses on six areas: patient safety, health care quality, care transitions, supervision, well-being, and professionalism.[3] CLER surveyor visits to hospitals or other clinical sites involve all departments, hospital leadership, nursing, and other support staff, emphasizing the multidisciplinary nature of trainee and patient interactions and their effects on patient care. QI depends on teams, which is why it is important that surgeons understand and support team-based care.

Surgical safety and quality initiatives have become a key priority in many health care settings.[5] Through investment in resident QI training and initiatives, health care entities can empower residents, both as individual trainees and as a group, to remedy problems within medical systems. Many problems that residents see or experience every day are within their purview or ability to solve. Becoming a surgeon aligns well with QI initiatives; after all, surgeons are inherently scientists trying to find answers and solve problems. In addition, training for and accomplishing QI goals not only yields immediate patient benefits and enhances team building, but it also can boost the young surgeon's career and goals. In a training program imbedded with QI, residents will have opportunities to solve problems and be a part of the solution. Ultimately, residents will find it gratifying to identify quality problems and develop QI projects to address those problems. Achieving recognizable QI will lead to further motivation and participation, and, ultimately, sustainable results.[6]

Residents can apply QI in all aspects of their training, not just to clinical problems. For example, residents could improve the parts of the curriculum or administrative processes that directly affect them and fellow residents. Promptly applying solutions rather than waiting for site visits or curriculum reform can immediately improve the training of residents.[7] Training residents in QI initiatives can also be incorporated into established hospital-wide QI initiatives, such as infection prevention. Although residents might have unique training requirements based on their specialty, QI training can be team-based and can help to foster collaboration and a shared vision for patient care improvement. Although residents are already on the front lines and work with many team members, QI fosters important relationships and teamwork between trainees and allows for mentorship between senior and junior residents for those collaborating on the same project.

Layers of Success

Training in QI is a valuable investment for faculty and health systems on several levels. Formal and dedicated education in quality methods equips trainees with tools to improve surgical outcomes during their residency training and can help to set the stage for lifelong learning. Furthermore, involvement in QI can lead to career opportunities in the rapidly evolving area of implementation science, which is the scientific study of methods and strategies that helps put evidence-based practice and research into regular use by practitioners and policymakers. QI experience for trainees can be both engaging and rewarding not only by improving patient care, but also by fulfilling training requirements and by providing educational and personal value, scholarships, and future career opportunities.

Ultimately, keys for successful QI initiatives for trainees include dedicated and educated faculty mentorship, alignment with hospital or health-system goals, and selection of projects with relevant, clear, and achievable goals.

QI training can also prepare trainees for the emergence of public reporting and value-based care, which is likely to affect surgical disciplines first. In this way, QI training will prepare today's residents for health care delivery tomorrow.

Teaching QI Techniques to Trainees

Instructional Methods and Implementation

Several outstanding curricular resources can help programs deliver QI education to trainees. The foundational content that should be included in any QI curriculum is the ACS *Optimal Resources for Surgical Quality and Safety*, the "Red Book." Similarly, The Royal College of Physicians and Surgeons of Canada have an e-book, *Teaching Quality Improvement in Residency Education*. A resident curriculum, the ACS National Surgical Quality Improvement Program (ACS NSQIP®) Quality In-Training Initiative (QITI) Primer is a good resource, as is The Institute for Healthcare Improvement Open School.[8,9] Programs should not assign online modules or readings to trainees without adequate support to ensure they understand the content and its relevance to their current and future practice. Learning that is experiential and involves solving problems that residents routinely face helps make the content relevant and memorable. Delivering the content through engaging instructional methods as well as incorporating this instruction into an already busy training program remain significant challenges.[10] In addition, the ultimate learning goal for trainees is to be able to apply QI principles to address "real" quality problems in their clinical environment. Leading a QI initiative helps trainees progress from "knows how" to "shows how," and ensures they leave their training program with the skills to apply what they have learned.[11]

QI may seem like just another box to check or extra work for many trainees. Programs should be dedicated to provide in-person instruction and interaction between faculty champions and residents.[12] Online modules and readings help, but instructional methods must include a didactic or small-group discussion component. These opportunities can be delivered in conjunction with an already established educational curricula, or through a separate didactic series. Some programs may also elect to deliver didactic/discussion sessions in a more concentrated and intensive fashion, such as through a multi-day workshop or during a specific clinical rotation within the program. The in-person component is crucial in gaining resident buy-in and ensuring learning goals are met.

In addition to delivering foundational content to develop residents' knowledge base, surgeon-educators will need to ensure that residents can apply what they have learned through leadership of or participation in QI projects.[13] Organizing and supporting this component of the curriculum can be logistically challenging because residents conduct QI projects in different clinical domains, on different rotations, and even at different clinical training sites. A basic QI and safety curriculum should include the nine standards in the ACS Red Book, which includes the cultural, leadership, committee structure, processes for case review and data use, and other features that help a QI program achieve a state of high reliability. Assigning trainees to quality problems of their own choosing that are identified, selected, and aligned with hospital priorities will expose them to hospital leadership, support personnel, and authentic data, allowing them to have firsthand experiences and develop buy-in and personal commitment to the project. Ultimately, the problem the resident is trying to solve should be appropriately scoped and aligned to help them succeed.

Incorporating a QI curriculum into any residency program needs to be somewhat program-/institution-specific, depending upon available resources and other programmatic constraints.[14] One proposed model includes QI education throughout the program, with junior residents learning core content, mid-level residents leading QI projects, and senior residents reviewing their own patient care outcomes (for example, through NSQIP) and even teaching the junior residents. This works well when the junior residents have had QI training in their undergraduate courses and come to residency with interest and engagement.[15] Some programs may deliver the entire QI curriculum, including QI projects, during a single postgraduate year. Another model incorporates QI education into a single rotation, such as an endoscopy rotation, that is not as taxing from a work-hours perspective, or during an academic development or research year. Ultimately, the timing of QI training must be customized to what the institution and program can support.

Resources Required

Faculty champions (at least one but preferably more) are critical in the support of a successful QI curriculum. Many teaching faculty members, who were trained before the focus on QI and patient safety, were not taught QI principles and skills during their own medical school and residency training. As a result, it is critically important to "train the trainers" to prepare the faculty to serve as effective QI teachers.

Residents will be new to QI fundamentals and will need someone to answer questions and guide them throughout the process. Although one faculty member can lead the didactic component of the QI curriculum, that faculty member should not be expected to serve as a mentor for each and every resident QI project. Additional faculty with QI knowledge and skills are needed to support residents in their QI projects. In addition, faculty can support residents in gaining access to data and other resources needed to conduct their project. Residents can also be supported by other faculty and resources found among faculty of different departments, which also supports multidisciplinary continuous improvement. Other team members who can support QI projects and learning may be found in nursing or hospital administration, particularly those with a QI department.[16,17]

Lack of access to data, one of the most significant barriers to completing QI projects for any clinician, is even more challenging for residents who do have the authority to prioritize their data requests. Simple check sheets can be used as data collection tools, but residents frequently need access to "big" data, such as the information gathered through the EHR, to address specific clinical problems. The more residents understand the importance of data, the better they will be able to leverage that information for QI purposes. Residents actively engaged in collecting and reviewing raw data will feel responsible for the data and it will motivate them to improve processes.[18]

Some programs may have access to hospital staff hired specifically to support QI efforts in the clinical environment. Health systems scientists and human factors engineers, who are increasingly part of health care systems across the country, have specific training and expertise in leading QI initiatives. Program leaders should ask their hospital administration and medical staff to find QI specialists within their system with whom they can explore collaboration opportunities. These partnerships support the trainees in their QI efforts and education and can lead to real clinical improvements that provide cost savings to the hospital.

Assessment and Evaluation

The fundamental goal of a QI curriculum is to develop trainees' knowledge and skills in QI. Unfortunately, assessment of learning in QI has yet to be well established. The ACGME Milestones include sub-competencies related to QI, which vary from specialty to specialty, and are generally quite broad, with anchors such as "the resident leads a QI initiative." Unfortunately, this situation further exacerbates the "check the box" mentality of doing a QI project as opposed to how well trainees learned and applied foundational QI concepts. The QI Knowledge Application Tool (QIKAT-R), a tool to assess foundational QI knowledge, has been validated by internal medicine residents.[19] Unfortunately, this tool has not been validated by other learner groups and uses the "Aim, Change, Measure" framework, as opposed to other more common models, such as DMAIC (Define, Measure, Analyze, Improve, and Control). Details regarding the DMAIC approach are presented later in this chapter.

Some programs try to evaluate the impact of QI curricula on the quality of patient care delivery and cost savings in the clinical environment. While residents' success with QI initiatives is likely to improve the delivery of quality care in their hospital system, this is not the fundamental goal of a QI curriculum. That said, the improved quality and cost-savings aspects of QI initiatives can support appeals for additional resources and support for a resident QI curriculum.

Sources of Information that Trainees Can Use to Identify a Quality Problem

Identifying a problem is one of the first steps in achieving better quality of surgical care. There are several reasons to help trainees identify quality challenges. First, trainees should understand and integrate the principles of quality evaluation and QI into their daily workload and education, starting with identifying improvement opportunities. Second, trainees, who are often at the front lines for much of the care of the surgical patient, play a vital role in identifying issues and QI opportunities. The ACS Red Book contains the "how to" aspects of quality evaluation and QI, including sections that address how to identify, define, and solve problems, and perform QI in both formal and informal ways.

As highlighted in the Red Book, many sources are available for trainees and others to identify potential problems and opportunities. These resources include databases and registries as well as event-reporting systems; the central source will be the resident's everyday clinical care activities. Learning clinical care requires the ability to identify a quality problem or a quality opportunity. For example, surgical trainees need to know about surgical site infections or when their patients have been readmitted. Teaching residents, fellows, and medical students rotating on surgical services to identify surgical problems should be a priority in their training and education. Training is the best time for faculty to teach and model the idea of continuous quality evaluation and QI.

Morbidity and mortality conferences often have already identified the surgical complications or problems, but studies show these types of conferences commonly underreport complications. This culture and practice of underreporting issues is a problem unto itself. It deprives trainees of the opportunity to understand a process that starts with the acknowledgement that a problem occurred in the delivery of care. Experiencing this process, which includes the "baring of the soul" of the surgeon, as well as the humility, intellectual debate, incorporation of evidence, and the possible change needed to make improvement, is an essential component of resident QI education. Furthermore, most problems in the surgical setting are system-based issues that focus on the complexities of how surgical care is delivered across the continuum—from the preoperative setting to the intraoperative and postoperative phases and then to postdischarge care. System of care includes standardization as well as innovation. It also includes the basic tenets of teamwork and leadership as well as communication and culture. These aspects are essential in the surgical trainee's education as well as the continued education of surgeons after training. It all starts with problem identification. Too often, this aspect of surgical education and training is underprioritized.

Next Steps

Once a quality problem has been identified, the hard work begins. Trainees should do an in-depth analysis of the quality problem before rushing to develop and implement an intervention to "fix" it. They must make sure the problem identified is really an issue and then find its causes. To illustrate the process, here are some "real-life" examples.

Are the Data Clean?

The first step is to define the problem. Make sure that the data are correct and clinically accurate and that the "problem" is truly a cause for concern. Many sources of data track specific metrics. Not all data are used for QI, so it is essential to understand the collection, analysis, and purpose of the data. Seven hundred institutions are ranked among the top 100 hospitals because it is completely dependent on the data, where the data analysis started, and what conclusions were reached. [20-22]

Consider a hypothetical situation. A trainee, who works in a health system that participates in the Vizient Quality and Accountability Program, finds their institution is a high outlier for Patient Safety Indicator (PSI) #5—Retained Surgical Item or Unretrieved Device Fragment Count. The report shows that the medical center has a high number of cases of retained foreign bodies and is one of the worst performing medical centers for this PSI. A retained foreign body after surgery is considered a "never event" by the National Quality Forum, so the resident is alarmed.

Before rushing off and implementing new checklists or changing workflows in the operating room to address the problem, the resident needs to understand the definition of the problem. In this case, the resident learns that the definition for a "retained foreign body left in during procedure" is quite broad and open for misinterpretation by the administrative coding team.

Next, the resident does an in-depth review of the "outlying cases" to determine if the cited cases meet the definition used to identify the problem. This requires the hard work of digging into the medical record. The trainee finds that the administrative coding team's broad interpretation of PSI #5 often includes packing of the abdomen to control intraoperative hemorrhage with the plan to return at a later date to remove the packing. The trainee also finds that other flagged cases included several endovascular cases where a vascular closure device sealed vessels as the vascular sheath was being removed. After this in-depth chart review, it is clear that the root cause of the problem for several of the flagged PSI #5 cases was a lack of clinical understanding on the part of the coding team. The trainee proposes an initial intervention, in which a physician liaison is assigned to work with the coding team to review each potential retained foreign body to determine whether it meets the definition and is a true clinical problem.[23]

Once the residents understand the definition of the problem and what informs that definition, they should conduct an in-depth analysis of the data to ensure that the perceived problem meets the definition and that the data are clean. This latter step is critical because if there is a data integrity issue, the only intervention that may be needed is to clean up the data extraction process. But if there is a clinical problem, this step is also important to ensure the data are reliable to accurately monitor the impact of any interventions that address the identified clinical problem.

When a Problem Is Real

In the above case, despite cleaning up the data and implementing the clinician/coder linkage solution, there were still several cases of PSI #5 where a retained sponge was believed to be clinically significant and harmful to the patient. In this scenario, the problem is now much more complex; to increase the likelihood of a successful intervention, a data-driven quality strategy should be used to identify root causes and prevent the QI team from skipping crucial steps. Two straightforward strategies to pinpoint the problem and help design a solution are using a fishbone diagram or the DMAIC framework.

A fishbone diagram, also known as an Ishikawa diagram, is a cause-and-effect diagram that providers can use to track down the reasons for deficiencies, variations, faults, or failures.[24] The diagram looks just like a fish skeleton with the problem under investigation at the head and its causes feeding into the spine like the ribs of a fish's skeleton. To better organize the process, the causes for most defects can be grouped into six major categories (people, process, equipment, materials, environment, and management) that facilitate discussion and identification of sources of variation. This technique has the advantage that it is a visual method geared for brainstorming sessions of multiple stakeholders; it can help quickly reveal possible root causes as participants bring them up; and the potential causes can be seen simultaneously. The fishbone diagram method has the disadvantage that complex problems may yield too many root causes, which clutter the visual and make it difficult to identify interrelationships between the causes, thereby hindering the drive to a solution.

DMAIC is an acronym for the five steps (define, measure, analyze, improve, and control) involved in this QI process.[25] Traditionally DMAIC has been associated with LEAN and Six Sigma initiatives in the automotive and aviation industries, but the process can be used to help identify problems and generate potential solutions in health care. The first step is to define the problem (and/or the improvement goal – such as our hypothetical example eliminating retained sponges) and list the key process inputs that need to be improved to reach the goal. "Measure" refers to the data collection step, which is critical to establish a baseline and to track any improvements after implementation of the proposed solution. This is followed by "Analyze," which refers to identifying the root causes for the problem. "Improve" means to design and implement solutions to address the root causes of the problem. Finally, "Control" is the process where the successful solutions are embedded in day-to-day work and the process is continuously monitored for sustainability.

Back to the hypothetical problem: For purposes of discussion, the fishbone diagram technique was used to identify multiple root causes for the problem, including inconsistent practices for the timing of the sponge count across ORs; circulating nurses who cite the pressures of end-of-case multitasking that are a distraction during the count; and, most concerning, the sponge count was reported to be complete in most of the cases of retained sponges.

To address these issues, two interventions were developed. First was to standardize the timing and conduct of the sponge count by invoking a "sterile cockpit rule," meaning that only activities focused on the sponge count could be carried out during the process and other nonessential activities were prohibited until after the completion of the count. In addition, because the costs of a retained surgical sponge are significant to patients and hospitals, and the manual counts are potentially inaccurate, the resident convinced the hospital administration that implementing a radiofrequency-labeled sponge detection system would be a cost-effective intervention. The result: several years without a retained sponge at the institution.

Identifying Key Stakeholders and Developing Consensus

Multidisciplinary teams must be developed that include the key stakeholders who are affected and/or have influence on improving surgical quality. Surgeons who lead these teams must identify the key stakeholders in surgical QI and what is important to each of those groups. Developing interventions that address factors important to the key stakeholders will increase their engagement and may help garner more resources to further improve the quality of care delivered.[26,27] Patients and their families, payors/insurance companies, employers, health care systems, and health care providers are all key stakeholders. When their interests are aligned, they can help to improve systems.[28]

Key stakeholders in the surgical QI process and the issues of most concern to them are as follows:

- *Patients and their families* want safe, highly reliable, and effective care when, where, and how it is most convenient.
- *Payors* are concerned with the cost of care provided to their insured members. Poor-quality surgical care, which is primarily driven by perioperative complications and variable follow-up care, significantly increases costs. Hence, payors may be willing to support initiatives or models that drive QI.
- *Employers* want high-quality care for their employees. Aside from concern for the health and welfare of their employees, they are driven by the desire to 1) get the most out of health care premiums, which are a tremendous expense; and 2) reduce the number of employees who go on medical leave due to poor-quality care, which adds cost and strains the workforce.
- *Health care systems and hospital administration leaders* want to offer high-quality care at a market competitive price. The increased cost associated with poor-quality care eats into already thin operating margins. In addition, poor quality increases hospital length of stay, which may limit the capacity for receiving new patients.
- *Surgeons and members of the surgical team* potentially have the greatest influence in the surgical QI process. Training residents in QI is important to their mission as medical professionals: to provide the highest standard of care to patients.

Measuring the Impact of QI Interventions

Once quality gaps are identified and addressed by interventions, trainees need to rigorously measure the effectiveness of those interventions. This process can help the QI team improve successful interventions and discontinue unsuccessful interventions. Weeding out unsuccessful interventions is important because it allows new interventions to be tried in their place, redirects resources and attention devoted to the intervention to more promising activities, and may prevent future harm by revealing that the intervention causes harm in unpredictable ways.

Quality Measurement Strategies

The standard approach to quality measurement follows the classic Donabedian model of structure, process, and outcomes (Table 1). Each type of measurement strategy has its advantages and disadvantages.[29] The correct measure to use on a given project will depend on the specific context.

Structural Measures

Measures of health care structure are fixed attributes that determine quality of care. For example, hospital volume, surgeon volume, hospital nurse staffing ratios, and surgeon specialty training are structural quality measures.[29] Most ACS Quality Verification Programs (Cancer, Trauma, Vascular, Thoracic, High-Risk Gastrointestinal, Bariatric, Pediatric, Geriatric, Rural Surgery, Strong for Surgery, and so on) use standards that are based on a model of structural requirements essential to deliver high-quality care. A strength of structural measures is that they are a straightforward way to measure and serve as an essential basis for quality, although not sufficient unto themselves. In certain contexts, they strongly correlate with important outcomes.[30] A weakness, however, is that these structural measures do not drive quality to certain outcomes, such as a lowered infection rate, or to outcomes important to patients. As a proxy measure, they do not perfectly correlate to outcomes. For example, hospital volume may be a proxy for better outcomes, yet some high-volume providers may have low quality and some medium-volume providers may have high quality.

Structural measures are not routinely used in all QI initiatives. However, compliance with a QI requirement based on structural measures can serve to define what is

Table 1. Approaches to measuring the quality of care for aortic surgery with advantages and disadvantages of each approach

Type of measure	Example	Advantages	Disadvantages
Structure	• Hospital or surgeon volume	• Inexpensive and readily available • Good proxy for outcomes	• Not very actionable for QI • Not good for discriminating among individual providers
Process	• Prophylactic antibiotics given on time • Adherence to venous thromboembolism prevention guidelines	• Actionable as targets for improvement • Less influenced by patient risk and random errors	• Known processes relate to unimportant or rare surgical outcomes • Very few "high leverage" processes of care are known
Outcomes	• Anastomotic leak rates with bariatric surgery • Wound infection with ventral hernia repair	• Seen as the bottom line of patient care • Enjoy good "buy-in" from surgeons	• Need for detailed data for risk adjustment • Sample sizes often too small at individual hospitals

referred to as conformance quality – conformance with basic, essential structural elements. Conformance quality does not necessarily equate with a level of excellence that an institution may wish to achieve.

Process of Care Measures

Process of care measures entail tracking specific details of the actual care delivered to the patient.[29] Process of care measures can include attributes of perioperative care (for example, timely delivery of preoperative antibiotics), specific aspects of technique associated with better outcomes (for example, laparoscopic approach for colectomy), or any other aspect of care shown to be associated with better outcomes.[31] Among the strengths of process of care measures are that they often can be directly measured with high fidelity and usually do not require risk adjustment. The rates of process adherence (greater than 50 percent) are usually higher than the rate of most adverse outcomes (greater than 10 percent), so sample size problems are encountered less often with process of care measures than with outcome measures. The weakness of process of care measures is that it is difficult to find processes that strongly correlate with outcomes.[32,33] For example, the Surgical Care Improvement Program (SCIP) combined several measures thought to be associated with surgical site infection.[34] However, numerous studies demonstrated that compliance with this "bundle" of process of care measures did not improve outcomes in a meaningful way.

Process of care measures are often used in QI projects. The goal of such projects should be to ensure that a process of care measure is selected that has a strong correlation with the desired outcome, whether it is a clinical outcome or a measure of efficiency.

Outcome Measures

Outcome measures directly measure the end results of care. Regarded as the QI gold standard, this approach is the most difficult to do correctly. Outcome measures include clinical outcomes (for example, mortality and morbidity), economic outcomes (such as health care costs), or patient-reported outcomes (for example, health-related quality of life).[29] A strength of outcome measures is that it is easier to achieve dependable buy-in from providers because these metrics are considered the gold standard.[35] On the other hand, outcomes are difficult to measure accurately and reliably.

With outcome measures, it is often important to take patient risk into account.[35] This process requires collecting detailed data on demographics, disease severity, and patient coexisting conditions, and creating risk-adjustment models. Risk-adjustment models are an extension of multivariate regression modeling, which is taught in most introductory statistics classes. In brief, a model is created that uses either linear (continuous outcome variables) or logistic (dichotomous outcome variables) regression to predict a particular outcome variable. The coefficients for each risk factor (independent models in the regression equation) are used to account for these differences across patients. The goal is to create a setting in which we are comparing outcomes across a level playing field, as if all surgeons or hospitals had operated on patients with similar risk profiles.

Risk adjustment is particularly important when comparing outcomes, or benchmarking, across hospitals or surgeons. However, when examining outcomes improvement within an individual hospital, risk adjustment may be less important. For example, if a hospital-level benchmarking suggests that the rate of readmissions is too high, and an effort to reduce readmissions is launched, it is appropriate to track unadjusted readmission rates (or whatever complication is under study). The reason is that the goal shifts from accurately identifying outlier performance (risk adjustment is important) to reducing the number of clinical events (risk adjustment is less important). Moreover, risk levels may differ across hospitals, but they are likely to be stable within a hospital over time.

Perhaps the biggest limitation of outcome measures is small sample size.[36] Although rigorous attention to sample size and statistical power is common in designing and conducting clinical trials, it is often overlooked when measuring outcomes. However, the same rules of statistics apply to measurement regardless of whether the outcome is from a trial or a QI initiative.[37,38] For example, although surgeons and residents know that large numbers of patients, especially for rare outcomes, are needed to avoid an underpowered trial,[9] they may present their 10 successful cases of a procedure without an adverse outcome as evidence of high quality. When applying a post hoc power calculation to zero events within 10 cases, the confidence interval goes from zero to more than 30 percent. Thus, when using outcomes to measure quality, always consider both the event rate and the sample size. Both should be relatively high (for example, wound infection after colectomy) if outcomes are to be a useful measure of performance.

Choosing the Right Measure

There is no "best" approach to quality measurement. In general, selecting the right approach depends on characteristics of the procedure and the specific goals of the QI project.

Consider certain characteristics of the surgical procedure when selecting a quality measure (Figure 1), such as the frequency of the outcome of interest (for example, how high is the complication rate?) and the volume of the procedure (in other words, how often is it performed?). For procedures that are both common and relatively high risk (for example, colectomy and gastric bypass), outcomes are reliable enough to be used as measures of quality (Figure 1, Quadrant I). For procedures that are common but low risk (for example, inguinal hernia repair), measures of the process of care or patient-reported outcomes are the best approach (Figure 1, Quadrant II). For procedures that are high risk but uncommon (for example, pancreatic and esophageal resection), structural measures such as hospital volume are likely the best approach (Figure 1 Quadrant IV). In fact, empirical data suggest that structural measures such as hospital volume are better predictors of future performance than direct outcome measures for these uncommon, high-risk operations.[25] Finally, for operations that are both uncommon and low risk (for example, Spigelian hernia repair), it is probably best to focus quality-measurement efforts on other, more high-leverage procedures (Figure 1, Quadrant III).

Choosing the right measure depends on the risk (high versus low), which is the vertical axis, and frequency (low versus high caseload), which is the horizontal axis. This figure shows which type of quality measure is most appropriate for each quadrant in the graph and includes examples.

Figure 1. Choosing the right measure

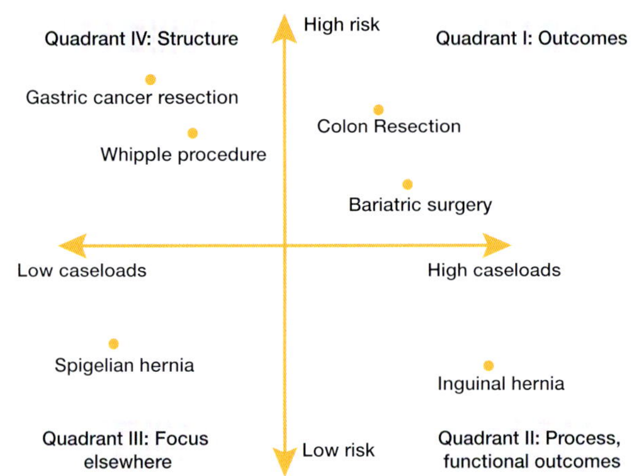

What We Have Learned from the ACS Quality Verification Programs

Part of a curriculum for residency training about quality should include the experience and essential elements that exist in ACS Quality Verification programs. The overall model includes: (1) creation of standards for a particular surgical program through evidence or consensus, (2) the structural implementation of the standards, (3) data measurement to assess performance of the standards, and (4) peer review and verification that a facility and the surgeons meet the standards.

All ACS Quality Verification programs define standards (structural and process), which include: (1) commitment and culture, (2) leadership and oversight responsibility, (3) specific personnel and equipment resources, (4) care delivery pathways and guidelines, (5) systematic case review and data analysis, (6) specific institutional resources necessary to improve identified problems, (7) ongoing measurement of corrective action and improvement loop closure, and (8) education and research responsibilities. Overall, the most important aspect of a quality verification program is to assess whether a hospital can identify and correct ongoing problems. Ultimately, surgeons use this verification process to meet their professional responsibility to serve the public and assure them that they have their interests foremost in mind.

Conclusion

Each type of measure—structure, process, and outcome—has strengths and weaknesses.[29] Structural measures are strongly related to outcomes for certain procedures but often cannot be adapted for QI projects. Process measures offer actionable steps for improvement, but often have a tenuous association with outcomes. Outcomes are the bottom line in surgery, but sample sizes must be high and risk-adjustment methods need to be considered, as appropriate. Ultimately, when choosing among the various approaches to define surgical quality, surgeons need to be flexible and consider the constraints of each type of measure and the specific goals of the project. In the journey to outcome-driven quality assessment, ACS Verification programs remain a critical step in overall health care delivery change management.

References

1. Moffatt-Bruce SD, Nguyen MC, Fann JI, Westaby S. Our new reality of public reporting: shame rather than blame? *Ann Thorac Surg*. 2016;101(4):1255-1261.
2. Accreditation Council for Graduate Medical Education. Common Program Requirements. Available at: www.acgme.org/Portals/0/PFAssets/ProgramRequirements/CPRResidency2019.pdf. Accessed June 16, 2021.
3. Institute of Medicine. *Crossing the quality chasm*. Washington DC: National Academies Press; 2003.
4. Accreditation Council for Graduate Medical Education. Clinical Learning Environment Review (CLER). Available at: www.acgme.org/Portals/0/PDFs/CLER/CLER_Brochure.pdf. Accessed January 23, 2021.
5. Royal College of Physicians and Surgeons of Canada. About CanMEDS. https://www.royalcollege.ca/rcsite/canmeds/about-canmeds-e. Accessed July 8, 2021.
6. Ingraham AM, Richards KE, Hall BL, Ko CY. QI in surgery: the American College of Surgeons National Surgical QI Program approach. *Advances in Surgery*. 2010;44(1):251-267.
7. Kelz RR, Sellers MM, Merkow R, Aggarwal R, Ko CY. Defining the content for a quality and safety in surgery curriculum using a nominal group technique. *J Surg Educ*. 2019;76(3):795-801.
8. Starr M, Sawyer T, Jones M, Batra M, McPhillips H. A simulation-based QI approach to improve pediatric resident competency with required procedures. *Cureus*. 2017;9(6):e1307.
9. Institute for Healthcare Improvement. Open School. Available at: www.ihi.org/education/ihiopenschool/Pages/default.aspx?gclid=Cj0KCQiAjKqABhDLARIsABbJrGlkj3ICL2e6P0qaUCllvMa-I6LKFE6Hpt3D2y6siH0M_T2jqWzF8L0aAkwWEALw_wcB. Accessed January 31, 2021.
10. Kelz RR, Sellers MM, Reinke CE, Medbery RL, Morris J, Ko C. Quality in-training initiative--a solution to the need for education in QI: results from a survey of program directors. *J Am Coll Surg*. 2013;217:1126-1132.
11. Malhotra N, Vavra AK, Glasgow R, Smith BK. Six steps to engage residents in QI education. *American College of Surgeons – Resources in Surgical Education*. Available at: www.facs.org/education/division-of-education/publications/rise/articles/six-steps. Accessed June 16, 2021.
12. Moffatt-Bruce SD, Lee ME, Kneuertz PJ. QI in cardiothoracic surgery residency: training in the culture of change. *J Thorac Cardiovasc Surg*. 2020 Nov;160(5):1255-1260.
13. Butler JM, Anderson KA, Supiano MA, Weir CR. "It feels like a lot of extra work": resident attitudes about QI and implications for an effective learning healthcare system. *Acad Med*. 2017;92(7):984-990.
14. Goldman J, Kuper A,Wong BM. How theory can inform our understanding of experiential learning in QI education. *Acad Med*. 2018;93(12):1784–1790.
15. Pender T, Urbik V, Boi L, Glasgow R, Smith BK. Implementation and evaluation of a novel high value care curriculum in a single academic department of surgery. *J Am Coll Surg*. 2021;232(1):81-90.
16. Bendermacher GWG, De Grave WS, Wolfhagen IHAP, Dolmans DHJM, Oude E. Shaping a culture for continuous QI in undergraduate medical education. *Acad Med*. 2020;95:1913-1920.
17. Hefner JL, Tripathi RS, Abel EE, Farneman M, Galloway J, Moffatt-Bruce SD. QI intervention to decrease prolonged mechanical ventilation after coronary artery bypass surgery. *Am J Crit Care*. 2016;25(5):423-430.
18. Chandrasekaran A, Anand G, Sharma L, Pesavento T, Hauenstein ML, Nguyen M, Gadkari M, Moffatt-Bruce S. Role of in-hospital care quality in reducing anxiety and readmissions of kidney transplant recipients. *J Surg Res*. 2016;205(1):252-259.
19. Gray DM 2nd, Hefner JL, Nguyen M, Eiferman D, Moffatt-Bruce SD. The link between clinically validated patient safety indicators and clinical outcomes. *Am J Med Qual*. 2017;32(6):583-590.
20. Singh MK, OGrinc G, Cox KR, Dolansky M, et al. The QI knowledge application tool revised (QIKAT-R). *Acad Med*. 2014;89:1386-1391.
21. Moffatt-Bruce SD. Public reporting: will this help inform what patients and families need to know? *J Thorac Cardiovasc Surg*. 2017;153(6):1623-1626.
22. Murray KR, Hilligoss B, Hefner JL, McAlearney AS, Huerta TR, Moffatt-Bruce SD. The quality reporting reality at a large academic medical center: reporting 1600 unique measures to 49 different sources. *Internat J Acad Med*. 2017;3(1):10-15.
23. Cua S, Moffatt-Bruce S, White S. Reputation and the best hospital rankings: what does it really mean? *Am J Med Qual*. 2017;32(6):632-637.
24. Nguyen MC, Moffatt-Bruce SD, Van Buren A, Gonsenhauser I, Eiferman DS. Daily review of AHRQ patient safety indicators has important impact on value-based purchasing, reimbursement, and performance scores. *Surgery*. 2018;163(3):542-546.
25. Ishikawa, K. *Guide to Quality Control*. JUSE:Tokyo, Japan;1968.

26. Betts, A. (2015) DMAIC Cycle. In J. Wiley (ed) *Encyclopedia of Management: Operations Management 3rd Edition*. Hoboken, New Jersey.
27. Moffatt-Bruce S, Clark S, DiMaio M, Fann J. Leadership oversight for patient safety programs: an essential element. *Ann Thorac Surg*. 2017;(17):31521-31527.
28. Moffatt-Bruce SD, Ellison EC. Celebrating human resilience to provide safe care. *Ann Surg*. 2012; 256(2):211-212.
29. Moffatt-Bruce SD, Funai EF, Nash M, Gabbe SG. Patient safety strategies: are we on the same team? *Obstet Gynecol*. 2012;120(4):743-745.
30. Birkmeyer JD, Dimick JB, Birkmeyer NJ. Measuring the quality of surgical care: structure, process, or outcomes? *J Am Coll Surg*. 2004;198(4):626-632.
31. Birkmeyer JD, Siewers AE, Finlayson EV, et al. Hospital volume and surgical mortality in the United States. *N Engl J Med*. 2002;346(15):1128-1137.
32. Haynes AB, Weiser TG, Berry WR, et al. A surgical safety checklist to reduce morbidity and mortality in a global population. *N Engl J Med*. 2009;360(5):491-499.
33. Hawn MT. Surgical care improvement: should performance measures have performance measures. *JAMA*. 2010;303(24):2527-2528.
34. Urbach DR, Govindarajan A, Saskin R, Wilton AS, Baxter NN. Introduction of surgical safety checklists in Ontario, Canada. *N Engl J Med*. 2014;370(11):1029-1038.
35. Stulberg JJ, Delaney CP, Neuhauser DV, Aron DC, Fu P, Koroukian SM. Adherence to surgical care improvement project measures and the association with postoperative infections. *JAMA*. 2010;303(24):2479-2485.
36. Khuri SF, Daley J, Henderson WG. The comparative assessment and improvement of quality of surgical care in the Department of Veterans Affairs. *Arch Surg*. 2002;137(1):20-27.
37. Dimick JB, Welch HG, Birkmeyer JD. Surgical mortality as an indicator of hospital quality: the problem with small sample size. *JAMA*. 2004;292(7):847-851.
38. Dimick JB, Welch HG. The zero mortality paradox in surgery. *J Am Coll Surg*. 2008;206(1):13-16.

AMERICAN C
SURGEONS A
OF SURGEON
COLLEGE OF
AMERICAN C
SURGEONS A
OF SURGEON
COLLEGE OF
AMERICAN C
SURGEONS A

CHAPTER 10
Curriculum: Business and Personal Financial Resource Management

Lead Authors

K. Craig Kent, MD, FACS, MAMSE

Mark Aeder, MD, MS, FACS

Co-Authors

William G. Cioffi, MD, FACS

Charles D. Mabry, MD, FACS

Michael F. Rotondo, MD, FACS

Selwyn M. Vickers, MD, FACS

CHAPTER 10

Curriculum: Business and Personal Financial Resource Management

Executive Summary

This chapter focuses on the economics of surgical practice—how surgeons get paid and how to enjoy a long and financially satisfying career and lifestyle. It seeks to answer the following questions:

- Why should residents be concerned with health care economics?
- How do government and other payors determine how surgeons will be compensated for services rendered?
- What is value-based care?
- What financial challenges are unique to private and academic practice?
- How can surgeons protect their personal finances?
- What resources are available to residents who want to learn more about health care financing and strategies for success?

Introduction

In addition to disruptions associated with the unforeseen emergencies such as the Coronavirus Disease 2019 (COVID-19) pandemic, residents also must deal with a rapidly changing business practice environment. Yet, despite these challenges, the practice of surgery can and should be satisfying, sustainable, and provide a lifetime of financial security, satisfaction, and enjoyment. In this chapter, we address the question of how we can best educate and prepare residents for their financial future.

Knowing how the business side of the practice of surgery is conducted, how surgeons earn money, how they are compensated, and what factors determine the success of a surgical practice are all key lessons to learn.

Why Is This Important?

When it comes to training surgeons, one topic is often ignored—the business of medicine. Once, not long ago, it was considered undignified for physicians to talk about money or politics. Today, providing adequate care to our patients requires surgeons to learn about business practices, cost effectiveness, and value-based care. The Accreditation Council for Graduate Medical Education (ACGME) requires residency programs to teach practice management. Moreover, three of the six ACGME education core competencies are systems-based practice, practice-based learning, and professionalism, which are all related to practice management. In addition, physicians often are unfamiliar with federal regulations for coding and billing even though the Centers for Medicare & Medicaid Services (CMS) require them to comply with these regulations. Finally, with the growing focus on cutting costs and improving patient outcomes, practicing physicians need a basic understanding of health care economics.

Although physicians are among the highest-earning professionals in the U.S., most medical students graduate with significant debt. The median debt of medical school graduates with loans has nearly tripled from $71,000 (in 2018 dollars) in 1986 to more than $200,000 in 2018. One in eight graduates now owes more than $300,000 in educational debt. Nonetheless, financial literacy is poor among physicians, and financial education is largely absent from medical school and residency curricula. This lack of preparation significantly affects physician well-being. The risk of physician burnout, which affects more than one in two clinicians, is associated with increasing debt and the lack of financial acumen.

Most medical schools and residency programs could do a better job preparing their graduates to manage their practices. Students graduate without being familiar with contract negotiation, conflict resolution, change management, and related topics. Consequently, young physicians frequently enter health care practice without knowing how to improve clinical workload to enhance productivity, critically evaluate the financial performance of a private practice, or manage their personal finances. For example, published data show that 75 percent of graduating radiation oncology residents feel unprepared to handle their future financial decisions.[1]

This knowledge gap is not new. In 1993, a large survey by Cantor and colleagues found that only 3 percent of respondents felt they received adequate financial education during residency and were well prepared to manage the business aspect of their practices.[2] Some specialties have responded to this education deficit. Family medicine has a 40-year history of practice management education. However, little has been done in surgery programs, at least according to a search of published studies. One of the few studies that could be found comes from 2008, in which Jones and colleagues found that a tightly focused curriculum that sought to improve accuracy of coding and documentation improved accuracy by more than 50 percent.[3]

This lack of attention to the financial literacy of surgical trainees comes despite a 2005 study by Lusco and colleagues that reported 87 percent of surgery program directors surveyed believed residents should get practice management training while only 8 percent believed that they did receive adequate training.[4] More than a decade later, Ahmad and colleagues assessed financial literacy among residents and fellows, finding deficits in knowledge regarding basic investing principles, the relationship between interest rates and bond prices, and other personal finance issues, including health insurance.[5] These residents also reported high debt levels and minimal retirement investments.

With finance education largely neglected by the medical education system, a cottage industry of financial advisors has developed to provide advice to physicians. Although many of these advisors are highly qualified, they often charge high service fees and encourage customers to buy inappropriate products. Physicians in training are at high risk for being victims of unscrupulous advisors. Thus, medical educators should help physicians understand their own personal finances as well as the business of medicine.

Surgery programs historically relied on informal methods for teaching these concepts, according to Mizell and colleagues.[6] In the past, surgeons learned these concepts by taking courses outside of practice despite busy schedules or through on-the-job training, which may lead to trial-and-error, lost revenue, and other unwanted outcomes. Thus, the 2012 Mizell study implemented and evaluated an evidence-based 18-hour curriculum drawing on several prior courses finding that residents thought the curriculum improved their understanding of personal financial and practice management—in part because they *did* understand these topics better.[6]

Other medical schools have tried to fill this gap by offering their students dual degrees in medicine and business administration. For example, the University of Arkansas for Medical Sciences, Little Rock, offers a business-of-medicine elective that covers billing and coding, taxes, investment and retirement planning, student loan management, contracts, estate planning, recruitment, and so on. This 20-hour course lasts 10 weeks, and has become increasingly popular, with less than one-third of students enrolling in its first year to more than 70 percent of students five years later. Upon course completion, most students thought themselves to be significantly more capable of managing their future personal finances; they felt the business aspects of medicine should be taught throughout medical school.

Personal financial literacy is an important aspect of physician well-being. A better understanding of the business of health care is needed for success in the ongoing struggle to balance cost and outcomes. Physicians need at least a basic understanding of relative value units (RVUs), funds flow models, and concepts such as time-driven activity-based costs and business and economic principles; medical schools and training programs should integrate these topics into their curriculum.

As we increase business education efforts, how should their effectiveness be assessed? Some possibilities include the yearly American Board of Surgery In-Training Examination (ABSITE) or the ABS Qualifying and Certifying Exams. Another possibility is for the American College of Surgeons (ACS) to create a course on physician business education similar to the Advanced Trauma Life Support® or Fundamentals of Laparoscopic Surgery® courses.

The U.S. Health Care System: The Economic Imperative for Change

Residents need firmer grounding in business and economic principles in large part because medicine has shifted from a cottage industry to a big business. In the context of the free-market economy, health systems in the U.S. have evolved into a highly complex and variable array of business relationships that color and define health care quality and costs. This evolution has been driven by myriad factors, including state and federal regulations, supply and demand conditions, and local culture and health literacy. Moreover, the interdependence of the elements of the health care system is further complicated by the differing economic characteristics and regulatory imbalance that exist between them. For example, whereas payment for services rendered to patients is highly regulated through the CMS and further modulated through the third-party payors, supply chain costs (pharmaceuticals, instruments, electronic equipment) are largely unregulated.

Furthermore, some episodes of care may be financially favorable to hospitals but not to physician practice. This makes it hard to align incentives between providers and hospitals. In addition, the free-market economy promotes competition for patients, creates pressure for clinical production, and leads many stakeholders to believe that unnecessary services are rendered simply to generate revenue. To many, these competing factors, the lack of care continuity and the complexity of health care, produce a system that has high costs and high variability.

The demographics of the service region of both hospitals and physician practices may be the key factor influencing financial sustainability. Historically, access to care has been highly correlated with the ability to pay. Well-insured patients generally pay only a fraction of the costs of their care.

Safety net hospitals evolved from the charity hospitals and public hospitals of the late 19th century to serve the uninsured. By the mid-20th century, public hospitals affiliated with universities, medical schools, and nursing schools had developed into significant biomedical research centers. Many early residency training programs were built on this infrastructure. Post-World War II prosperity drove people to the suburbs, and employment benefits provided them with access to affordable health insurance. As a result, interest in and tax revenue to support public hospitals began to diminish, and the loss of insured patients threatened the financial viability of safety net hospitals.

By the mid-1960s, the public hospital system was under duress. President Lyndon Johnson's Great Society, the War on Poverty, and the advent of Medicaid and Medicare were the first attempts to address the financial dilemma of the public safety net hospital system. From the start, the Medicaid and Medicare programs fell short in enrolling the patients for whom they were designed and adequately covering the true cost of care. In the 20 years after these programs were established, per-bed hospital costs rose disproportionately to the consumer price index, and public hospitals were once again in jeopardy.

In 1980, the National Association of Public Hospitals (NAPH) was established as an umbrella advocacy group; one of its early legislative victories was to win recognition for the disproportionate burden borne by hospitals that serve low-income patients, leading to public hospitals receiving billions of dollars in funding.

It is now recognized that safety net hospitals remain committed to the challenged communities they serve through inpatient and outpatient services, including HIV/AIDS care, substance-abuse counseling, prenatal and high-risk obstetric services, and Level I trauma care. In most markets, given the current reimbursement structure, however, these services do not produce enough profits for them to sustain their missions; the system is still under economic duress.

The U.S. has a complex health care system that mixes public and private financing, for-profit and not-for-profit hospitals, academic and community-based medical centers, independent and employed providers, and federal, state, and local agencies (Figure 1).

Figure 1. Organization of the health system in the United States[7]

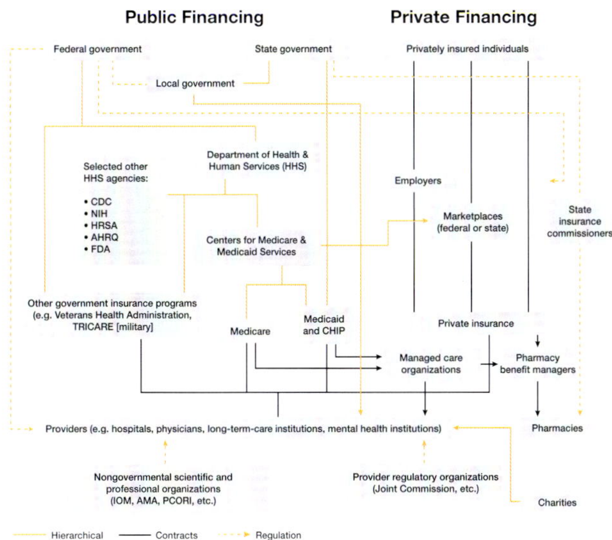

Note: CDC = Centers for Disease Control and Prevention; NIH = National Institutes of Health; HRSA = Health Resources and Services Administration; AHRQ = Agency for Healthcare Research and Quality; FDA = Food and Drug Administration; CHIP = Children's Health Insurance Program; IOM = Institute of Medicine; AMA = American Medical Association; PCORI = Patient-Centered Outcomes Research Institute.

The most recent attempt to address access for uninsured patients was created under the Obama Administration in 2010. The Affordable Care Act (ACA) of 2010 includes a variety of health care policies intended to extend health insurance coverage to uninsured Americans. The ACA expanded Medicaid eligibility, created health insurance exchanges, and prevented insurance companies from denying coverage or charging more for preexisting conditions. It also allowed children to remain on their parents' insurance plan until age 26 and offered lower-income families extra savings through premium tax credits and cost-sharing reductions. A controversial part of the ACA was the individual mandate, which required all Americans to have health care coverage or face increasingly stiff tax penalties. This mandate served the dual purpose of extending health care to uninsured Americans and ensuring a sufficiently broad pool of insured individuals to support health insurance payouts. ACA has undergone, and is still experiencing, numerous challenges. While the constitutionality of the mandate was upheld by the U.S. Supreme Court in 2012, Congress reduced the penalty to $0 in 2017.

Before the ACA, the conceptual framework of value-based care, advanced by Michael Porter, PhD, and Thomas Lee, PhD, began to emerge. Both government and corporate purchasers of health care began to adopt policies correlating the "quality" of health care to the "cost" of health care. The value-based imperative for the transformation of the U.S. health care delivery system began to take hold. In this context, Porter has advocated for an intrinsic and relational concept of value, writing in the *New England Journal of Medicine* that "achieving high value for patients must become the overarching goal of health care delivery, with value defined as the health outcomes achieved per dollar spent."[8]

However, the application of the value proposition to health care delivery in the U.S. has proven difficult for many reasons. Some challenges are inherent to the nature of health care itself; others are more endemic to the U.S. At the root of the value-based conundrum is the fundamental problem of developing working definitions of quality and cost. A recent collaboration between the American College of Surgeons and the Harvard Business School (THRIVE [Transforming Health care Resources to Increase Value and Efficiency]) is exploring the measuring of value by determining the costs of production using TDABC (Time Driven Activity-Based Costing). More about this program can be found at *www.facs.org/quality-programs/acs-thrive.*

These political, social, economic, and cultural factors have focused the debate on the cost of our delivery system as it relates to overall health, as opposed to access to care and the provision of services. In 2008, Berwick and colleagues introduced the Triple Aim strategy to advance health care reform in the U.S. by improving the individual experience of care and the health of populations, and reducing per capita costs of care.[9] The question is, does the cost of delivering services directly relate to the overall health of our population? Hence, the focus on so-called population health.

This concept has driven the federal government and health systems to explore ways in which the overall health of a given population could be measured with respect to cost, quality, and patient satisfaction. From a regulatory perspective, the movement toward value-based care has resulted in a transition from traditional fee-for-service revenue to bundled payments with financial incentives for providers who can demonstrate optimal outcomes at the lowest cost. This has led to, among other things, standardizing care, a rapid rise in the number of employed physicians in an attempt to align incentives, and the aggregation of health care business entities.

These trends likely reflect the need to have larger patient cohorts over which to distribute risk. By aggregating patients into large networks and using a data-driven approach, optimal care management can be applied to achieve the most favorable outcomes for the lowest cost for a given condition or for a given cohort of patients. Perhaps most importantly, this better aligns, at least theoretically, providers and health systems.

The Payment System: How Surgeons Get Paid

In theory, fully aligned population health focus appears to be fiscally prudent and socially responsible; however, there are significant impediments to implementing such a system given the tenets of population health and the principles of public health. Chief among these barriers is the fact that financial models do not reward health care delivery systems for making meaningful investments in the health of geographic populations. This is a significant problem. Despite the movement to employed physician models, physician reimbursement is still based on a fee-for-service Relative Value Unit (RVU) scheme, and hospitals are still reimbursed based on Diagnosis Related Groups (DRGs) established by CMS. The Alternate Payment Models (APMs) that CMS has proposed and implemented have done little so far to shift the fundamental economics of the system.

CMS developed the Resource-Based Relative Value Scale (RBRVS) for physician payment, which decouples the price of services from the medical decision-making process and links it to resource costs, including the amount of work (w), practice expense (pe), and professional liability (pl) for more than 7,500 different services. Hence the equation:

TOTAL RVU = wRVU + peRVU + plRVU

Work RVUs (wRVU) are determined by the time, effort, skill, and intensity needed to provide the service considering the mental effort, stress, and amortized training expense. The wRVU has three separate components: preservice (preoperative preparation), intra-service (operation), and post-service (postoperative care). Practice expense RVUs (peRVU) and professional liability RVU (plRVU) refer to the cost of running a practice and purchasing liability coverage, respectively. CMS adjusts the total RVU for differences across geographic areas of the U.S. and assigns a dollar amount (conversion factor) for each RVU.

Physician services also are described using the Current Procedural Terminology (CPT) codes and Healthcare Common Procedure Coding System (HCPCS) codes, which range from those that require considerable physician time and effort, clinical staff, and specialized equipment, to those that require little, if any, physician time or resources. The ACS Relative Value Scale Update Committee (RUC), which meets annually, estimates RVUs for each CPT code and new services developed, and sends recommendations to CMS for consideration and a final decision. The role of the RUC has been challenged recently, but at present remains the basis of surgeon payment from CMS.

CMS pays for hospitalizations based on the DRG payment system—a patient classification system that standardizes a prospective fixed payment to hospitals with the intent of containing cost. Upon patient discharge, a DRG is assigned based on the primary diagnosis, and the hospital is paid a fixed amount for that DRG, regardless of the actual cost to render care during that episode. This was the first attempt by payors to transfer financial risk to the providers and hold them accountable for delivering services within a capitated payment model. If a hospital can effectively provide the care for less money than Medicare pays for the DRG, then the hospital generates a profit margin on that hospitalization. If the hospital spends more money than Medicare pays for the DRG, then the hospital loses money on that hospitalization. At present, the margin is often negative, with Medicare payments falling short of meeting true, measured costs.

Clinical Integration and Consolidation of Markets

From a business perspective, it makes sense for physicians and hospitals to join forces around driving clinical margins, and that health systems aggregate and consolidate to meet the challenges of Berwick's Triple Aim, population health management, and public health imperatives. However, some federal regulations, intending to promote competitive behavior and protect patients, impede development of a fully aligned and aggregated business model.

The Federal Trade Commission (FTC) is tasked with ensuring that all markets remain competitive, so that consumers benefit from lower costs, better care, and more innovation. The FTC enforces antitrust laws in health care markets to prevent anticompetitive conduct that would harm consumers. The agency offers guidance to all participants in the health care market—including physicians and other health professionals, hospitals and other institutional providers, pharmaceutical companies and other sellers of health care products, and insurers—to help them comply with U.S. antitrust laws.

Several laws and regulations that prevent health systems and providers from engaging in anticompetitive behaviors also protect patients from unscrupulous business practices. The most important federal fraud and abuse laws that apply to physicians are the False Claims Act, the Anti-Kickback Statute, the Physician Self-Referral Law (Stark law), the Exclusion Authorities, and the Civil Monetary Penalties Law. Government agencies, including the Department of Justice, the Department of Health & Human Services (HHS), the Office of Inspector General, and CMS, are charged with enforcing these laws.

Despite these efforts, the trend in health care delivery for the last several decades has been toward mergers and consolidation, allowing for more coordinated care as a means of improving outcomes, controlling costs, and improving access for underserved patients. Some key terms to understand are as follows:

- *Accountable Care Organizations (ACOs)* are groups of physicians, hospitals, and other health care providers who collaborate to offer coordinated, high-quality care to Medicare patients. The goal of coordinated care is to ensure that patients get the right care at the right time, while avoiding unnecessary duplication of services and preventing medical errors. When an ACO succeeds both in delivering high-quality care and controlling spending, it shares in the savings it achieves for the Medicare program. To date, this experiment has had mixed results in terms of lowering costs.
- *Value-based contracts,* also known as risk-sharing agreements or outcomes-based contracts, are an alternative payment model that brings together two key stakeholders—for example, health care payors and physician organizations—to deliver care to patients.
- In *narrow network plans*, insurers work with a smaller pool of physicians, hospitals, and treatment centers that agree to a lower price for services with the expectation that they will have greater patient volume, which can, in turn, lower the cost of insurance premiums.
- *Time-driven activity-based costing* (TDABC) is a methodology that calculates the costs of health care resources used as a patient moves through an episode of care. Limited data exist on the application of TDABC from the perspective of the health care provider.
- A *professional service agreement* (PSA) is generally defined as a financial relationship between a physician practice and a hospital in which the physician practice remains autonomous, but the physicians receive compensation from the hospital at the fair market rate. These agreements are necessary for physicians to render services in concert with a health system and remain in a safe harbor relative to fraud and abuse.

Challenges Unique to Academic Health Care Systems

It is challenging enough to make the economics work for delivering care and services to patients; but for academic medical centers (AMCs), there are the extremely expensive concomitant missions of education and research. Moreover, AMCs are particularly complex in their internal business structures as they play host to the university, the medical school, the teaching hospital, and the faculty practice. While all elements play a vital role in satisfying all three missions—education, research, and patient care—each academic medical center has its own business model imperatives.

The clinical operating margin is the economic engine for most U.S. AMCs because of an array of compounding market factors over the last decade. This economic reality, coupled with increasing competition from lower-cost nonacademic health systems and a highly volatile market, has resulted in academic health systems (AHSs) becoming increasingly integrated operationally and financially—most notably among faculty practices and primary teaching hospitals. The need to align the strategic and financial interests of the faculty practice and teaching hospital/health system to sustain the three-part mission of AMCs has become a significant trend in academic medicine. With consideration given to the AMC's organizational design, financial condition, public/private status, culture, and other factors, the approach required to achieve this alignment varies.

Some AMCs, such as the University of Utah, Salt Lake City, have adopted a mission-based management (MBM) approach. MBM is a process for organizational decision-making that:

- Is mission-driven
- Assures internal accountability
- Distributes resources in alignment with organization-wide goals
- Is based on timely, open, and accurate information

MBM is a resource for the health sciences, which aids in infrastructure for financial/data analysis, system/process development, and is a forum for discussion and decision-making related to policy and planning.

Although they share characteristics and themes, each AMC in the U.S. has a unique organizational structure and operating model. In the last five years, AMCs have tried to make their clinical enterprise more responsive to the health care market and to increase investment in the academic enterprise. These changes include merging entities, governance structures changes, new leadership/management models, and new approaches to funds flow.

With the convergence of economic factors, including cuts in federal, state, and commercial health care reimbursement, National Institutes of Health (NIH) funding, GME-related funding, and rising competition for high-caliber faculty, AMCs must develop and maintain a high-performing clinical enterprise to provide a source of investment to sustain the three-part mission. Studies and industry literature in recent years[2,3] affirm that the basic components of AMCs are inextricably interdependent; therefore, these components must become more integrated in the face of challenging market factors. AMCs are under tremendous pressure to make bold changes and spend political capital to find ways to act as one unified AMC.

While some worry that focusing on clinical enterprise performance could jeopardize an AMC's medical education and research missions, economic and market factors suggest the opposite is true. AMCs that focus on the academic enterprise without a well-aligned and high-performing AHS are more likely to fall behind in the market. AMCs need to examine their three-part portfolio through a single lens to ensure that maximum value is generated from the clinical enterprise to make resources available, consider trade-offs, and prioritize strategic goals. Greater integration between the teaching hospital and physician organizations can yield benefits, including the following:

- Higher-performing, cost-efficient infrastructure for physician organizations and hospitals
- Collaborative strategic planning and prioritization
- Joint operating and capital planning
- Proactive program development/planning
- Joint workforce planning, including recruitment and retention of top talent
- Improved payor contracts, including both fee-for-service and risk arrangements
- More conducive environments to build and sustain major service lines/centers
- More responsive and informed decision-making and clearer points of accountability
- A more engaged physician leadership model that fosters a dyad reporting relationship between physician leader and administrators
- Alignment of compensation with health system performance

The teaching hospitals and physician organizations of AMCs have been active participants in corporate restructuring in recent years. The Association of American Medical Colleges (AAMC) represents this realignment as a new funds flow approach that aggregates all the clinical funding, whether health system or practice based, to develop the system overall and support the academic mission (Figure 2).[10] That said, the political complexities of AMCs make achieving such arrangements challenging, especially in the current economically stressed environment.

Figure 2. Current funds flow views: Grow clinical to fund academics[10]

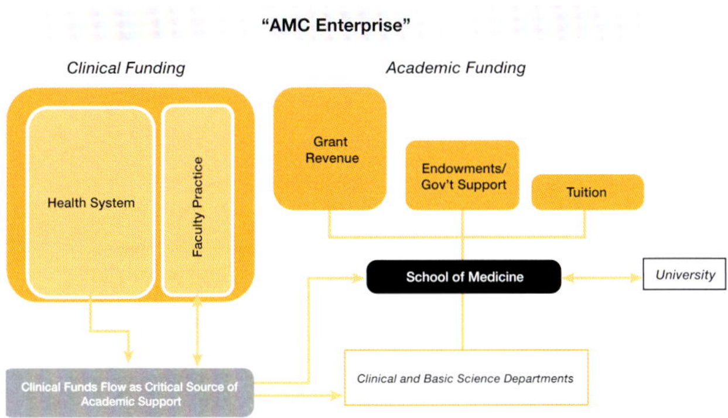

AMCs should lead population health improvement for a variety of reasons, including the growing focus on population-oriented payment mechanisms, the plethora of unanswered research questions regarding effective and financially stable models of care, the need to train health professions in new paradigms, and the fundamental social mission of AMCs. But the major challenge to this imperative lies in the limited infrastructure and human capital within AMCs and the lack of organized effort at the state or federal level to support these activities.

Tangible and Intangible Value: Garnering Resources
In the current health care environment, the best way to garner resources is to identify initiatives that add value across the missions of the institution and align with its top strategic priorities. For the purposes of this discussion, one might classify value in two main categories:

- Tangible value: An initiative that brings revenue to the institution and generates a margin, either directly or indirectly.
- Intangible value: An initiative that advances the research and education mission and/or advances the reputation of the organization.

Development proposals most likely to get support include those that:

- Align with institutional culture, values, and active strategic priorities
- Align with all aspects of the institutional mission
- Support multiple aspects of the mission and bring both tangible and intangible value to the goals of the institution
- Carry with them a cogent, well-conceived business plan that calibrates up-front investment with tangible timely returns and limits frontend loading of support
- Are melded with and contribute intangible value for the clinical, research, or educational missions
- Are supported across disciplines and elements of the institution, many of which have vetted the plan and have contributed to it
- Work within the existing governance, leadership, and management structure
- Don't create an internal competitive conflict that leads to a series of no-win choices for leadership
- Are proposed and led by a credible, proven, trusted leader with responsible management skills

So, in a highly competitive environment with complex organizational dynamics and tight resources, it takes vision, careful planning, and the ability to develop collaborators and coalitions of support to advance new initiatives within a health care institution.

Academic and Private Practice Management

Few aspects of medicine have evolved more than professional finance models. These changes have been driven by economic pressures and the continued growth of the cost curve for health care in our country. The U.S. clearly stands out in this area of medical expenditures, as 16 percent of its gross domestic product (GDP) is spent on health care. For the last several years, health care has been one of the largest industries in the country, and costs have risen annually. All these factors affect funding for academic medicine and private practice.

The key factors driving significant change in practice management are:

- The need to bend the cost curve in overall health care expenditures.
- Ongoing cuts in physician reimbursement and a drive toward value-based, bundled payments.
- Contracts, hospitals, and health systems have had significant profit margin erosion because of growing labor expenses.
- Faculty practice plans depend more than ever on facility and technical fee revenue from hospitals due to declining professional reimbursement.
- The growth of research programs and the drive toward innovation and translational research, as well as education, is vital to the mission to attract and retain top talent in academic medicine. However, for every extramural research dollar, an additional 50 cents from clinical revenue must be invested to sustain the programs.
- Nonacademic medical centers, the at-large community, and for-profit corporate hospitals are affected by the increasing focus on reducing costs and meeting quality metrics, and by decreasing reimbursement from competitive third-party contracts.

AMCs and practice management plans are positioned and primed to create more integrated funds flow models. When creating an integrated funds flow model, several key issues must be addressed, starting with topline revenue (total expected revenue from all sources). Tackling this issue often requires a plan consistent with a cost containment culture, the need to invest in increasingly expensive research infrastructure, and the increased scrutiny of quality and outcomes.

Practice plans, which are core income generators for hospitals, need to evolve. The history of academic practice plans includes periods of high reimbursements with indemnity insurance, independent practice corporations for clinical departments that managed separate billing, and professional contracts with payors. In their day, these entities submitted separate bills for their own collections and effectively functioned as separate corporations. Now practice plans provide a direct link to physicians to create incentives physicians need to support their salaries.

Although clinical departments were part of a practice plan well into the 1990s, they were not a multidisciplinary integrated practice plan with mutually accountable financial standards. Most of the models functioned as if each department had little accountability for the financial outcomes of the other departments. Consequently, there was little incentive to prevent or to bail out the deficits of another department's revenue loss.

In the early 2000s, however, a trend to centralized billing was driven by insurance companies, a centralized focus on contracts, new government rules regarding the electronic health record (EHR), a need for efficiency, and the ACA. In addition, the continued decline in reimbursement to physicians and the loss of technical fees to the hospital threatened the viability of the previous models. This trend was also the result of:

- Decentralized processes for billing, which resulted in payors receiving dozens of separate bills from the same hospitalization and high patient dissatisfaction
- Lack of collective power among providers to negotiate with payors because they were all independent practice plans
- No available mechanism to collect central expenses from departments to allow the overall institution mission to grow, such as a dean's tax or subsidies to support the clinical practice infrastructure

Thus, most medical center funding models have moved to a more integrated platform.

These funds flow models require the engagement of faculty practice plans, which are either separate 501(c)3 organizations or are fully integrated into the health system as a practice group with an employed status with academic appointments in medical schools. In these models, departments still are accountable for their finances; however, incentives and mechanisms for mutual support and accountability, as well as ongoing central reviews of each department's finance, are available. This model helps maintain a department's reserves. In some cases, however, departments may become cost centers requiring central approval of annual clinical and academic budgets. These funds flow models may allow for shared or central reserves, as well as the development of funds to support strategic clinical initiatives for the academic institution or the practice.

In addition, the more highly integrated model collects revenues, such as a dean's tax, to cover centralized expenses, such as those of the overall school infrastructure, the departments, and the faculty. Centralized billing is more efficient and enables a practice group or institution to bargain for improved contracts. This integrated funds flow model also provides a cross subsidy for those areas, particularly primary care, that frequently require subsidization under the current reimbursement structures. Finally, this model creates institutional alignment and a strategic fund for specific clinical hires and initiatives. In many cases, specific funds can be created to invest in research and research infrastructure. At some institutions, it is called the academic enrichment fund.

Some basic principles for designing these funds flow models should include:

- Clear evaluation of revenue, income, and expenses to identify prior subsidies, revenue capacity within the system, and where the organization can provide broader support to the clinical and academic mission
- A dedicated group of individuals to manage the funds flow process by looking at how professional fees and technical fees combine to support an academic clinical practice
- A strong economic alignment between a hospital and physicians anchored in a common strategic plan with common growth goals across the clinical mission
- A culture that understands that academic and clinical growth work best when occurring in parallel with each other and that success will require ongoing investment
- A plan that is simple, transparent, and accompanied by a market-driven, competitive compensation plan
- Ongoing flexibility, review, renewal, and revisions necessary to create sustainability

Private practice and independent business models are also changing. In integrated delivery systems with employed physicians and in AMCs, most professional medical financial models integrate physician professional fees, hospital technical fees, and collections. To be sustainable, the clinical, research, and educational missions must be aligned to support the AMC. Integrated models will be a critical component of ongoing health care delivery in the U.S. An integrated system that delivers measurable outcomes with price transparency is the most cost-effective way to deliver care in the future. This will require a gradual conversion of payment from fee-for-service to bundled, capitated payment. Physicians and hospitals working together will be able to reduce the risk associated with this payment method and, in so doing, deliver lower cost and increased value to the whole population. This transition is the biggest challenge facing health care delivery today.

Personal Financial Management

As surgeons we have spent many years learning and perfecting our craft, becoming experts in disease and diagnosis, performance of surgical procedures, postoperative follow-up and long-term treatment. Maintaining our surgical literacy is a never-ending challenge to keep up with the changing landscape, new procedures and products, and best practices. We have dedicated countless hours to developing our professional life, anticipating a long and successful career. Our professional life is only one side of our existence. We also have our personal life, one in which we have to consider the needs of those close to us—spouses, families, significant others, partners, and friends. This is the social half, the one where we retreat after our professional responsibilities are concluded for the day.

There is a close association between these two lives—the professional life and the personal life. Having a successful and rewarding surgical career while maintaining an enjoyable time away from work is the best of both worlds. This situation would, under ideal circumstances, lead to personal happiness and good mental and physical health. When one or both of these two lives is not going well, if there are stresses and difficulties, then the emotional strain can be carried from one to the other with significant psychological and physical consequences.

A key factor in a healthy personal life is overall personal financial health. For many couples, finances are the leading cause of disagreements that may upset personal relationships. There are many strains on the surgeon's personal finances, especially as many of them carry significant educational loan obligations from college and medical school, have growing families as the residency years progress, and are still receiving relatively limited salary support for a number of years in training. This situation is amplified because surgeons often have a limited educational background in personal financial management, topics that are rarely discussed, if at all, during the medical school or college years.

The key to having a good perspective of personal fiscal management is to develop a basic knowledge of how to approach your personal financial situation. Having a competency in the basic concepts, knowing what questions to ask, having an idea of where to go for good impartial advice, and learning to avoid the missteps and errors that physicians have historically made will start physicians on the right path to a good financial plan. This counsel should come from an impartial source, not someone who is trying to sell a product and gain one's business.

The following sections form a broad outline of items to address, especially early in one's career, as the sooner the financial aspects are considered and addressed, the more benefit they will provide as the years progress. This overview is not meant to be comprehensive as each topic would require a text of its own, but rather to lay the foundation for future growth and education. The important thing is to understand the basic principles and build a team to plan for your future. The topics discussed subsequently can be incorporated as a formal component of the residency program educational curriculum.

Savings

Saving some income is the most critical tool to start building a financial nest egg. After years of college and medical school, receiving first paychecks, even as a resident, can make you feel better as a little cash accrues in your account, and the pent-up desire to finally start to spend more freely becomes a real temptation. This will especially escalate with the first paychecks after residency when the salary really starts to climb. It is a good idea to wrest control over the situation before you miss some opportunities.

A dollar saved in a person's 20s and 30s will be worth approximately four times that of a dollar saved in the 50s or 60s. The time value of money is significant. Before we get into the principles of investing, the important thing to remember is that the returns on any savings will be compounded significantly if safely put away, reinvested, and allowed to grow.

Fortunately, a number of federal savings programs are designed to encourage retirement savings and building for the future. Although each may have different tax consequences, the fundamental principles are similar. The money is saved in a regulated account with an authorized financial fiduciary (bank, investment firm, and so forth), cannot be withdrawn without penalty or under defined extenuating circumstances until age 59.5 years, and some require a certain percentage be withdrawn by age 72.5 years. There are also allowances for additional contributions starting at age 50. Although that seems like a long time in the future, it is important to begin to build these accounts early in a surgical career to achieve the maximal benefits. Let's look at the options.

The most common retirement account is an Individual Retirement Account, an IRA, which can be opened at any income level. The money may be invested in a range of options and remains yours until withdrawal. The limits vary year to year and are presently set (2021) at $6,000 annually. There are two types of IRAs, the traditional IRA and a Roth IRA.

A fundamental concept for everyone to understand is the basic terminology. If an item is paid for or contributed pretax, it means that the amount is deducted from the total tax bill that an individual owes, and no taxes are paid on that amount. If the same funds were paid or contributed post-tax, like many of our daily expenses, the taxes have already been paid on this money. An account that is tax-deferred means that no taxes are due on any of the transactions within that account as long as the money remains in the account. This is how most retirement accounts are structured.

The traditional IRA has been in place for more than 50 years. The contribution made, up to the maximum, is with pretax dollars. Hence, the amount of funds within the account are allowed to grow tax-deferred, and the money withdrawn is then taxed as ordinary income. Taxes on all the withdrawals are paid at the current tax rate when the money is withdrawn. For example, if over the years deposits of $100,000 are placed into a traditional IRA account, and the account grows to $500,000, upon withdrawal, all $500,000 will be taxable as ordinary income.

A Roth IRA is structured differently. The contributions are made with post-tax funds, meaning that tax had been already paid on this contribution; therefore, the account will grow tax-free and taxes are not due on this money when funds are withdrawn. Using the above example, if you funded your Roth IRA with $100,000 and it grew to $500,000, none of the monies withdrawn would be taxable. The Roth does have total income restrictions for eligibility, but overall, it is a great advantage for tax-free growth of your savings. However, the tax nuances are complex, especially for higher wage earners, and a good accountant will be needed.

While anyone with an income can open and contribute to an IRA account, there are important employer-sponsored retirement accounts as well. The two most well-known are a 401k if you work for a for-profit company, and a 403b, which is offered for not-for-profit companies, including many hospitals and universities. The restrictions and tax-deferred growth within accounts are similar to the traditional IRA, and all withdrawals are taxed as ordinary income. The differences are that the employer controls the investment options and may have a matching contribution to an account that provides a financial bonus. This additional contribution cannot be underestimated because once vested in the program, this is free money for the owner. The amount of one's contribution is choice based and reaches a maximum, which changes annually. For 2021, the maximum allowable is $19,500. If this account is maximally funded and combined with an IRA contribution, $25,500 can be easily saved each year to grow tax deferred.

Depending on one's employment situation, other tax-deferred investment accounts may be available, such as a 457 or a Health Savings Account, but these vary by employer, contract, and other considerations. Be sure to look for these opportunities. The points are to maximize retirement accounts to gain that tax-deferred benefit, to take advantage of any matching opportunities, and to always remember to avoid using retirement funds early as they are almost always protected from creditors and you may be charged a penalty for early withdrawal.

Another key tax-deferred vehicle to be used for educational expenses is a 529 account. These are personally established with the naming of a beneficiary, typically of one's children, although there is a fair degree of latitude for the owner to transfer them to other beneficiaries if the proceeds are used for educational expenses, such as college tuition. All states have different rules and may have additional incentives, such as state income tax credits, to promote their use. There are limits to the contributions, but a 529 account is another excellent investment opportunity.

Table 1. Main points for savings

- Start as early as possible
- Maximize contributions to your retirement accounts to generate years of tax-deferred or tax-free growth
- Pay yourself first: Save by having money taken from your paycheck before you see it
- Check your retirement investments and consider readjusting them once a year
- Prioritize your savings, even if you have significant debt

Other Savings—Your Life's Fund

It is important to budget disposable income each month to allow for the creation of a daily savings account. In the financial vernacular, this would be disposable cash on hand. It is important to fund this account with the same attention as retirement accounts, as it will initially provide a buffer for unexpected expenses and may even be used for discretionary spending for enjoyment and relaxation. Following are the basic tools to get this account started.

It begins with a budget. The concept of budgeting is important for addressing all the financial factors in one's personal life. The important thing to realize is that everyone's budget is different as each person, each couple, and each family has different priorities, depending on circumstances and responsibilities. The mirror component of this is debt and obligations. As basic as it sounds, a simple monthly budget is the best tool for understanding your financial situation. On a spreadsheet, the total monthly take-home income from all sources (including spouse, partner, significant other as applicable) will be placed at the top. This figure indicates how much capital you must work with for that month. The rows down the side should include all monthly expenses. Start with fixed expenses, such as mortgage/rent, auto loan/lease, loan repayments, insurance costs, utilities, and work down to the ones that are more variable for estimation, such as food, clothing, maintenance and upkeep, and so on. The remainder of the sheet comprises the most discretionary expenses, such as entertainment, dining out, memberships—items that are not essential but would be nice. The total of these on a monthly basis are called debits, and when this number is subtracted from the total income, this represents your net or disposable income. This is the amount of money you have each month to save for other events or a "rainy day." Even reducing home costs and/or car expenses by a few hundred dollars a month can add up to an increase of thousands of dollars in disposable income each year. For a good benchmark, put aside about 10 percent of one's total paycheck income each month (some months will be better than others) into a disposable income fund to build your personal savings account. Part of this might be an education fund for children or a vacation fund but there should be an amount that can be held back in reserve. Pay yourself first.

Table 2. Keys for a budget

- There are fixed expenses each month and must be paid on time
- You can modify your fixed expenses by not outspending your income
- There are discretionary expenses that can be modified monthly to enhance cash flow
- If you anticipate major expenses, such as a child's education or a life event, it is beneficial to start saving for this as early as possible
- House ownership is expensive—do not buy more than you need
- Keep your auto costs reasonable

Debt

One of the basic concepts to managing debt is understanding that all debt is not created equal. There are different types of debt, some are long term, others exist for a short period, and they may have contrasting functions. Each debt contract signed will have varying terms, obligations, and interest rates. The key financial consideration is to understand your debt and, in some ways, how to have it work to your advantage.

What Is Debt?

Financial debt is funds that have been given to you or used to cover a financial obligation that one has incurred. The debtor has the obligation to reimburse the lender for their money and other costs, such as interest, within a defined period of time. Most people take on two main types of debt: extremely large financial obligations, which cannot be paid off in total and need to be spread out in repayments over a longer period of time; and shorter-term debt incurred by borrowing funds to cover expenses from spending.

Examples of the first category are educational loans or home mortgages. In many cases, these loans are hundreds of thousands of dollars, and few people are able to pay these costs in full upfront. These loans contribute to the debt load, accumulating interest, and affecting lifestyle. The short-term debt, often from use of a credit card, is generally spending debt and is much more controllable. Sometimes credit is extended for approximately 30 days without penalty or interest, such as the restaurant meal or trip to the store that ends up on one's credit card. Other times it may be an item paid for over a few months.

To understand your debt, loans and general spending should be looked at separately, categorizing each by the number of months remaining to pay the debt off and the interest rate. Debt can be subdivided into "good debt" and "bad debt," which is defined later. The basic principle is that not all debt is bad. In fact, sometimes taking on debt can actually accelerate financial gains. The key is knowing what defines as bad debt and eliminating it as soon as possible.

The next division is whether the debt is structured, meaning that it has a defined obligation at a defined time period (such as a mortgage obligation), is unstructured (meaning that the payment can be variable over different time periods), such as a line of credit, or is open-ended, with no distinct deadline for repayment, such as many family loans. The latter may be the most flexible both with respect to terms and repayment scheduling.

Finally, there are two other categories that are helpful when approaching the budgeting considerations of debt load—those debts that are fixed obligations or uncontrollable and those that more discretionary. Debt or payment obligations that are uncontrollable are those that recur on a timed basis and are linked to everyday living functions. Obviously large loans, such as educational payments or mortgage or rent bills are consistent on a monthly basis. There are also other recurring obligations including electric, insurance, or cell phone bills. These will regularly appear at various times during the month for payment, but the amounts can vary with each invoice. This will give some, but not complete flexibility, in debt management, and will be incorporated into the budget process. Controllable debt includes the discretionary spending that may occur monthly, such as dining out, subscriptions, and memberships. Carefully controlling such spending can save thousands of dollars a year.

Bad and Good Debt

Typically, long-term debt taken on to buy a house or fund an education is considered "good," as the interest rate is relatively low, and its purpose is to acquire an asset. In contrast, credit card debt used to pay for discretionary spending is considered "bad" because it carries a high rate of interest and, some would argue, does not result in the acquisition of something with lasting value.

Review debt and the interest rates. The worst debt most people carry is balances on their credit cards. Often the interest on these balances is 18 percent or more. Credit cards are a convenient way to defer payments and avoid the use of cash (not to mention accruing rewards benefits and other purchase protections), but the balance should be paid off by the credit card cycle due date. If you do not have the funds to afford the purchase, you should question whether it is really necessary. If you do, there are generally other options for you to finance through the vendor with much more competitive terms.

Consider paying off other high interest loans in your portfolio, particularly those with rates that are well above the current market rate. Often it makes sense to pay off the highest rate loans first, but in some cases, it may make sense to pay off a smaller loan to eliminate the burden of a monthly payment.

Good debt is money owed that carries an interest rate below what one's investments may earn. In 2021, mortgage rates were near all-time lows, about 3 percent, but inflation was creeping up to approximately 5 percent, and investments in a moderately aggressive equity account was returning more than 10 percent. Finance any major purchases at special deals if they are offered, such as a car at 0-2 percent, leaving little cash in the car and more left to put into savings and investments.

Table 3. Keys to debt management

- Understand the difference between good and bad debt
- Pay off the highest rate debt as quickly as possible, especially credit card debt
- Keep the good debt, with low interest rates, to their full term
- If a purchase cannot be paid within the billing cycle, avoid buying it
- Budget for expensive items and vacations
- Never miss a payment due date (set up automatic payments) and never default on a loan

Credit Score

An individual's savings, debt, the debt payment history, and credit use have a huge impact on the credit score and the credit score affects the ability to not only borrow money, but also the interest rates that will be charged for loan. It can also affect insurance premium payments as well as eligibility for certain preferred programs. To see the effect, examine the main components of the score.

The most important factor is the payment history (35 percent), and even one missed payment can affect the score. Set up automatic payments before due dates to try and avoid interest, penalties, and a reduced score.

The next important factor is the credit usage (30 percent), which is the amount of credit use compared with the total amount of credit extended. If, for example, a credit card has a $10,000 limit, and the balance is $1,000.00, then the credit use is 10 percent. The credit usage totals all the available credit and the balance due on the accounts. Keeping the balance below 30 percent will result in a higher credit score.

The third component is the credit history length (15 percent), the total age of all the credit accounts with the best scores given for the longest credit history. Fourth is the credit mix (10 percent), which is diversity of the credit accounts and the ability to manage a range of credit products (that is, credit cards, student loans, mortgage, auto loan). The final component is recent or new credit (10 percent), which looks at recent hard inquiries to the credit record. Too many inquiries can indicate an increased risk and lower the credit score.

What Is a Good Credit Score?

Credit scores are measured on a continuum from 300 to 850. Although they can be subdivided by various lenders and underwriters differently, scores above 800 are considered exceptional, and those between 300 and 600 are viewed as credit risks. The closer to a 740 score, the better for most professionals with regards to obtaining credit at the best interest rates. Many services and credit cards permit checking credit scores (these are soft inquiries) so status can be monitored, and any possible credit record errors can be corrected.

Investing

To understand investing, you have to appreciate the many ways to make, and lose, money. Having the true breadth of the potential markets requires an extensive knowledge base, similar to someone knowing everything related to all fields of medicine in exquisite and up-to-date detail. The basic equation is that the amount of money earned on an investment is the return on investment (ROI).

When looking at the standard financial markets, there are types of investments which, by their nature, may fluctuate in value. Some values consistently go up, such as money put in a certificate of deposit (CD); however, with the current rates of return at less than 1 to 2 percent in most cases, even if the dollar amount increases, the spending value of that amount decreases because of inflation, which may be 4 percent or more. Super safe investments may return a higher total dollar amount, although by the time you get your money back, it may be worth less in spending value. Given the current low rates of return on bonds, not much more than CDs at this time, safe or conservative investments may generate too little capital growth for financial growth. These investments are low risk, but the ROI is extremely low as well.

A good way to understand investment is to subdivide them into two main categories—liquid and illiquid. Liquid investments can be accessed quickly, such as cash, or sold easily, such as a stock (also called equity as one has part ownership of the company by holding its stock). Most mutual funds are composed of multiple equities or just may be tracking an index and are run by an investment firm. These investments are relatively easy to sell to raise cash.

Illiquid investments are ones that are more difficult to leave or "cash out," as money is tied up until a buyer is found. A house is an illiquid asset, one that is purchased and owned, which may have increased in value, but whose value cannot be realized until it is sold. When thinking about illiquid investment, think about real estate, artwork, collectibles, private business ownership—any investment in which the funds are unavailable until a buyer is found for investment holding.

Most people rely on liquid asset investing, such as stocks (equities). There are different ways to own these equities. Shares can be purchased in an individual, publicly traded company, for example, Company A. If the value of Company A increases (more people want to buy a share), an investment will be worth more. Investing in a single company can have more upsides if it is doing well, and also more risk if the management or products perform poorly, and it goes down. A knowledgeable financial advisor can provide the best insights into the choices of buying or selling a single company. If managed well, the returns can be rewarding.

A mutual fund is the pooled investments of many people into a fund that is directed by a fund manager. The manager will assess the market and buy large quantities of shares in companies that they believe are likely to be good financial investments. You own a portion of each position the fund has, and there may be dozens of equities in each mutual fund. Some of the equities will do well and some may lose, and it is the fund manager's job to try and achieve the best possible returns for the fund.

In addition to the gains and losses in each fund, there are other considerations. Every fund has a management fee, which is taken out of the calculated share price. Some funds may charge an entrance and/or exit fee (called a load), which is a percentage of the amount invested or withdrawn. Also, as the fund will buy and sell different equity positions throughout the year, the gains are taxed (either short- or long-term capital gains), which will have to be reported when filing income taxes. An advantage of a tax-deferred retirement account is that no yearly tax payments are required, and any gains are rolled into the investment total.

Another more specific type of fund possibly encountered is called an exchange traded fund or ETF. These funds generally are more specific than other mutual funds and trade more like an equity. These funds are not actively traded by the manager, and there are no capital gains to pay taxes on until it is sold. There are no loads for these funds and often a reduced management fee but may have some trading costs. Finally, many investors own an array of equities in their stock portfolios. Stock selection is important and will have a huge impact on your total return. Unfortunately, the ROI depends not just on which stocks you own, but when you buy or sell them. Therefore, many investors use a professional advisor to guide their accounts.

For years, the standard teaching in financial advisement has been to have a balanced or diversified investment portfolio. Depending on age, there are variable percentages which include investments in higher-risk products such as equities; conservative investments, such as bonds, which pay a certain amount each year; and cash. With the near-decade long decline in interest rates, this weighting system has generally been replaced by a strategy of more high-growth equities balanced with a percentage of value-based equities, especially those with a good dividend, and a small amount of cash. Most bonds now are a poor money-growth proposition as the rates are low, and, following taxes and fees and accounting for inflation, may result in less capital than initially invested. Also, bond values fluctuate inversely with the market interest rate—the principal value goes down when interest rates rise and rise when interest rates fall. Especially for younger investors, it may make sense to be relatively aggressive in choosing investments, since even if the stock market goes down significantly, the chances are excellent the prices will recover in value over time. A defensive investment position tends to work better for older or retired investors, who prefer to be safe in times of economic uncertainty and are more focused on a fixed income than portfolio growth.

Table 4. Keys for investing

- Follow your accounts regularly and discuss possible changes with your advisor
- Your invested amounts will grow based on time and the rate of return
- Do not be too conservative or you will lose growth
- Rule of 72: Years to doubling investment = 72/annual rate of return
- Avoid having mutual funds in your taxable accounts
- Avoid believing that you know more than the investment professionals

Insurance

Insurance is a way to protect oneself against the various risks that everyone faces in life. These risks include such events as getting sued, being unable to work due to illness or injury, damage to home or car, or dying. Insurance companies typically price their products based on their projections of how much, how likely, and when they would have to pay. Consider life insurance. The insurance company must assess how long the buyer is likely to live. The rates are adjusted for different factors, such as health history, lifestyle, and so on; generally speaking, the longer the buyer is likely to live, the lower the premiums. A healthy 30-year-old would be expected to have at least 50 years of life ahead, so the premium rate would be based on that. As the person ages and health issues arise, the premium rates for a new policy would rise. Typically, it makes sense to buy a long-term life insurance policy at a fixed premium rate when you are young and healthy.

Some basic insurance products that most people should have, regardless of profession, include homeowners' or rental insurance for coverage of personal items and structural issues; auto insurance for an owned or leased car (as required in many states); and health insurance. These policies have various limitations, conditions, and riders, and coverage should be adjusted to fit your circumstances. In addition, most surgeons have professional liability insurance. Four other insurance coverage priorities every surgeon should consider include life, disability, umbrella, and long-term care insurance.

Life Insurance

Life insurance protects your family against loss of income that would result from one's unexpected death. Although the risks are relatively low for most residents and practicing surgeons, this insurance serves as a buffer against an unexpected accident or illness. A relatively inexpensive term life insurance policy for approximately five times annual income (minimum of $500,000) should be established while healthy to take advantage of the most favorable rates.

As your career develops and you take on other responsibilities, such as establishing a family, your coverage needs will likely change as short- and long-term financial responsibilities will have grown. A sudden death at this time would be devastating for your family's future, including its financial future. A term life insurance policy, with its relatively low cost, would help protect your family against such an event. Good coverage here would be at least eight times the yearly take-home salary, plus tax-deferred contributions. For most surgeons this total would be in the $2 million range. Invested well and spent judiciously, the amount would help cover your family through the early to mid-growth years and fund education expenses.

As a surgeon enters their mid-practice years, expenses likely peak because of lifestyle, housing, college education, travel, and other events. Again the risk of death is still relatively low, but this phase is when other insurance options should be explored. Multiple products, which historically had been called whole-life or variable-life products, should be considered. Depending on locale, health and finances, and with the assistance of a financial advisor and accountant, these policies may be good options for further tax-deferred growth with the insurance component. At this stage of life, you have insurance to help your family maintain their lifestyle and preserve assets for retirement or even future generations.

Whether you keep or cash out your life insurance policies in retirement is a decision that should be evaluated with your financial advisor and accountant. Tax consequences, inheritance considerations, and opportunities for improved cash flow are unique for every individual situation. It is important, though, to keep abreast of the financial status of your insurance products, make certain all the payments are on time, and to reevaluate as financial situations change.

A note about an employer-provided life insurance policy: This option will probably be offered as part of your package. Base coverage is usually two or three times base salary up to a limit, and the opportunity to buy more insurance (following a physical exam) at a preferred rate. Certainly it is prudent to accept the free coverage, but remember that if you leave your employer, the free coverage will be lost as well as the preferred rate. Any new life insurance you get through a new employer – either the price or whether it is even offered –

would be likely be affected by any changes to your health. Considered buying insurance on your own and carrying it throughout your life. Once a person is insured, no matter what health issues develop, the policy will remain in force.

Table 5. Keys for life insurance

- Own your policy and carry it with you
- Obtain a policy while you are healthy
- Term life insurance policies are relatively inexpensive for young healthy people and a good option
- Know why you have the policy and adjust the amounts (five to 10 times take-home income) as needed
- Accept employer-offered policies but as a supplement to your own policy

Disability Insurance

Disability insurance is the most important income protection product that you can own. During a career, there is approximately a 50 percent chance that a surgeon will experience a disability that precludes performing surgery for at least 90 days or more. More than 90 percent of long-term disabilities are the result of physical illness, infection, or malignancy. The expenses involved in care and rehabilitation can be significant and place marked financial and emotional strains on families. Having a good long-term disability insurance policy can help to mitigate some of these stressors.

Short-term disability insurance often is provided by the employer. It generally has a coverage period of up to 90 days and can cover an uncomplicated postoperative period or a lingering illness. After the coverage period, the surgeon must return to work or file for long-term disability. Most policies have a waiting period of at least 90 days, and it can be months before the claim insurer has completed the evaluation and outlined the benefits.

Surgeons should buy a long-term disability insurance product as soon as possible, even in residency. The monthly benefit amount is capped as a percentage of the total salary, so this product needs to be evaluated as income increases.

The nuances of the long-term disability insurance are critical to understand. All available products from reputable insurance companies with excellent financial stability should be considered. It is important to understand the process of buying disability insurance and to ask the right questions. An independent medical insurance broker can help in this evaluation. The key provisions to understand about a policy include whether the policy is specialty-specific (for example, if you can no longer work as a vascular surgeon but can still perform other duties as a doctor, you will still want the claim to be paid); whether it pays up to a certain age or for life (preferably, the latter); whether it has an available cost of living rider (hopefully, yes); and if it is affected by another source of income (hopefully, no).

The second major factor pertains to the payment of policies with after-tax dollars. If all taxes are paid on the money before you need to use it, then no taxes are due on any of the benefits received. It should be treated not as a business deduction, but rather as personal protection coverage, just like homeowners' or rental insurance. Insure yourself for the maximal monthly benefit allowed or that which can be afforded. The carrier will impose a limit, such as 50 to 60 percent of the maximal monthly income. Once owned, the policyholder should carry it throughout their entire professional life. Again, the best rates will be available while you are healthy.

Employers may offer long-term insurance coverage for a minimal amount (for example, $1,000 a month, taxable) as a benefit with the opportunity to buy up to a higher benefit. This plan should be viewed as a supplement to the insurance already owned; it should not be viewed as the primary disability policy. Often times these are income replacement policies and have time limits. As with life insurance, the policy is only good as long as you work for that employer, and you would start over with any change.

Table 6. Disability insurance

- It is important to buy a policy from a financially stable company; use a broker to help
- Buy the maximum limit you can afford
- Increase coverage to the maximum allowable within your budget
- Buy it before any health issues; once insured it will remain in force
- Carefully compare terms, riders, stipulations, and so on; make it specialty-specific and avoid termination limits (x years); add cost of living increase options
- Pay premiums with after-tax dollars
- Own your policy and supplement with employer's policy

Umbrella Insurance

This is insurance that every high-income family should purchase. Like most insurance products, it is a hedge against an unanticipated financial claim. This insurance is an "umbrella" over the personal liability limitations outlined in the automobile and homeowners' insurance policies. Many of the standard limitations of these policies are a few hundred thousand dollars at most and can quickly be attached should the policyholder or someone in their family have an adverse incident. Understanding the potential financial responsibilities that would be encountered if someone is injured at your home or by any member of your family in a motor vehicle collision is important. The umbrella policies would protect the policyholder from paying out of pocket a large award to the plaintiff. Relatively inexpensive compared with the coverage (again because the likelihood of ever needing it is small), a policy that covers an additional $3 million to $5 million should be part of the financial portfolio.

Your Professional Financial Team

There are so many complexities associated with a medical practice and career that it requires nearly 10 years of medical school and training before a physician can start seeing patients independently. Your professional financial team should also be well-trained. Building your professional team of consultants is vital to not only maximize your financial success but also for the safety of your work in the years ahead. Besides a financial advisor, you should also have an accountant and an attorney to anchor your financial team.

Selecting a Financial Advisor

The financial advisor should be the quarterback of all financial investments. This individual should have a deep understanding of your goals, where and how all your funds are invested, anticipated sources of income, and see the entire distributive playing field for your opportunities.

Before selecting a financial advisor, have a good outline of your goals. Discuss them with your spouse, life partner, or whomever you have a lifetime bond. Carefully map out your timeframes, priorities, and needs.

Develop a list of recommended advisors and schedule interviews. They should have questions for you about your thoughts and goals. They should be a good listener – you want someone who you feel understands you and your family's unique situation. A good advisor may not have all the answers for you right away but will follow up with some excellent planning ideas. You should feel comfortable with the conversations. It would be expected that they check in with you for a review at least twice a year. Interview as many candidates necessary to find the best fit.

It is important who you choose as your financial advisor. Care and thought should be dedicated to find someone who understands you and your financial goals. Everyone's situation is unique, so take your time with this process.

Just as you should not choose a friend as your physician or surgeon, avoid individuals with whom you have a personal relationship. An investment loss, which is inevitable in the ups and downs of the stock market, may strain your relationship. It is best to have someone who is objective.

Watch for red flags, such as anyone who appears to have all the answers for you before you have had a chance to explain your situation; those who tell you that all the physicians in the area are clients, so they know what you need; or those who suggest they can achieve certain annual rates of return on your investments. A steak dinner or group seminar is not necessary to find your ideal advisor. Remember, you are looking to add a key member to your life team.

Sometimes, you may have access to a top-flight financial advisor through a direct referral from one of their clients. But most new investors do not have enough assets to have access to some financial advisors, such as those who may require a certain minimum to open an account with them. For new investors, some of the best options are not the privately held investment groups but the larger financial institutions such as Morgan Stanley, Merrill Lynch, or Schwab, which give a full range of options.

Refer to Table 7 for highlights. If things are not working as anticipated after a few years, it is important to reevaluate and, if necessary, change advisors by repeating the process. The following sites provide background on potential advisors:

- *Barrons.com/articles/top-1200-financial-advisors-america*
- *Brokercheck.finra.org*
- *Sec.gov*

Table 7. Selecting a financial advisor

- Selecting an advisor is one of the most important decisions of your life—discuss at home first
- Avoid selecting a family member or a good friend
- Have an outline of your unique situation and your goals
- Interview as many advisors as you need to feel comfortable – feel their passion
  - There is no acknowledged "Advisor Group for Physicians"
- Any recommendation should be someone with at least one financial cycle
- Do your due diligence—this is an important decision

Selecting an Accountant

Tax laws are complex, with the tax codes comprising thousands of pages. Add in the aspects of state and local taxes, personal considerations, and opportunities and you will quickly appreciate the importance of establishing a long-term relationship with an experienced accountant. It goes beyond just filing the returns once a year; rather it entails a year-round assessment of tax planning and reevaluation. Many opportunities to rearrange your accounts to maximize the tax benefits are available, keeping in mind that they can be affected by different state laws and limitations. Your accountant should be aware of potential deductions that you may not have considered. Your accountant also will know deadlines that must be met to avoid costly penalty and interest payments. Similar to selecting a financial advisor, choosing an accountant requires due diligence. Developing a long-term relationship and choosing someone who will be a good partner are important. If you have circumstances that require even more specialized input, such as dealing with foreign funds or the dissolution of family properties, then there may be an advantage to having someone associated with a larger firm, which generally has partners with specific expertise in these areas. The key point is that a good working relationship with a knowledgeable accountant will be vital to long-term financial success.

Selecting an Attorney

An attorney is the third key member of the team, not so much for day-to-day operations but rather if questions arise. Unlike the other members of the "A team," this individual may be a family member or friend. For legal questions, the primary attorney may be able to deal with the issue directly, but if not, might have a partner or a colleague for referral. Even early in your career, you should have a basic will to keep your estate out of probate and to direct assets as well as to answer questions about your wishes. Every employment contract offered should be vetted by an attorney who is well-versed in employment laws, which can vary from state to state. Even documents such as agreements with contractors for home improvement, hiring a household employee for childcare, or creating a lease document if you are renting out property should be examined for completeness and conformity with current statutes. An attorney can make these situations much easier and help avert a costly error.

Other professionals may also play specific roles at different times on your financial team, such as an independent insurance agent or someone to appraise property and valuables.

Having a strong financial team will safely provide and efficiently manage your assets. While many physicians try to manage their finances themselves, they often fall short; the adage that you get what you pay for applies here. Depending on the amount under management and the various accounts to follow, a financial advisor may cost approximately 1 to 1.5 percent annually of the amount managed. Depending on the complexity of your tax considerations and the number of forms to be filed and the hours involved, accounting fees over the year can vary from $700 to a few thousand dollars a year. Attorneys charge by the hour, so prepare everything ahead of time to keep the billings low.

Remember that taking the time to build your financial team will result in greater returns and ensure that issues are well handled, allowing more time to dedicate to practice and other interests.

Other Items to Address

There are a few items necessary to ensure protection of personal assets, note future directions, and define personal instructions.

Regardless of age, family status, health, or assets, everyone should have three basic documents. The first is an advanced directive to clarify a specific set of parameters of what an individual wants at the end of life. Life-altering events can arise that will add to the stress of an already anxious situation.

The second document is a health care power of attorney (POA). If an individual is unable to make health care decisions, then the designated surrogate will be called upon to act on their behalf and will ease and coordinate decision-making at a difficult time. The desires and parameters should be well defined for the individual who will have the POA.

The third form names a general POA to act on behalf of someone who is incapable of preforming legal or financial decisions on their own. This is an important role, often left to a close relative, who will have full access to all of the individual resources and is expected to manage them to the benefit of the incapacitated individual.

In addition, a full inventory of all the assets should be taken, including the accounts, deeds, insurance papers, and documents so the possessions can be accessed. Even items not usually considered, such as airline miles or credit card points, can be worth thousands of dollars. Other assets could include property, autos, artwork, and jewelry. Having a full list safely stored but available will help in case of an emergency. Someone should have access to all the passwords to e-mail accounts, computers, phones, and devices and all programs, cards, services, and so on, not only to keep track of valuable items (such as pictures and documents stored in the cloud), but also to redeem assets before they are lost. If these items are held in a safe or safes, the POA should have access to the combinations; they should also know about and have access to all safety deposit boxes.

There should be a list of all debts and other unfulfilled obligations, so these can be promptly addressed and satisfied. Similarly, all other major documents, digitized and physical, should be organized for easy access and password-protected. The will should be readily available, as it may outline specific instructions in case of sudden death.

Although most young surgeons and professionals may believe their life to be relatively simple in financial scope; in reality, it is often complex. Paying attention to financial health is key to a stable personal life and a productive professional career (Figure 3). It will provide security and the resources to achieve personal goals while building a nest egg for retirement. Financial stability reduces stress, reduces life's uncertainty, and provides a base for growth and future success.

Figure 3. Financial health affects quality of life

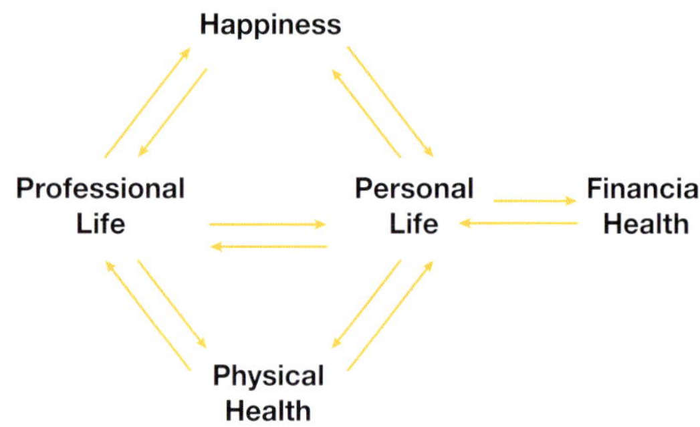

Resources to Prepare Today's Trainees for Practice

So, how do we best prepare surgical residents to face the challenges of the future? Following are suggested educational resources, as well as a series of important skills and perspectives that all residents should know and understand in order to succeed in today's environment.

Resources for Understanding the Changing Health Care Environment Today

If this chapter had been written 15 years or even 10 years ago, a third or more of surgical residents would plan to go into private practice, with the rest entering some type of employment. Today, most surgery residents seek some form of employed practice, and 60 percent to 75 percent of surgeons are employed. Roughly half of the employed surgeons are now employees of institutions or in academics, and the other half are employed by large groups of physicians.

This shift has occurred for multiple reasons, but the three main drivers are:

- **Burdens placed on surgical practices.** The challenges to maintaining a surgical practice have grown exponentially. The expense of the EHR, federal and state regulations, publicly reported quality metrics, the demands for prior approval, and challenges to recruiting new surgeons all have combined to make life in private practice more challenging. These factors, combined with the recent trend toward hospital and practice consolidations and mergers, have led to fewer surgical residents choosing to enter private practice.
- **Financial incentives now favor hospital-based practice.** Physician reimbursement from commercial and government insurers has not kept up with inflation over the last 20 years. This effect, complicated by the rising costs of running a practice, has resulted in less money for the practicing surgeon's salary and for essential resources to run a practice. In contrast, hospital reimbursement has kept pace with inflation. As a result, money that used to stay in a surgeon's practice is migrating into the coffers of health care institutions. This extra revenue then allows institutions to pay for surgeons based upon their value to the organization and competitive market forces rather than based on reimbursement for professional services.
- **Work-life balance.** Today's young surgeon wants a balance between work and personal time, preferably with some type of schedule and reasonable call expectations. Although it is possible to achieve this balance in private practice, it is easier to join a larger group of surgeons offering some form of employment.

There are many protected coves and harbors of private practice in which surgeons can and do flourish successfully. However, these niches are the exception rather than the rule today for most surgical residents.

Regardless of whether a resident picks private practice or employment, some common skills are essential to know and master in order to succeed. Understanding the business side of surgery is just as important for surgeons in employed practices as for those in private practice.

Educational Resources on Practice Management

The ACS has developed three powerful practice management resources that should form the foundation of any resident education regarding the business side of their new careers. They are as follows:

- *ACS Resources for the Practicing Surgeon, Volume I: The Employed Surgeon* (Figure 4)
- *ACS Resources for the Practicing Surgeon, Volume II: The Private Practice Surgeon* (Figure 5)
- *ACS Practice Protection Committee: Economic Survival Strategies in the COVID World*

Figure 4. ACS Resources for the Practicing Surgeon, Volume I: The Employed Surgeon

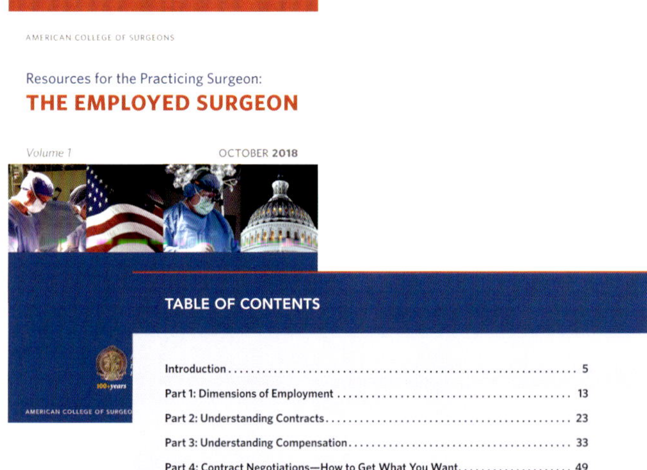

Figure 5. ACS Resources for the Practicing Surgeon, Volume II: The Private Practice Surgeon

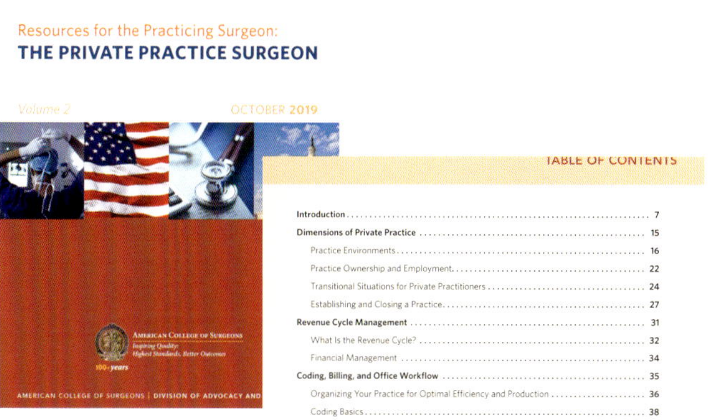
AMERICAN COLLEGE OF SURGEONS

Resources for the Practicing Surgeon:
THE PRIVATE PRACTICE SURGEON

Volume 2 OCTOBER 2019

AMERICAN COLLEGE OF SURGEONS
Inspiring Quality: Highest Standards, Better Outcomes
100+ years

AMERICAN COLLEGE OF SURGEONS | DIVISION OF ADVOCACY AND

TABLE OF CONTENTS

The first two resources describe what it is like to practice in an employed and private-practice environment and has helpful chapters on how to survive and thrive in these two different practice arrangements. No practice will be truly successful if the surgeon has financial difficulties because of poor financial planning and practices. This section incorporates information from the first two references, while the last reference outlines time-tested recommendations on how to thrive financially and professionally, especially in times of stress.

In addition, there are important and helpful resources on the ACS Division of Advocacy and Health Policy page of the ACS website. All these resources are free, available at a click of the mouse, and a benefit of your membership in the College (Table 8).

Table 8. ACS advocacy and practice management resources

- CPT coding *Bulletin* articles
- On-demand CPT coding courses
- COVID-19 practice management resources
- 2021 office/outpatient E/M visit coding changes
- ICD-10 coding
- 2020 Physicians as Assistants at Surgery Report
- ACS Coding Hotline
- Webinars
- Primers and compendiums
- Quality payment program

Where Can Residents and New Graduates Get Help with Billing and Coding?

Knowing the proper codes for both diagnoses and procedures is essential for an office or an institution. It is an error to dismiss the importance of proper documentation, what CPT code to use, or selecting the best International Classification of Diseases (ICD)-10 diagnosis code.

These skills are important for proper billing, to avoid denials, audits, and even liability issues. Chapters 2 and 3 of the *ACS Resources for the Practicing Surgeon, Volume II: The Private Practice Surgeon* include a lengthy discussion of revenue cycle, billing, and coding, which help improve understanding of how all of these critical gears work.

The ACS produces and sponsors excellent CPT and ICD-10 coding courses and publishes frequent coding updates and coding tips in the *Bulletin of the American College of Surgeons.*[11] A summary of available resources is located on the ACS website under Advocacy (Table 9). While the coding courses are fee-based, many resources, including the Coding Hotline, are offered free of charge to ACS members. Residents should be encouraged to take advantage of these resources.

Table 9. *Bulletin of the American College of Surgeons* coding articles

- Abdomen, stomach, liver, gallbladder
- Hernia
- Intestines, rectum, anus
- Breast
- Lymphatic system
- Skin, integumentary system
- Trauma and critical care
- Vascular system
- Modifiers
- Evaluation and management
- ICD-10
- Practice management

Understanding Contracts, Contract Negotiations, and Compensation Plans

Here are some common questions that residents often ask, along with suggested responses.

Q. I am considering starting practice as an employee. What do I need to know before I start looking for a place to practice?
A. There are several critical areas to know about and understand as you near the end of your surgical residency. To become employed, residents will have to search for and consider prospects, secure an offer, and then negotiate and sign a contract. Large institutions will have a fixed contract and consistent with all starting physician placements across the enterprise. Smaller institutions and group practices will typically offer more flexibility regarding some terms of the contract.

Q. What can I expect for a salary?
A. Compensation plans can vary greatly from employer to employer and from location to location; however, most plans share certain similarities across the compensation spectrum. Are you starting out with a flat salary, a base-plus-production bonus, or a pure production compensation plan? Knowing the difference between these, and then picking the right details within each type, are essential to choose an employer.

Q: How do I negotiate with a prospective employer?
A. What is a fair salary, and what should you do if they offer too little in terms of a salary, benefits, or a bonus plan? Knowing how to start—and end—negotiations will be essential to finalize a fair and equitable contract. Knowing how to ask for what you want and how to recognize what is nonnegotiable are two important skills to master before starting a job search. You should first determine nonnegotiable "asks" you have before signing a contract. You need to understand the market and be reasonable with your requests.

Q. What about benefits, retirement plans, and liability, disability, and health insurance?
A. Each institution and contracts within that institution may have a wide variability in how they address an overall benefit package for an employee. Some retirement plans are fixed, whereas others offer multiple plans. Liability insurance is a key item to ask about, especially in regard to whether or not you will need to buy "tail insurance" if you leave employment. Tail insurance is purchased to cover responsibilities for care to a patient well after the period of employment; understanding who pays for this insurance if employment ends is important. Disability insurance in a group plan is often under the control of the institution and not the employee, and many factors should be considered if you begin at one hospital and later decide to change. Some surgeons may want to consider having both a personal and a group disability plan in some circumstances.

Answers to all these questions and more are covered in parts two, three, and four of the *ACS Resources for the Practicing Surgeon, Volume I: The Employed Surgeon* as well as in the *ACS Practice Protection Committee: Economic Survival Strategies in the COVID World* monograph.

Conclusion

Understanding the complex history that has shaped the current business environment and financial landscape of surgical practice is essential to an optimal curriculum in surgery residency training. In this chapter, we presented a comprehensive overview of fundamental topics such as the U.S. health care system; academic and private practice management, including the physician payment system; personal financial management, including best practices in managing debt, savings, and investments; and various resources pertaining to the changing health care environment, billing and coding, contracts, negotiations, and compensation. It is critical for trainees to have an understanding of the larger health systems within which they operate. Equally important are sound personal financial management strategies to safeguard their earnings and financial well-being.

Suggested Readings

America's Essential Hospitals. Challenges in a changing marketplace: 1930–1965. Available at: http://essentialhospitals. org/about-americas-essential-hospitals/history-of-public-hospitals-in-the-united-states/challenges-in-a-changing-marketplace-1930-1965/. Accessed October 8, 2021.

Anderman T. What to know about narrow network health insurance plans. Consumer Reports. Available at: https://www. consumerreports.org/health-insurance/what-to-know-about-narrow-network-health-insurance-plans/. Accessed August 25, 2021.

Anderson SR, Kaplan RS. Time-driven activity-based costing. Harvard Business Review. Available at: https://hbr.org/2004/11/time-driven-activity-based-costing. Accessed August 25, 2021.

Association of American Medical Colleges. Medical school graduation questionnaire 2018 all schools summary report. Available at: https://www.aamc.org/download/490454/data/2018gqallschoolssummaryreport.pdf. Accessed October 8, 2021.

Barker SJ. Lord or vassal? Academic anesthesiology finances in 2000. *Anesthes and Analges*. 2001;93(2):294-300.

Barnes J, Abrams KJ. Funds flow in academic medical centers: moving toward a transparent and equitable funding model. Available at: https://www2.deloitte.com/content/dam/Deloitte/us/Documents/risk/us-risk-funds-flow-in-academic-medical-centers.pdf. Accessed October 8, 2021.

Becker's Hospital Review. 7 things hospitals should know about professional services agreements. Available at: https://www.beckershospitalreview.com/hospital-physician-relationships/7-things-hospitals-should-know-about-professional-services-agreements.html. Accessed August 26, 2021.

Centers for Medicare & Medicaid Services. Accountable care organizations (ACOs). Available at: https://www. cms.gov/Medicare/Medicare-Fee-for-Service-Payment/ACO. Accessed August 25, 2021.

Enders T, Conroy J. Advancing the academic health system for the future. Association of American Medical Colleges. Available at: https://www.manatt.com/uploadedFiles/Content/2_Our_People/Enders,_Thomas/AdvancingtheAcademicHealthSystemfortheFuture_AAMC_ Accessed August 26, 2021.

Gottlieb G, Dzau V, Lipstein S, Schlichting N, Washington E. Essential stewardship priorities for academic health systems. National Academy of Medicine. Available at: https://nam.edu/perspectives-2013-essential-stewardship-priorities-for-academic-health-systems/. Published June 11, 2020. Accessed August 26, 2021.

Gourevitch MN, Thorpe LE. Advancing population health at academic medical centers: a case study and framework for an emerging field. *Acad Med*. 2019;94(6):813-818.

Hauge LS, Frischknecht AC, Gauger PG, Hirshfield LE, Harkins D, Butz DA, Taheri PA. Web-based curriculum improves residents' knowledge of health care business. *J Am Coll Surg*. 2010;211(6):777-783.

Health Research & Educational Trust and Kaufman, Hall & Associates, Inc. Value-based contracting. American Hospital Association. Available at: https://www.aha.org/system/files/hpoe/Reports- HPOE/Value-Based_Contracting_KaufHall_2013.pdf. Accessed August 25, 2021.

Kenton W. Affordable Care Act (ACA). Investopedia. Available at: https://www.investopedia.com/terms/a/affordable-care-act.asp. Accessed August 25, 2021.

Kibbe MR, Troppmann C, Barnett CC Jr., et al. Effects of educational dept on career and quality of life among academic surgeons. *Ann Surg*. 2009;249(2):342-348.

Kolva DE, Barzee KA, Morley CP. Practice management residency curricula: a systematic literature review. *Fam Med Actions*. 2009;41(6):411-419.

MD Content. The Business of Health Care. Available from http://mdcontent.com. Accessed October 8, 2021.

Mizell JS, Thrush CR, Susan Steelman S. The business of medicine: a course to address the deficit in financial knowledge of fourth-year medical students. *Journal of Medical Practice Management*. 2019;34(6):344.

National Health Policy Forum. The basics: relative value units (RVUs). Available at: https://www.nhpf.org/library/details.cfm/2720. Accessed October 13, 2021.

Office of Inspector General. U.S. Department of Health and Human Services. A roadmap for new physicians: fraud & abuse laws. Available at: https://oig.hhs.gov/compliance/physician-education/. Accessed October 13, 2021.

Rotondo MF, Stites SW, Collins CT. The inevitable call for integrated academic health systems. *Becker's Hospital Review*. Available at: https://www.beckershospitalreview.com/hospital-management-administration/the-inevitable-call-for-integrated-academic-health-systems.html. Accessed August 26, 2021.

Satiani B. Business knowledge in surgeons. *Am J Surg*. 2004;188(1):13-16.

Tsai MH, Urman RD. Using time-driven activity-based costing as a key component of the value platform: a pilot analysis of colonoscopy, aortic valve replacement and carpal tunnel release procedures. *J Clin Med Res*. 2018;10(4):314-320.

University of Utah Health Sciences. What is MBM? Available at: https://www.uofuhealth.utah.edu/mbm/about.php#:~:text=MBM%20is%20a%20process%20for%20organizational%20decision-making%20that,4%20Based%20on%20timely%2C%20open%2C%20and%20accurate%20information. Accessed August 26, 2021.

What is value-based healthcare? *NEJM Catalyst*. Available at: https://catalyst.nejm.org/doi/full/10.1056/CAT.17.0558. Accessed August 25, 2021.

White FJ. Can the value proposition work in health care? *Inquiries Journal*. Available at: http://www.inquiriesjournal.com/articles/1743/can-the-value-proposition-work-in-health-care. Accessed August 25, 2021.

References

1. Royce TJ, Davenport KT, Dahle JM. A burnout reduction and wellness strategy: personal financial health for the medical trainee and early career radiation oncologist. *Pract Radiat Oncol*. 2019;9(4):231-238.
2. Cantor JC, Baker LC, Hughes RG. Preparedness for practice. Young physicians' views of their professional education. *JAMA*. 1993;270(9):1035-1040.
3. Jones K, Lebron RA, Mangram A, Dunn E. Practice management education during surgical residency. *Am J Surg*. 2008;196(6):878-881; discussion 881-882.
4. Lusco VC, Martinez SA, Polk HC Jr. Program directors in surgery agree that residents should be formally trained in business and practice management. *Am J Surg*. 2005;189(1):11-13.
5. Ahmad FA, White AJ, Hiller KA, Amini R, Jeffe DB. An assessment of residents' and fellows' personal finance literacy: an unmet medical education need. *Int J Med Educ*. 2017;29(8):192-204.
6. Mizell JS, Berry KS, Kimbrough MK, Bentley FR, Clardy JA, Turnage RH. Money matters: a resident curriculum for financial management. *J Surg Res*. 2014;192(2):348-355.
7. Rice T, et al. United States of America: health system review. *Health Systems in Translation*. 2013;15(3):27.
8. Porter ME. What is value in healthcare? *N Engl J Med*. 2010;363:2477-2481.
9. Berwick DM, Nolan TW, Whittington J. The triple aim: care, health, and cost. *Health Aff* (Millwood). 2008;27(3):759-769.
10. Association of American Medical Colleges and Manatt Health. *Next-Generation Funds Flow Models: Enhancing Academic Health System Alignment*. October 2018.
11. American College of Surgeons. CPT coding *Bulletin* articles. Available at: https://www.facs.org/advocacy/practmanagement/cpt. Accessed October 8, 2021.

AMERICAN C
SURGEONS A
OF SURGEON
COLLEGE OF
AMERICAN C
SURGEONS A
OF SURGEON
COLLEGE OF
AMERICAN C
SURGEONS A

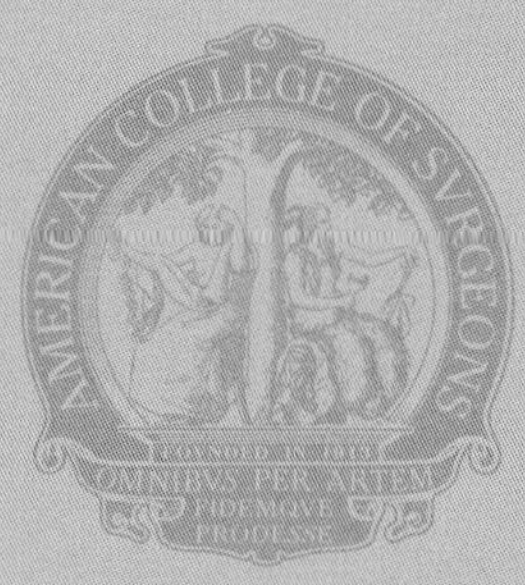

CHAPTER 11
The Surgeon as Advocate

Lead Author

Andrew L. Warshaw, MD, FACS, FRCSEd(Hon), MAMSE

Co-Authors

Patrick V. Bailey, MD, MLS, FACS

Frank G. Opelka, MD, FACS

Amy E. Liepert, MD, FACS

Christian Shalgian

Gary L. Timmerman, MD, FACS, MAMSE

CHAPTER 11

The Surgeon as Advocate

Executive Summary

This chapter explains why surgeon advocacy training has become essential in today's health care environment. The content is designed to present the critical curricular elements for trainers and trainees. Herein, we answer the following questions:

- What is surgeon advocacy, and what are some examples?
- How does research affect the development of public policy?
- How does the American College of Surgeons (ACS) develop its policy positions and legislative agenda?
- How does the government implement policy?
- What is the role of surgeon advocates?
- What resources are available to surgeon advocates?

What Is Surgeon Advocacy?

Physician advocacy has been defined as an action that a physician takes to promote those social, economic, educational, and political changes that ameliorate the suffering and threats to human health and well-being that are identified through professional work and expertise. Surgical advocacy is an act of support or recommendation for a particular policy or cause by an individual or group to have a preferred policy adopted. To support a position, an advocate should know the relevant health policy and the public officials who make the rules related to that policy. To influence the policy outcome, an advocate should understand the position of those parties with competing interests and disparate goals and be open to bargaining with them to arrive at a meaningful compromise.

Historically, physicians considered involvement in politics inappropriate, bordering on unprofessional. However, in recent decades, greater involvement from professionals has become imperative to promoting access to care, quality of care, and patient safety. Decisions made by policymakers, those who set regulations, or by those who draft and pass legislation, cannot be fully informed without input from the people who are most directly involved in the care and medical decision-making of the patients—the providers.

Today, an integral part of a surgeon's professional responsibility is to advocate on behalf of patients. Paramount to the surgeon's mission is to ensure patient access to quality surgical care in an environment conducive to the practice of surgery. To accomplish this goal, surgeons have a responsibility to advocate for the necessary health policies. It is that simple.

Although effective surgeon advocacy has many components, the unifying thread is to build relationships with other surgeons, other medical professionals (and their organizations), payors, state and federal legislators and regulators, members of the state and federal executive agencies, and the media (Table 1).

Table 1. Advocacy as a spectrum

- Patient Advocacy
  - Optimal care of an individual patient or family
- Local Advocacy
  - Addressing a hospital system or community issue, such as fall prevention and immunization
- State Advocacy
  - State laws, budgets, such as health funding and scope of practice
- Federal Advocacy
  - National issues, such as Medicare, physician payment, Medicaid, and expansion of the Affordable Care Act

Examples of Advocacy Efforts at Different Levels
Example 1. J. Patrick Walker, MD, FACS, a Texas surgeon, helped to pass the Uniform Emergency Volunteer Health Act (UEVHA) in his state. States enacting this bill recognize the licensure of physicians and health practitioners from other states during a declared emergency if those health care professionals have registered with a public or private registration system. Dr. Walker's efforts were conducted over the course of three legislative cycles, and included visiting regularly with legislators, answering questions from the governor's office and state agency heads, and identifying an excellent legislator to champion the bill.

Example 2. Lenworth M. Jacobs, Jr., MD, FACS, a trauma surgeon in Connecticut, recognized deficiencies in the initial response to the 2012 mass shooting of children at Sandy Hook Elementary School. Existing procedures called for immediate cordoning off the site, which limited first responder access to the wounded, potentially delaying lifesaving care. He formed a coalition of medical first responders, surgeons, law enforcement representatives, and military trauma experts, which helped develop an improved approach to managing a mass shooting event with an active shooter. This led to the question of what could be done before first responders arrive. The coalition's answer, a program to teach laypeople how to stop bleeding before paramedics arrive, was viewed as analogous to teaching cardiopulmonary resuscitation to ordinary citizens. This led to a national STOP THE BLEED® campaign led by the American College of Surgeons (ACS) Committee on Trauma, to provide training for the public and elected officials on methods to control hemorrhage following injury.

Example 3. In its effort to control the growth of Medicare spending for physician services, Congress enacted the Sustainable Growth Rate (SGR) as part of the Balanced Budget Act of 1997. Though designed to anticipate some increases in fee-for-service payments to physicians and a rise in the number of Medicare beneficiaries, the overall goal of the policy was to reduce fee-for-service physician payment rates. For most of the following 17 years, the growth rate of Medicare expenditures exceeded the target as outlined under the SGR. As a result, the Centers for Medicare & Medicaid Services (CMS) consistently sought to reduce Medicare fee-for-service payment rates for physician services. However, concerns about reduced reimbursement for physicians and reduced access to care for patients led to political pressure brought to bear each year by the ACS, other physician groups, and patient/beneficiary organizations, which resulted in Congress enacting a series of temporary reimbursement adjustments ("doc fixes") to prevent the cuts from taking effect. Because the annual "fix" did not alter the underlying SGR formula, the divergence between "doc fixes" payments and those called for by the formula continued to widen, ultimately leading to potential payment reductions of more than 20 percent. For more than a decade, SGR repeal was the top priority issue for the ACS and most other physician groups; this persistent, specific advocacy, which included working with congressional champions, including the House "Doc Caucus", ultimately led Congress to repeal the SGR in 2015.

Development of ACS Health Policy Positions and Legislative Agenda

The ACS has long been a leader for the surgical profession when it comes to health care advocacy.

The ACS Division of Advocacy and Health Policy (DAHP) was created to address rapidly changing and increasingly expensive health care, and to develop and influence policies and endeavors affecting surgeons and surgical patients. This came at a time of congressional efforts to impose greater financial regulation and initiatives to create managed health care networks and/or national health care systems. The division is staffed with a director, two medical directors, a regulatory affairs section, a quality section, health policy expertise, and lobbyists who work with federal legislative and regulatory staff, as well as a state affairs team that supports state-level legislative and regulatory efforts.

To ensure strategic direction and input from ACS fellows and leadership, the Health Policy and Advocacy Group (HPAG) is composed of ACS fellows, governors, and regents. HPAG scrutinizes and sets targeted priorities and goals on many topics broadly related to health care and the profession of surgery, from E/M (evaluation and management) codes to the federal Affordable Care Act (ACA) to telemedicine. Integral with HPAG is the Legislative Committee, which is responsible for identifying, evaluating, and recommending positions on federal legislation and policy issues before Congress that may affect the needs, interests, and roles of surgeons and surgical patients.

Because so many topics are still "local," the ACS formed the Health Policy and Advisory Council (HPAC) to address state legislation and policy issues. This committee helps direct a grassroots advocacy network throughout the ACS membership and state chapters. Councilors from this committee convey the message of the ACS to Fellows and members using their firsthand expertise on local/regional legislation, politics, and regulatory issues and then convey responses from the local Fellows back to the College.

Under the ACS structure, the Regents, Governors, Advisory Councils, Young Fellows Association (YFA), and Resident and Associate Society (RAS) all contribute to advocacy efforts. Each group has health policy committees that work with DAHP and HPAG.

Advocacy is one of five pillars, or principal activities, of the ACS Governors. ACS Fellows serve as advocates for their patients, practice, and community. The ACS often asks Fellows to contact their local and federal legislators, especially those with whom they have a personal relationship.

Legislative teams in DAHP are led by a surgeon medical director with a background in interpreting and writing legislation. These team members are registered lobbyists who understand the legislative structure, processes, the committees and calendars, as well as consensus building. Their roles are tied to the legislative and oversight functions of the Congress with work in both the House and the Senate. Each chamber has its own, distinct legislative process and follows its own intricate rules and procedures. To stay informed on which topics may arise as part of the legislative process, ACS staff members rely on their relationships with congressional committee staffs.

Stopping unfavorable legislation is as important as supporting favorable legislation. With each election the majority party may shift, which may change leadership and control of congressional committees and the overall legislative agenda. As a result, the ACS legislative team must appear party-neutral to maintain access to the congressional staff and to effectively represent surgeons and surgical patients.

To further resolve and commit to the College's political agenda, the ACS Professional Association (ACSPA) created a political action committee (PAC). The ACSPA-*Surgeons*PAC provides financial support to elect congressional candidates who support and can advocate for the College's legislative issues. Because it is difficult for elected representatives or senators to track, comprehend, and take a position on all the issues before them, congressional staffers keep them informed about the legislative agenda. As a result, relationships with the congressional staffers are vital to the ACS legislative team. The ACS uses various means to encourage its members to become involved in advocacy. One of the most prominent is offering the ACS Leadership & Advocacy Summit each spring in Washington, DC. Over the course of several days, members, as well as congressional staff, government leaders from health care agencies, and members of Congress are exposed to a robust program on surgical leadership and an informative and thought-provoking advocacy agenda. The Advocacy Summit culminates in prearranged visits on Capitol Hill to the offices of representatives and senators from the states of each attending member. The summit is also an opportunity to meet and network with other ACS Fellows.

Research and Development of Health Policy Positions

Health policy and health services research informs federal and state agencies as they craft the legislative and regulatory aspects of U.S. health care, serving as the basis for developing the legislation, rules, and regulations needed to manage health care (Table 2).

Table 2. Policy domains

- Payment
- Health insurance
- Quality
- Data: interoperability and curation
- Price transparency
- Professional liability
- Workforce burnout
- Privacy
- Care models
- Employment of physicians

As a result, health policy affects almost every aspect of health care delivery. Policy implications manifest in clinical domains, such as the funding for cancer research, trauma centers, bariatric surgery centers, alternative payment models, and so forth. Policy affects the availability for screening and prevention efforts. Policy defines the resources used in care models and the care environment. Policy has an impact on the data models used to track and inform care. Policy addresses the affordability of care. Policy calls out the importance of patient goals of care and end-of-life decisions. Policy and advocacy go hand in hand to define and support optimal care.

Each new medical advance creates issues of cost, access to care, quality, and appropriateness of care. Because organizations and individuals often oppose policies that affect the delivery of care, surgeons must understand the interaction between policy, the processes for achieving policy goals, and the methods for implementing them.

- **Key definitions**
  - **Policy** is a course or principle of action adopted or proposed by a government, political party, business or other interest group, or an individual.
  - **Process** is a series of actions or steps to achieve an end goal, such as formulating public policy. Policymaking typically involves interaction between social groups and political institutions or between political leadership and public opinion.

- **Politics** are the activities associated with governance that involves the competition or relations among individuals or parties with different overall priorities or perspectives on issues, or between individuals or parties that aspire to achieve power. Politics is the means of affecting the process to realize a policy goal.

Policy development begins with defining the issues that need consideration and prioritizing them. Research is then used to clarify and deepen understanding of key health policy issues and frame them for action. A well-framed issue or problem becomes a strategic initiative, which may then require more research. It also can serve as the foundation for creating a policy position and public statement. Policy positions and public statements can help frame further action either through regulatory or legislative action. Moving a proposed policy into action requires a detailed concept design, which includes defining what success looks like, and an implementation strategy, which includes measuring the impact of the policy if it is successfully implemented. Successful implementation requires that barriers and burdens be lifted or moved. Thus, good policymaking is more than just a statement—it is a process.

Policy research and development are intense academic exercises that require significant resources to be effective. Once a law becomes statute, it is published in the *Federal Register* and is interpreted by federal policymakers, who advise how the statute can be implemented through rules. These rules are the legal implementation of the statute; essentially, they are the law. Proposed rules are published and public comment is solicited before they become a final rule. The comments are tabulated, and each receives a published response in the final rule. Regulatory personnel track several federal agencies, typically those in the Department of Health and Human Services (HHS), that publish these rules and prepare comments pertinent to surgical patients and surgeons. These agencies include the Centers for Medicare & Medicaid Services (CMS), the Centers for Disease Control and Prevention (CDC), the Food and Drug Administration (FDA), the Office of the National Coordinator (ONC), the National Institutes of Health (NIH), and the Agency for Health Research and Quality (AHRQ). The topics covered include care models; insurance coverage; access to care; quality; payment; health information technology (IT); research; clinical areas of focus, such as cancer or trauma; implantable devices; and medications. Rules range from broad generalities about health policy to health care informatics.

Policy institutes and academic centers at major universities help inform health policy. Policy institutes abound in Washington, DC, and many focus on health care, quality, or economics. Examples include the Commonwealth Fund, the Kaiser Foundation, the Peterson Foundation, and the Robert Wood Johnson Foundation. Some of these entities hire research analysts, whereas others award grants to analysts. Some entities are quasi-government organizations receiving most of their support from federal funds, such as the National Quality Forum. In addition, the role of the health care sector in our economy is an area of interest for major universities, including Harvard, Brandeis, Johns Hopkins, Duke, Stanford, and Northwestern universities. Large health care delivery systems also sponsor policy centers or institutes, such as the Mayo Clinic's Kern Center.

These institutes and centers offer grants to explore specific areas of health policy research. They sponsor educational symposia and publish articles and reports about major challenges and solutions in health care.

How Advocates Choose Their Battles

ACS Fellows may find specific issues important depending on whether they are employed or self-employed, work at an academic medical center or a community hospital, and so on. But core issues that affect all surgeons and their patients should always be kept in focus. Surgeons also should be willing to act on behalf of other surgeon specialties and practice arrangements even if the issue does not affect their specialty or practice model. In addition, the ACS and other surgical societies may ask surgeons to advocate for a view that contradicts that of their institution or employer. If a surgeon's personal political views differ with the politics of an employer or academic institution, the surgeon should choose a position carefully.

At its best, politics is the art of reaching a compromise suitable to both sides of an issue or concern. Skilled legislators attempt to achieve their party's or constituents' goals through negotiation, debate, and, ultimately, consensus. The endpoint of deliberations is a compromise acceptable to both sides, not one in which one side wins to the detriment of the other. Furthermore, goals achieved through negotiations often serve as starting points for future opportunities or next steps. In the end, the outcome should reflect true compromise that maintains the ongoing mutual respect between the participants.

Extreme partisanship in recent years has made such compromise increasingly rare, but it is still possible. The ACS recently took on the politically charged, divisive issue of gun ownership versus gun control. One side argues that guns equal personal freedom and safety, whereas the other maintains that guns limit personal freedom and represent violence. Given that firearm injuries directly affect surgeons and their patients, the ACS deliberated its role in the debate about firearm injury prevention, considering the following advocacy options:

- Defend and support Second Amendment rights and gun owners
- Promote increased gun control measures
- Remain tacit on the topic
- Seek consensus or compromise on this controversial issue

The College chose to seek consensus based on the principle that all surgeons could accept—reduce firearm injury and death. ACS leadership on both sides of the issue authored a list of nine potential action steps and conducted three separate surveys with the COT, the Board of Governors, and the Fellows of the College. Although ACS Fellows surveyed had opposing views on personal gun ownership, much like the public, most agreed on more than half of the nine proposals. Then a Firearm Strategic Taskforce (FAST) group, comprising firearm-owning surgeons, was created to deliberate on firearm-related injuries and prevention. The conclusions of the FAST workgroup and the ACS leadership initiatives resulted in open and constructive dialogue, leading to support for increased public safety, safer firearm storage with enhanced personal responsibility for gun owners, greater awareness and enforcement of existing gun laws and regulations, and the promotion of innovation and greater weapon safety technology. The collective result fostered consensus recommendations regarding "strategies and tactics to increase firearm safety, reduce the probability of mass shootings, reduce firearm-associated violence, address mental health factors, and encourage federally funded firearm injury research while preserving the right to own and use a firearm."[1] Both sides agreed that their interests were well represented.

Government Implementation of New Policy

Government develops and implements health care policy through Congress and its key committees and government agencies tasked with rulemaking. Following is a description of how that process works.

How Congress Enacts and Oversees Health Care Policy

Health care-related legislation in Congress comes under the primary jurisdiction of five committees—two in the Senate and three in the House of Representatives. They are the Senate Finance Committee, the Senate Health, Education, Labor and Pensions Committee (HELP), the House Committee on Ways and Means, the House Committee on Energy and Commerce, and the House Committee on Education and Labor.

All health care-related legislation passes through at least one House committee and one Senate committee before being considered by each entire body. Many times, the content of the legislation and overlapping jurisdictions based on that content requires committees in the House and the Senate to hold hearings.

In addition to holding hearings and passing legislation, the committees also oversee executive branch agencies (HHS, and so on) that implement legislation. These committees of jurisdiction frequently hold oversight hearings in which members of the administration testify. Here is a brief description of each of the five committees and their specific jurisdiction related to health care matters:

- **The Senate Finance Committee** focuses on taxation and other revenue measures generally; bonded debt of U.S. Customs; reciprocal trade agreements; tariff and import quotas and related matters; the deposit of public funds and health programs under the Social Security Act, including Medicare, Medicaid, as well as the Social Security program itself; the Children's Health Insurance Program (CHIP); Temporary Assistance to Needy Families (TANF); and other HHS programs financed by a specific tax or trust fund.
- **The Senate HELP Committee** has jurisdiction over most of the agencies, institutes, and programs of the HHS, including the FDA, CDC, NIH, the Administration on Aging, the Substance Abuse and Mental Health Services Administration, and AHRQ. The HELP Committee's jurisdiction also includes most federal labor and employment laws, including the Employee Retirement Income Security Act (ERISA) which governs most health benefits provided through employers.
- **The House Committee on Ways and Means** is the chief tax-writing committee in the House of Representatives. The committee derives much of its jurisdiction from Article I, Section VII of the U.S. Constitution, which declares, "All Bills for raising Revenue shall originate in the House of Representatives." In addition to revenue, it exercises jurisdiction over tariffs, reciprocal trade agreements, the bonded debt of the U.S., and revenue-related aspects of the Social Security and Medicare programs.
- **The House Committee on Energy and Commerce** has the broadest jurisdiction of any authorizing committee in Congress. It legislates and provides oversight on a range of issues, including health care; mental health and substance abuse; health insurance (including Medicare and Medicaid); biomedical research; and food, drug, device, and cosmetic safety. Other related issues in this committee range from environmental protection to interstate and foreign commerce.
- **The House Committee on Education and Labor** oversees education and workforce programs from job training through retirement, including relationships between employers and employees such as the National Labor Relations Act, the Bureau of Labor Statistics, and employment-related health and retirement security, including but not limited to pension benefits, health insurance, and the Employee Retirement Income Security Act (ERISA).

Hence, surgeon advocates need to develop personal relationships with lawmakers and the congressional staff who serve on these committees to bring issues important to surgeons and patients forward.

How Government Agencies Implement Health Policy
Many government agencies are responsible for implementing health policy. Most of these entities fall under the jurisdiction of HHS, including CMS, CDC, FDA, ONC, NIH, and AHRQ. These agencies are funded through the budget process. The process begins with the executive branch. Each agency proposes a budget as part of an overall federal budget. The federal budget undergoes Senate and House review and often is amended before a final budget is passed and signed by the president.

The House Appropriations Committee determines the level of funding, up to the maximum expenditure of the authorized budget. Each HHS agency has its own budgetary authority and appropriations process, with the Senate and House determining the final amount authorized for each agency. Finally, the House approves the expenditure by releasing funds through its appropriations responsibility.

For those who track health care policies, these agencies are the main sources of information. Specifically, information on policies related to payment and access to care comes from CMS; implantable devices and medication, FDA; population health and disease prevention, CDC; and federal research grants, NIH.

Each year, these agencies sponsor several open forums and listening sessions related to their policy areas. Successful advocates build relationships with deputies and directors within these agencies. By working with agency staff to define challenges and problems and frame possible solutions before a rule or regulation becomes final, these relationships help advocates be proactive rather than reactive to policy.

How States Implement Health Policy
States have departments of health that report to the governor. Like those at the federal level, state policies, rules, and regulations begin in a legislative body. The statutes are framed into rules and regulations published in each state. In addition, states control the regulations for commercial insurance products for health care. To handle the complexities of health care and the interface between federal and state programs, states typically have a specialist, such as a state health insurance commissioner.

States work closely with federal programs, particularly on Medicaid expansion under the ACA. Some states have relatively few uninsured patients, and their Medicaid programs are well-funded, whereas other states overflow with uninsured (or underinsured) patients and lack the resources for an adequate Medicaid program. Surgeon advocates support policy actions that provide the most support for patients and their physicians while respecting the limits of the state resources.

States can serve as a testing ground for federal legislation. For example, the Massachusetts Health Care Reform law developed by then-Gov. Mitt Romney was a precursor to the ACA. Other policy actions deal with scope of practice for nonphysician providers, such as optometrists seeking expanded privileges under their licenses or nurse anesthetists seeking independence from anesthesiologists. Once a policy is enacted in one state, other states often track the impact and consider their own actions.

As a result, surgeon advocates should develop relationships with state lawmakers and the staff who serve on these committees, as well as the state agencies relevant to health care policymaking.

Rulemaking: Putting Policy into Effect
Once Congress has passed and the president has signed a law, it is up to the various agencies within the executive branch to develop rules and regulations to put the new legislation into effect. The Administrative Procedure Act (APA), enacted in 1946, governs the process in which federal agencies propose, develop, and issue regulations. It also grants federal courts oversight over actions taken by federal agencies.

The APA applies both to federal executive departments and independent agencies, serving as a "constitution" for administrative law and a "bill of rights" for those parties who are regulated by the federal government. Under the APA, the public must be kept informed about the organization, procedures, and rules of federal agencies, and individuals and public entities must have the opportunity to provide written comments on an agency's proposed rules and rulemaking process. The APA allows people or organizations to ask for judicial review regarding adverse impact of agency actions, including the issuance of policy statements, licenses, and permits.

Rulemaking Activities
The Federal Register, originated in 1936, is generally divided into three large sections: Rules and Regulations, Proposed Rules, and Notices. It publishes rules and regulations promulgated by federal agencies, proposed rules and regulations, all presidential proclamations and executive orders, and other documents, such as notices of meetings, agency collection activities, applications, and policy statements.

As a result, surgeon advocates have the opportunity to get involved in the rulemaking process as early as possible. For example, the College's DAHP submits formal written comments to various federal agencies in response to proposed rules. These comments cover health policy topics spanning physician reimbursement, quality, price transparency, hospital policies that affect surgery, privacy, digital health, and more. DAHP staff and medical directors also develop relationships with representatives from federal agencies to influence policies before, during, and after they are formally proposed. DAHP staff work closely with ACS committees and Fellows to understand the membership's needs and to effectively advocate on their behalf with federal administrators.

Surgeon advocates can achieve success either through reaching a desired legislative or regulatory goal or by preventing an unfavorable policy, regulation, or law. For example, through a long-maintained campaign, the ACS convinced CMS to sustain the 90-day global fees that pay for surgical procedures.

Lobbying: How It Works

Sean's Law: How a Surgeon Advocate and a Grieving Family Help Pass an ATV Law

A Personal Story from Dr. Peter Masiakos

In late October 2006, eight-year-old Sean Kearney sustained a severe brain injury in an all-terrain vehicle (ATV) accident and died three days later.

His parents, Mark and Katie Kearny, asked Sean's physician, Peter Masiakos, MD, FACS, a pediatric general and thoracic surgeon at Mass General, for help to enact legislation that would prevent children from incurring the injuries Sean sustained. Dr. Masiakos agreed.

First, the Kearneys and Dr. Masiakos searched for evidence to illustrate why this was an important problem. They found that in 2004–2005, 935 pediatric ATV-related injuries were recorded in Massachusetts—approximately 30 percent of all reported ATV injuries, according to the Massachusetts Department of Public Health. The average age of the injured child was just older than 13 years of age. Of these injuries, 309 required surgery and 206 required intensive care unit (ICU) admissions. Hospital charges for the 35 severe head injuries totaled $2.3 million, which included only the acute costs.

Next, faced with strong industry opposition to new legislation, surgeon advocates needed to educate the legislators about the dangers that ATVs pose to children and to dispel the misinformation circulated by the ATV lobby. The medical literature was used to inform legislators about how injury prevention would not only save lives, but also save a great deal of money.

By the summer of 2008, the family and Dr. Masiakos had met with key state legislators, including the President of the Senate and the Chair of the Joint Committee on Transportation. Together, they drafted a comprehensive bill that improved rider safety, protected private property and public land, and safeguarded sensitive natural resources.

Over the next few years, the Kearneys and Dr. Masiakos met with almost every member of the state legislature to tell Sean's story. By the end of 2008, every major medical center in Massachusetts, the state medical society, the Massachusetts Chapter of the ACS, the American Academy of Pediatrics, the American Academy of Orthopaedic Surgeons, Safe Kids USA, the Brain Injury Association of Massachusetts, and the Massachusetts Association of Health Plans had endorsed this legislation. By the summer of 2009, the ATV bill had bipartisan support in the state House, with 22 members in both branches of government and in both parties cosponsoring it.

On July 31, 2010, after nearly four years and two legislative sessions, an act to regulate the use of off-highway and recreation vehicles, or "Sean's Law" as it would be known, was passed. It provides stricter safeguards for the use of ATVs by prohibiting children under the age of 14 from operating ATVs.

Since inadequately treated concussion causes potential long-term cognitive and medical consequences, a second law followed, An Act Relative to Safety Regulations for School Athletic Programs. Further, high school athletic programs now must have staff trained in concussion awareness. Students suspected of having a concussion will need written medical clearance before returning to play.

Lobbying

Lobbying is the use of persuasive communication by special interest groups to influence actions, policies or decisions of legislators, congressional staff, regulators, and other government actors. Lobbying for health care issues may be done by individual surgeons or by professional organizations, such as the ACS.

The ACS sometimes hires professional lobbyists in its advocacy efforts. These lobbyists, who are often former congressional staff, communicate on a daily basis with congressional staff of committees or of members of the House and Senate. Their activities are closely regulated by the Lobbying Disclosure Act of 1995, which requires quarterly reports detailing who the individual lobbyist spoke to, what they discussed, and related expenses.

Those who promote change or advance an idea through legislation must understand the audience most affected by it if they are to be effective. Therefore, local or regional issues are addressed by grassroots or local advocates, whereas grand or sweeping initiatives are often better considered by federal or national advocates.

If knowledgeable invested experts, such as surgeons, do not help inform the decisions of legislators and regulators, health care will be adversely affected. Hence, surgeons, who are respected and esteemed as experts, have a prime opportunity to influence policy. Communication with legislators' offices can directly influence their actions. Although direct personal contact is most effective, phones calls, letters, or electronic messages can influence lawmakers because they are typically entered into a database that tabulates positions taken by constituents. Legislative offices use these data to gauge constituent interest and positions.

Effective surgeon advocates engage lawmakers and their staffers regularly over a long time. These relationships cannot develop when a specific crisis arises. Also, although it is good to visit the Capitol Hill offices of individual representatives and senators as part of the ACS Leadership & Advocacy Summit each spring, more is needed to establish a relationship with lawmakers and staffers that is akin to a relationship with colleagues and friends. Ultimately, lawmakers and staff should view the surgeon advocate as a constituent who is a reliable resource and expert on health care-related issues.

To influence someone, it is necessary to understand their perspective and what motivates them. To do this, surgeons must draw out and listen to the views of legislators and their staff and incorporate that knowledge into their "pitch" or "ask."

Aside from attending the ACS Leadership & Advocacy Summit, other ways to stay in contact with representatives and their staff include sending e-mails, making phone calls, and arranging personal visits. Also, most legislators host regular in-district meetings and fundraisers throughout the year, at which constituents can actively engage with legislators. Surgeons should encourage others to participate in these events with them. Through these opportunities, surgeons can develop a relationship with lawmakers and staff, who will view them as a valuable resource.

After contacting legislators, surgeons should inform the staff in the ACS DAHP of the contact, what was said, and what was learned. This feedback will help ACS lobbyists tailor their message and gain the support of representatives and senators.

Tools and Resources

Building a Coalition

One of the most effective ways to advocate for an issue is to find common ground with other organizations and build a coalition around those common interests. The ACS has led many efforts in this regard, recently organizing the Surgical Care Coalition, which actively campaigned and successfully curtailed reimbursement cuts that directly threatened provider finances and patient access to care. Critical to coalition success are the reputations of coalition members among legislators or regulators. As an organization, the ACS is extraordinarily effective as measured by respect, access, and credibility. Surgeons concerned about local or regional issues should consider developing or joining a coalition at the local level.

ACS Resources

The ACS regularly provides information about legislative issues relevant to surgeons through online communications including the Advocacy Community (daily), *Bulletin Brief* (each Tuesday), the *Advocacy Brief* (every other Thursday), and the monthly *Bulletin*. Perhaps the easiest way to get involved is online with *Surgeons*Voice.org. This comprehensive website educates surgeons about the issues and how to take action by contacting their individual members of the House and Senate. The electronic communications sent through SurgeonsVoice.org have an impact, usually receiving a response from the relevant senator and representative.

Periodically, the ACS requests members to express support of ACS policy positions to their congressional representatives and senators. This semi-automated process may require only e-mailing a prepared message or calling the legislator's office. The more members who participate in this process, the greater the impact.

The RAS-ACS, the YFA, and local ACS state chapters offer numerous opportunities for involvement. The RAS Advocacy and Issues Committee meets monthly to offer their perspectives or raise concerns to the College. They also sponsor an annual essay competition that culminates in a RAS Symposium yearly at ACS Clinical Congress. Surgical specialty societies (such as the Society for Surgery of the Alimentary Tract) also have legislative committees to address health care concerns and may work with ACS and other societies as part of a surgical coalition.

Local ACS chapter meetings enable surgeon advocates to discuss state and federal advocacy issues with chapter leaders, who are often well-versed in the issues. Residents or young surgeons may find opportunities for leadership positions in the RAS and YFA sections of their state chapter or the national subcommittees. Local ACS chapters often have relationships with their state medical society, which may serve as the voice of medical community at-large. Acting with the state medical society amplifies influence on state and federal representatives. In addition, state chapters and/or medical societies often host physician-specific legislative action days at the state capitol, providing an opportunity to participate with colleagues on local and state advocacy agendas. The ACS provides grants to support state legislative action days.

Another opportunity exists for surgeons to invite their state and federal legislators to tour their hospital or facility during an in-district work period. Senators and representatives often welcome the opportunity to tour a hospital or facility in their area, as does the hospital administration, which will help arrange them. The visits, which may include a tour of the trauma center, the burn unit, the surgical ICU, the operating room facilities, or the clinic, offer surgeons a significant amount of time to interact with their elected official, offering them the chance to frame and deliver their message. Surgeons interested in learning about advocacy should identify a mentor who is typically open to collaborating with surgeons interested in health policy and advocacy.

Levels of Advocacy Engagement

There are several levels of advocacy engagement.

- Engaged:
  - Partial active: Read summarized info provided by experts, make limited legislative contact through calls, e-mails. May schedule in-district meetings. PAC contributor.
  - Full active: Engage in the above activities and seeks primary sources of information. Make personal contact with legislators through in-district meetings, fundraisers, personal contact, and legislative resource. Invite or encourage others to participate. Provide feedback at organizational level (ACS and/or corporate). Approach and engage others.
- Passive: Write letters (automatic e-mails), phone calls, may attend meetings. May make PAC contribution.
- Absent (lack of engagement): Aware advocacy is happening but does not participate.
- Disengaged: Purposefully avoids, may criticize, or detract.

Political Advocacy in a Nutshell

- It's a marathon (not a sprint)
- Expect opposition (different agendas)
- Base credibility on values (not rewards)
- Use stories (with emotional impact)
- Build relationships (find allies)
- Be realistic (set realistic expectations about outcomes)

Conclusion

Until recent years, surgeons and trainees considered involvement in political activities to be a personal rather than a professional obligation. However, as the health care sector grew from a cottage industry to an industrial complex with a greater impact on the U.S. economy, all stakeholders, including the government, physicians, patients, private payors, medical centers, and more, began seeking innovative ways to control health care spending while expanding access to quality care. It became increasingly apparent that if your voice was not heard, it would be much more difficult to sustain a viable practice.

The ACS DAHP has grown into a well-respected, proactive advocacy organization that represents all surgical specialties and the interests of surgical patients. But health care policymakers need to hear the stories of surgeon and surgical patient advocates who deal with the day-to-day realities of how surgical care is delivered.

Surgical educators are strongly encouraged to expose trainees to the advocacy process and the fundamentals of how our government works. The ACS offers stipends for residents and fellows who are interested in attending the Leadership & Advocacy Summit and a scholarship for individuals interested in attending an immersive program at Brandeis University. Together, we can ensure that surgical patients receive the care they deserve and that surgeons are properly represented in Washington, DC.

Reference

1. Talley CL, Campbell BT, Jenkins DH, et al. Recommendations from the American College of Surgeons Committee on Trauma's Firearm Strategy Team (FAST) Workgroup: Chicago Consensus I. *J Am Coll Surg*. 2019;228(2):198-206.

AMERICAN C
SURGEONS A
OF SURGEON
COLLEGE OF
AMERICAN C
SURGEONS A
OF SURGEON
COLLEGE OF
AMERICAN C
SURGEONS A

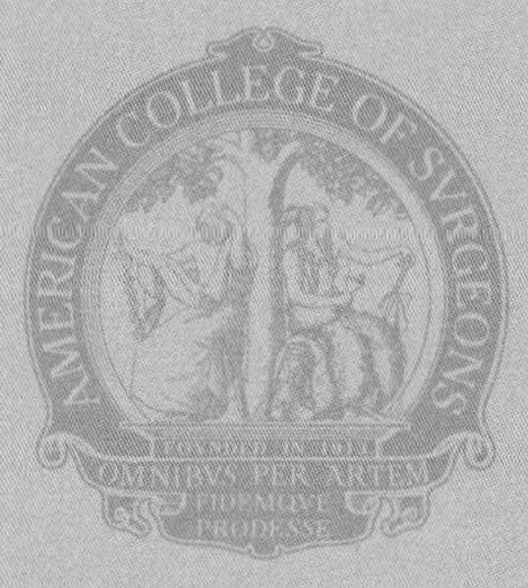

CHAPTER 12
Curriculum: Assessment and Evaluation Resources

Lead Author
John D. Mellinger, MD, FACS

Co-Authors
Thomas H. Cogbill, MD, FACS
Gerald M. Fried, MD, FACS, FRCSC, FCAHS, MCS
Paola Fata, MD
Daniel J. Vargo, MD, FACS

CHAPTER 12

Curriculum: Assessment and Evaluation Resources

Executive Summary

This chapter explores new strategies for assessing the progress residents are making in advancing their surgical technical skills, cognitive abilities, and professional competencies. The authors answer the following questions, among others:

- How are residency programs structured to ensure graduates are ready for independent practice?
- What strategies can program directors and faculty use to assess resident performance?
- What strategies can be used to evaluate training programs?
- What predictions can we make about the future of resident training based on the new technologies available in surgical education?

Introduction

To discuss strategies to implement curricula and assess curricular and resident performance for general surgery residencies, it is important to recognize several background themes.

First, surgical education is the fiduciary or stewardship responsibility of surgeons, whom the public and societal authorities have entrusted with considerable self-regulatory freedom. Honoring the public trust is an essential condition of any strategy to train the next generation of surgical providers. Hence, curricular and assessment structures are not simply a way to organize work and sequence trainee promotion; rather, they are the way the surgical profession fulfills its commitment to patient service and the public good. Educational stewardship is fundamental to being a professional and underscores for residents what it means to garner and preserve the trust on which professional privilege is founded.

Other important background themes include defining the scope of general surgical practice, outlining a process to inform curricular needs and priorities, and addressing the adult learning theory maxims that inform the educational process. The latter includes describing what learners need to know as defined by whom, how educators determine if the learner has attained the necessary skills and knowledge, and, critical for autonomous function, how do learners determine if they know what they need to know. Identifying the measures most predictive of performance is the key to execution in education. Clearly, curricular and assessment structure must address key learning theory questions in a professional development process and direct the educators' and learners' attention.

Designing curricular and assessment structures is more than a hierarchical exercise; it relies on a partnership between learners and educators. Otherwise, it will be harder to help residents acquire reflection, lifelong learning skill, judgment, and autonomy. The surgeon-educator must establish a covenant with the learner in which both sides commit themselves to outcomes and to the common good.

This chapter aims to provide educators with a model for designing and implementing the educational components of general surgery residency and to offer details on specific assessment strategies. The latter includes strategies to assess, formatively and summatively, each resident's performance and evaluate each program's performance with relevant, defined metrics. These themes are explored, with discussion of how professional and regulatory requirements and modern cognition science affect a program's educational structure. Specific curricular structures and methods are reviewed, including associated technologies, faculty development and competency, and autonomy-focused training. A detailed outline of tools and strategies to assess residents and evaluate programs will be offered, incorporating the competencies residents need to develop, such as medical knowledge, technical skill, and non-technical and behavioral capabilities. Remediation strategies also are described. Finally, with a view to the future, the chapter concludes with a discussion of competency-based resident education, Entrustable Professional Activities (EPAs), globalization, online and remote learning, video-based assessment, artificial intelligence, and the importance of training for lifelong learning and mastery.

Program Structure

Scope and Sequence of Curricular Topics

Understanding optimal program design starts with identifying the desired product. A surgical residency has two types of overall goals—practical and aspirational. The practical goals are to maintain full Accreditation Council for Graduate Medical Education (ACGME) accreditation for the residency and to ensure that residents qualify for the American Board of Surgery (ABS) certification process. Aspirational goals center on producing graduates who are prepared to enter independent general surgery practice or a subspecialty fellowship program. For either path, the public must be assured that the graduates are well-trained, ethical, professional, and competent. The five-year residency curriculum should produce a common pathway to meet these goals. For graduates entering practice, training needs to be broad-based (Table 1). Although most residents will enter a narrow field of practice, such as abdominal surgery, many areas of ABS content, such as orthopaedics, otolaryngology, urology, surgical obstetrics, and gynecology will never be practiced. A surgeon's scope of practice is determined by institution/community needs, hospital resources, and the specific skill sets they have mastered.

Table 1. American Board of Surgery content areas comprising essentials of general surgery

- Alimentary tract
- Abdomen and its contents
- Breast, skin, and soft tissue
- Endocrine system
- Solid organ transplantation
- Pediatric surgery
- Surgical critical care
- Surgical oncology (including head and neck)
- Trauma and emergency surgery
- Vascular surgery

The ABS has identified 10 content areas that comprise the essentials of general surgery (Table 1). The knowledge and experience expected in each area include the following five elements:

- Technical proficiency to perform core operations and familiarity with more complex, uncommon operations
- Knowledge of the anatomy, physiology, clinical presentation, and pathology of surgical conditions
- Knowledge of anesthesia, biostatistics, evaluation of evidence, minimally invasive techniques, transfusion, and coagulation disorders
- Knowledge of wound healing, infection, fluid management, shock and resuscitation, immunology, metabolism, pain, and nutrition
- Experience with clinical evaluation, stabilization and referral, preoperative care, management of comorbidities and complications, and use/interpretation of diagnostic imaging

The ABS Surgical Council on Resident Education (SCORE) curriculum outline for general surgery was initiated in 2006 by representatives of the ABS, the American College of Surgeons (ACS), Association of Program Directors in Surgery (APDS), American Surgical Association (ASA), Association for Surgical Education (ASE), Review Committee (RC) for Surgery, and the Society of American Gastrointestinal and Endoscopic Surgeons (SAGES). The outline consists of topics, grouped by ACGME competencies, to be included in a five-year general surgery curriculum. Patient care modules are divided into 27 categories for general surgery. Each module is further designated as a "core" or "advanced" topic for general surgery and covers either a disease/condition or an operation/procedure. Modules on the SCORE portal contain learning objectives, conference preparation, and self-assessment quizzes written by surgical faculty. Textbook chapters, practice guidelines, procedure guidelines, and operative videos provide additional support for comprehensive study. Open-ended questions are offered to stimulate group discussions. Many ABS examinations, such as the ABS In-Training Examination (ABSITE) and the General Surgery Qualifying Examination, include content that is aligned with SCORE's curriculum to streamline the learning experience.

Public Accountability

The public understands that surgeons need training and experience. However, as a result of increasing patient safety concerns in teaching hospitals, the public must be assured that attending surgeons are involved in all key elements of care, and residents are appropriately supervised; trainees are subject to ACGME duty-hour restrictions; patients are informed about the identity and role of who is caring for them; and surgical resident training stresses patient safety.

Regulatory Requirements

A variety of bodies establish surgical training requirements, including the ACGME, RC for Surgery, and ABS. The ACS-accredited Education Institutes (ACS-AEIs) establish requirements for skills acquisition training centers. We describe them below.

The *ACGME* establishes educational requirements for sponsoring institutions and common requirements for all graduate medical education (GME) residency programs. The common requirements at the top of the list for each specialty include duty-hour restrictions and workplace environment details. Overarching comments include the composition of Clinical Competency Committees and the Milestones semiannual reports.

The *RC for Surgery* establishes program requirements for general surgery residencies and performs initial accreditation and reaccreditation reviews of each program. Program requirements are listed by the RC for Surgery (*https://www.acgme.org/Portals/0/PFAssets/ProgramRequirements/440_GeneralSurgery_2020.pdf?ver=2020-06-22-085958-260*) for the following: oversight; personnel, including the program director (PD), program coordinator, and faculty; resident appointments; educational program, including scholarly activity; evaluation; and learning and work environment.

The RC for Surgery also requires each resident to submit a list of their operative experience in individual case logs. Program requirements for operative experience are created along with the ABS' individual requirements for board certification in surgery. Accreditation decisions are based on review of compliance with all ACGME and RC for Surgery program requirements, review of program operative experience in each of the case defined categories (Table 2), and five-year program first-time pass rates on the ABS Qualifying and Certifying Examinations.

Table 2. General surgery case log defined categories

- Skin, soft tissue
- Breast
- Head and neck
- Alimentary tract
- Abdominal
- Vascular
- Endocrine
- Operative trauma
- Nonoperative trauma
- Thoracic surgery
- Pediatric surgery
- Plastic surgery
- Surgical critical care
- Basic laparoscopic
- Complex laparoscopic
- Endoscopy

The *ABS* establishes the requirements for individuals to receive ABS board certification in general surgery as published in *The ABS Booklet of Information-Surgery* (*https://www.absurgery.org/xfer/BookletofInfo-Surgery.pdf*). Requirements for certification include a minimum of five years of progressive residency education in an accredited residency program; experience in all 10 essential content areas; PD approval; acceptable professional, ethical, and moral status; completion of Advanced Cardiac Life Support (ACLS), Advanced Trauma Life Support® (ATLS®), Fundamentals of Laparoscopic Surgery (FLS), Fundamentals of Endoscopic Surgery (FES); and operative experience. Operative experience requires cases in each essential area and a minimum of 850 cases as surgeon, 200 cases in chief year as surgeon or teaching assistant, 40 critical care cases, and 25 cases as teaching assistant.

The *ACS-AEIs* educate and train practicing surgeons, surgical residents, medical students, and members of the surgical team. The ACS-AEI program's goal is to promote patient safety by using simulation, to develop new modes of education technology, identify best practices, and promote research and collaboration among institutes. Both Comprehensive and Focused Education Institutes must meet rigorous standards for accreditation. Compared to Focused Education Institutes, Comprehensive Education Institutes must also have the following capabilities:

- Serve a wider range of learners, with a broader scope of education and training programs
- Develop original curricula, offer faculty development programs and courses, and evaluate their education and training programs' impact on patient outcomes and safety
- Have adequate space and staff to accommodate the higher volume of learners and scope of educational activities
- Engage in research or other scholarly activities that advance the field of surgical education and training

Cognitive Science-Based Strategies and Their Curricular Implications

Cognitive science-based strategies are essential to planning a residency education curriculum. Modern cognitive science views knowledge as a web of information that serves as the infrastructure for how an individual thinks. Clinical educators favor cognitive learning theories that focus on how learners acquire and process information to generate knowledge. Cognitive-based strategies focus on the learning processes and how they help develop mental models and knowledge structure. To enable learners to efficiently acquire knowledge, teaching these strategies is as important as teaching higher-level functions, such as analysis, synthesis, and evaluation.

Knowledge enables learners to effectively use higher-level skills, such as evaluating the patient and decision-making. Key knowledge elements are domain-specific, analogous to surgical expertise. Cognitive architecture is composed of working memory and long-term memory. Domain-specific knowledge is held in long-term memory. For example, resolving a clinical problem in surgery requires the resident to retrieve information into working memory from long-term memory. The more knowledge stored, linked, and automatized in long-term memory, the more space available in working memory, especially to handle challenging or unfamiliar clinical problems. Cognitive theory suggests memory is enhanced more through active practice than passive observation.

Understanding and integrating cognitive theories into instruction strategically affects teaching and learning. Spaced or distributed learning transforms new knowledge into long-term memory through short learning bursts combined with planned mental breaks to assimilate new knowledge. To promote retention, key learning objectives are revisited at periodic intervals through questions or tests. Organizing content into smaller chunks of information is key to an effective spaced learning strategy.

The chunking hypothesis suggests that during repeated exposure, information is organized into increasingly larger chunks. When first encountering new information, each item may be coded as an individual chunk, but after repeated exposure, several items may be coded together as one chunk. This theory suggests learning involves constantly monitoring and assimilating information into increasingly larger chunks of knowledge. The chunking strategy regulates the amount of knowledge that an individual can process at any one time.

Interleaving is a more recent cognitive learning theory that allows the learner to form connections to previously taught information by linking topics. The links and connections formed by interleaving, or mixing, clinical material or tasks can improve the consolidation phase of knowledge.

Modern cognitive science focuses on learning processes and recognizes how these processes interact to enhance learning. Combining the spacing effect to boost memory and chunking to process larger quantities of knowledge synergistically boost learning. Recognizing that practice is more effective when spaced out, interleaving boosts inductive category learning and increases connections to previously taught information. Together, spacing and interleaving can facilitate retention and result in a deeper understanding of new material.

Because the curriculum forms the resource base that residents draw upon when approaching clinical problems, it requires thoughtful design. This curriculum design needs to adopt cognitive-based learning strategies to help the learner build knowledge structures and mental models.

Knowledge is foundational to a learner's long-term memory. To become adept critical thinkers and problem solvers, learners must acquire knowledge. The more a learner knows, the better the learner can think (the Matthew Effect). By the end of residency, surgeons should not only have a robust and powerful knowledge base that enables them to make sound clinical decisions, but they should also be motivated to pursue lifelong learning.

Cognitive science's model of knowledge consists of schemata, or webs of interconnected pieces of knowledge. When residents begin surgical training, they have few schemata; that is, they have limited knowledge with few connections. The goal of training is to acquire well-linked and well-organized schemata, such as high-quality knowledge and domain-specific skills. Because schemata build over time, both time and content are critical elements of effective curriculum planning.

Effective schemata are strong and accessible. Spaced retrieval practice must be included throughout the curriculum, so residents can draw upon previous learning. Spaced practice, in which the revision of learned material is split up and spaced, is an effective method to strengthen retrieval. By planning the curriculum in detail and properly using interleaving, links can be made to content already covered in the curriculum, reinforcing concepts, making connections between concepts, and enabling a deeper understanding of new content by linking it to old content. Reflection is a powerful strategy to achieve transfer of knowledge and interleaving capability. Creating time and opportunity for learner reflection in a curriculum is important to identify gaps in knowledge and establish connections.

Evidence from cognitive theory suggests that repetition alone does not improve performance. Self-reflection, combined with structured and focused practice, is integral to a balanced curriculum. Learning objectives should be provided for learners, along with the necessary feedback or coaching to achieve them.

In cognitive theory models of learning, students actively participate in their education, which fosters the accountability and autonomy required for "self-directed learning"—a fundamental principle of both cognitive theory and adult learning. Personal goals and motivation for learning drive growth in this model. Self-directed learning is the foundation for lifelong learning and, ultimately, translates into improved patient care and outcomes.

Space, Time, and Personnel Requirements

These cognitive theory models of learning show that students and residents need infrastructure to develop into high-functioning physicians. Such structure should be established in all aspects of training so that students efficiently achieve competency and, ultimately, mastery. When designing curriculum, apply cognitive theory principles that allow for reinforcement and multivantage exposure to key content, whether for a clinical rotation, specialization experience, or the entire training program.

As technology has advanced, so have the requirements for implementing and assessing an educational program. As online content and virtual interaction capabilities have grown, the need for physical space has shrunk. In addition, as many institutions have added clinical faculty members and education specialists, more individuals are attuned to learning theory and curriculum design to shape the learner's educational experience. This approach does not replace the one-on-one teaching with faculty, but it integrates an optimal educational strategy into the overall curriculum.

When considering space, time, and personnel requirements, think about the specific content delivery systems and techniques that will be used within those systems. This instructional design element delivers information optimally and efficiently to the trainee.

For the purposes of discussion, content delivery will be broken down into in-person and online instruction. Learners can either participate in an activity simultaneously (synchronous instruction) or access content individually (asynchronous instruction).

Curricular Vehicles

For decades, large-group conferences and small-group discussions have delivered content. These approaches are reviewed with an eye toward their required space, preparation time, and pros and cons.

Grand Rounds

Grand rounds, a traditional format for medical education, once focused on an actual patient with a disease. This forum has evolved into a content expert lecturing about the patient with a disease, which may require a large room. Most grand rounds take place monthly or weekly.

An effective grand rounds program requires the educator to know who is attending and to develop content accordingly. This format can be challenging if the audience represents a broad spectrum of expertise. It can be a challenge to hold the attention of such an audience, given that some attendees, such as medical students or junior residents, may feel they are in over their heads, whereas other participants may find parts of the talk repetitive.

Furthermore, large lectures rarely deliver content efficiently. This format limits questions, is difficult to adapt to the audience, and yields low long-term memory retention among learners. On the other hand, this format allows novice learners to anticipate what is expected of them as they progress in the discipline, whereas more experienced students can learn about advances in the field. Grand rounds also can be a team-building exercise, allowing bonds to form between students and developing a community of learning that spans the group's range of collective experience.

Morbidity and Mortality Conference

Morbidity and mortality (M&M) conferences can take place as a service-based or small-group conference, although they are more typically conducted as larger conferences requiring more space. Topics discussed may be broad, depending on the cases discussed and the level of learners who attend.

The success of these conferences depends on having a moderator who knows the topics, keeps the discussion at the appropriate level for the students being questioned, prevents a hostile learning environment, and summarizes key teaching points from each case. Educators can be trained to become effective moderators for these conferences.

Unique to the M&M conference is the presenter, who provides background on the topic (usually a case presentation) and often leads the discussion with the moderator. The quality of the presenter can greatly influence the quality of an M&M conference.

Learning at these conferences depends on interaction. For example, students who are called upon will have a higher level of learning and retention. Unfortunately, these conferences do not efficiently teach because of the wide range of learners and relatively low level of overall involvement. Also like grand rounds, M&M conferences provide socialization and role modeling opportunities, and if the moderator facilitates appropriate interactions with learners of different levels, these sessions can be effective learning opportunities.

Service-Based Conferences

Service-based conferences may include: service education, M&M, case review, preoperative indications, treatment, operative planning, or even service-based administrative discussions. These conferences are smaller and require less space than grand rounds or M&M conferences and are often held weekly. A conference moderator establishes the flow of the meeting and, sometimes, delivers the content.

These conferences may use a variety of teaching techniques, such as flipped classroom, jigsaw puzzle, or forced debate. Students retain more when required to prepare and deliver content, making connections that incorporate the content into long-term memory or larger chunks of association. Service-based conferences are often used for real-time assessment of students' progress and to determine if they are completing assigned aspects of the curriculum.

Journal Club

Journal clubs deliver updated, high-impact information on a specific topic and, more importantly, provide foundational knowledge on research design and interpretation of results. As a smaller group activity, it has pros and cons like service-based conferences, except the educator must be well-versed in study design and assessment. Critical assessment of the literature can be taught by adding specific tools for interpreting various types of evidence-based scientific studies.

Virtual Content Delivery

Although content delivery activities are traditionally in person and synchronous, the advent of virtual content delivery, in which content is streamed and recorded, enables these programs to be offered asynchronously. Podcasts, online videos, and other streaming content expand the curricular elements offered to students.

Although synchronous virtual content delivery eliminates space requirements, students still need to read, prepare, and engage in the activity, and educators still need to know their audience and develop relevant content. Larger virtual meetings do not allow the educator or moderator to view the entire audience. Students may engage in other tasks with little risk of detection, making an inefficient activity even less efficient. For smaller meetings, educators can change teaching techniques, gauge the involvement of the students, and assess the students' knowledge in the virtual setting.

There are ways to increase the efficiency and participatory nature of virtual synchronous learning. Larger groups can be broken up into smaller "pods," with each pod having a leader who is responsible for keeping the group engaged. Asking questions and using the chat function allows pod leaders to increase engagement and monitor students.

Asynchronous learning, which can be either individual- or group-based, offers students access to content developed in advance. Asynchronous content delivery typically includes virtual conferences or reading programs. This type of delivery allows learners to participate on their own schedule and to review material multiple times. In addition, educators improve the material or revise it with new information.

Asynchronous content delivery is a good fit with many cognitive learning theories. Content can be broken into pieces appropriate for the student's level. The ability to repeat activities means that more of the information can be processed into long-term memory. Recall, critically important for knowledge application, also is improved, as is chunking of information and developing interconnections and context between bits of information. Finally, the ability to build on previously learned information is more consistent with asynchronous content delivery than with other content delivery systems.

Asynchronous learning still requires an educator to answer questions, assess learners, and provide appropriate context to the student.

Novel Technologies: Artificial Intelligence, Augmented, and Mixed Reality

Teaching and learning surgical skills can be enabled by recent technologic advancements. Surgical videos are a valuable source of data. Harnessing these data using artificial intelligence (AI), especially computer vision, which enables computers and systems to derive meaningful information from digital images, videos, and other visual inputs, can lead to valuable educational products. For example, AI algorithms can autonomously break down an operation into its elements, so the learner can review specific steps. Learners can view clips from multiple operations to observe a particular step being done well or needing improvement. The algorithms also can identify "events," such as bleeding, bile or stone spillage, which is particularly valuable for learning how to deal with intraoperative complications. By embedding evaluations directly into these annotated videos, critiques can be more focused and formative. Comments also can be tagged to specific steps of the procedure, allowing a supervisor to mentor the student more efficiently in a debriefing session.

Augmented reality systems are less expensive and more readily available. Headsets allow the learner to be coached while they see the anatomy and interact with a three-dimensional hologram. As programming becomes simplified, this technology can be an effective and efficient addition to the educational paradigm. When combined with actual structures, virtual patients, or products, this type of learning becomes mixed reality. For assessment, the student may be asked to identify anatomic structures or troubleshoot surgical devices in a realistic, yet standardized, setting.

Rotation and Clinical Settings

The goal of training in surgery is for learners to attain competence then excellence, as described by Miller's Pyramid (see Chapter 2). Progress toward this goal is greatly influenced by the curriculum. Instructional design decides when, where, and to whom to deliver the curriculum. The design must factor in the resources that are available to deliver the curriculum. Because surgical education has many pieces, varying from simple to complex, it is difficult to design an overarching curriculum that fits every program.

In designing a curriculum, several basic principles should be followed:

- Assess the knowledge level of the students who are entering the program. One assessment tool is the ACS Fundamentals of Surgery Curriculum® (ACS FSC), a modular program that assesses foundational knowledge in patient care. Another ACS tool is the Entering Resident Readiness Assessment (ACS ERRA), an online test that assesses the entering resident's knowledge by evaluating a variety of surgical problems. Finally, the ACS Objective Structured Clinical Examination (OSCE) uses standardized patients to assess care in 10 different situations, which enables a program to create a more personalized early learning plan to help a resident fill knowledge gaps.
- Develop the learner's foundational knowledge, both cognitive and technical. Cognitive content involves not just patient care, but also ethics, legal issues, nonbiased care, and so on. This aspect of training should ensure a resident knows the answer and why it is correct. These cognitive and technical aspects should build on previously learned material. In addition, validated assessment tools, such as FLS and FES, can check if students are making appropriate progress. Deficiency must be addressed by a specific training plan separate from clinical rotation or the clinical material presented to the learner.
- Design clinical rotations to enable the learner to attain foundational knowledge and specific knowledge related to their practice. Again, knowledge should be built incrementally, and appropriate tools should assess progress.

As the learner progresses, specific cognitive and technical skills should morph into more complex thinking processes. In patient care, this involves generating a differential diagnosis and developing care plans that anticipate a decision's ramifications, potential outcomes, and attendant resource costs. Hence, the learner must have autonomy to make decisions both in clinical care and in the operating room (OR). Use validated assessment tools to assess learners, such as team training in a simulated trauma environment.

Lastly, learners should be able to teach these various skills. Teaching shows the highest level of understanding of a cognitive or technical principle, especially if the learner can explain why an activity or assessment is performed.

Simulation
The ACGME has a section on simulation in its program requirements for GME in general surgery. In addition, the ACS has developed a program for medical students using simulation as an educational tool. Numerous studies show that simulation helps students learn clinical and technical material. All surgical education curricula should include simulation.

Simulation is not simply a resident using a knot-tying board or practicing for FLS. Simulation entails clinical skills, technical skills, interpersonal skills, and team training. Tools range in cost and sophistication from inexpensive simulation equipment appropriate for novice learners to high-fidelity simulators for more advanced surgeons. Surgery programs must enable residents to practice the skills needed to pass FLS or FES as elements required for ABS certification. Standardized patients may be used to help teach cognitive skills and interpersonal skills. Team training can run the gamut from low-fidelity mannikins to high-fidelity, fully simulated patient care areas.

At present, there is no certification requirement for simulation programs. The ACGME program requires that simulation be part of the curriculum and simulation activities to be actively managed by a simulation champion, which means that a program could meet ACGME requirements by having a bare minimum of space and equipment and a single simulation manager.

The ACS-AEI has a more rigorous simulation program that offers two levels, Focused and Comprehensive, each requiring space, equipment, and staffing levels, as well as an institute director and a surgical simulation director. The ACS-AEI Accreditation Committee reviews the program and determines accreditation, a rigorous process that requires submission of program curricula, types of learners engaged in the simulation activity, and evaluation of the program. Simulation education needs dedicated simulation instructors. Although many basic tasks can be taught by someone trained to use checklists, some simulation activities require educators well versed in education theory. The development of simulation curricular elements can be a complex process ranging from needs assessment to program evaluation.

Simulation enables programs to address the needs of their residents. Simulation can improve basic skills without putting patients at risk. It provides learners needed context and allows them to practice skills or behaviors until they are easily recalled from long-term memory, which in turn opens their minds for other learning opportunities while performing these tasks. Simulation also can be used to teach important skills rarely encountered in routine clinical contexts, such as specific operative techniques.

Programs must have simulation in their curriculum. Simulation should be tiered, with basic activities for medical students and junior residents progressing to complex tasks and team training for senior learners. The activities should match a learner's level of development or their participation in a specific rotation. For example, a postgraduate year one (PGY1) resident may complete the cognitive aspect of FLS during their month on minimally invasive surgery and then complete the FLS technical exam before starting a high-volume general surgery rotation involving laparoscopy.

Lastly, practicing surgeons use simulation to maintain their skills. Comprehensive ACS-AEIs are required to train practicing physicians and trainers, such as specifically skilled simulation educators.

Committee and Oversight Strategies for Curricular Monitoring and Management
Oversight and review of the activities within the curriculum can take many different forms, including academic standards and quality/efficiency.

Directors must ensure that all medical schools, residency programs, and fellowships meet academic standards. To assess academic standards, in smaller programs the PD often oversees requirement compliance, whereas larger programs typically establish a PD-chaired committee of educators well versed in the judgment criteria. This process can include ensuring all faculty members meet their teaching requirements, all activities are assessed, and the program is evaluated. This topic is discussed in greater detail at the end of this chapter.

In addition, programs should establish a separate committee to implement, assess, and update their curricula. Because the goal of a curriculum is to efficiently present high-quality material to learners, each element must be evaluated. One approach to evaluation is to ask a committee of learners and teachers what works best and what needs improvement. This shared ownership allows more educators to administer and improve the program, motivating them to ensure a quality product and easing the PD's burden. This committee meets regularly, reviews evaluations, and determines if adjustments are needed. Additionally, the committee can perform an initial review of any new programs and help decide timing and implementation.

Faculty Development Requirements and Related Issues

Residency programs need faculty members with different teaching styles and varied areas of expertise. Teaching faculty members need not be equally adept in all areas of instruction.

Patient teachers of basic surgical techniques are as valuable as faculty with advanced teaching techniques. Some faculty excel in small-group discussions, whereas others are best at lecturing. Each program needs staff members who can teach the principles of research and patient safety as well as those who can help residents to learn effective communication, professionalism, and leadership. Faculty development should capitalize on the strengths of each surgical educator while reinforcing common principles that focus on the educational environment, various teaching methods, and performance assessment.

As former students, surgical faculty members usually recognize if an instructor is effective or ineffective. However, few faculty analyze effective teaching techniques, study the education principles used to design optimal learning experiences for surgical residents, or get a timely assessment of their teaching strengths and weaknesses. Faculty development can fill these experience gaps.

Educators cite many motivations for teaching residents: a sense of responsibility to train future surgeons, an intrinsic joy of teaching, a chance to interact with younger colleagues, and/or an opportunity to mentor a young colleague. Some say that teaching is a great way to stay current in an area of knowledge.

Barriers to effective teaching include unclear curricular goals, negative student and faculty attitudes, lack of protected time for education, and lack of educational resources. Faculty members feel pressure to perform financially rewarding clinical and research activities as opposed to teaching activities that offer no clear financial rewards. Even in an academic setting, teaching excellence is often undervalued as a consideration in promotion. Furthermore, often too few faculty development opportunities are available to enhance teaching performance.

The ACGME requires faculty development for all medical and surgical residencies. Most institutions that sponsor residencies and fellowships offer, through their medical education departments, generic conferences on education principles and skills. Topics specific to surgical educators are chosen by the surgery department members based on departmental needs assessments from the PD. Non-surgeon instructors from the sponsoring institution or an area university may be available to offer valuable seminars to review education principles and effective lecture and discussion skills. Key teaching faculty also may benefit from attending one or more face-to-face interactive courses (see Table 3). The ACS Surgeons as Educators course is a six-day program that focuses on teaching skills, curriculum development, educational administration and leadership, and performance evaluation. The ACS ATLS Instructors Course, which is not limited to trauma surgeons, is a 2.5-day course including many practical sessions that reinforce basic educational principles. The APDS New Program Director Workshop is a two-day course designed to cover topics essential to surgery residency PDs and key faculty.

Table 3. Faculty development courses and workshops

- American College of Surgeons - Surgeons as Educators Course
- American College of Surgeons Advanced Trauma Life Support Instructors Course
- Association for Program Directors in Surgery New Program Director Workshop
- Association for Program Directors in Surgery/ Association for Surgical Education annual meeting workshops
- Royal College of Surgeons of England Training the Trainers Course

Content for faculty development lectures and discussions cover a variety of topics, such as:

- Preparing a didactic lecture
- Effective use of audiovisual techniques and contemporary principles of adult education have proven effective for surgical education (see Table 4)
- Establishing a safe, effective teaching environment focuses on physical and psychological elements
- Being intentional and efficient given time constraints
- Why deliberation and reflection in the OR have replaced experience by blind repetition
- Teaching to competence rather than relying on numbers as surrogates for experience
- How focus on the faculty-resident relationship has reshaped the understanding of knowledge and skill acquisition
- How mentoring and emphasis on lifelong learning can help build strong career foundations

Assessment of teaching skills and behaviors provides essential feedback for faculty development. The department chair, residency PD, senior faculty mentor, and non-surgeon educators should conduct regular performance reviews. Most important, each faculty member should be assessed by surgery residents, with residents given strict anonymity to avoid the risk of reprisal. The assessments must include the evaluation of teaching environment, techniques, behaviors, knowledge base, and opportunities for autonomy. All results must be shared with the faculty member in an unvarnished fashion, preferably in a face-to-face session with the PD. Only in this way can the faculty members learn their strengths and weaknesses as teachers.

Table 4. Surgical residency adult educational principles for faculty development

- Establish an educational environment of psychological safety
- Training should be intentional: each activity with an attainable goal
- Training must be more efficient
- Faculty entrustment and resident entrustability are inextricably intertwined
- Deliberate practice and reflection are more important than repetition
  - Briefing, instruction, debriefing
- Promote progressive autonomy
- Teach to competence with competency-based assessment and advancement
  - Surgery milestones
  - Entrustable professional activities
  - Credentialing during residency
- Teach lifelong learning strategies
  - Clinical research
  - Surgical outcomes
  - Patient safety
  - Practice management
- Importance of mentoring

Role models are valuable for careers in surgery. For members of the teaching faculty, mentoring is important at two levels. Young teaching faculty can benefit from the advice and example of senior staff members with effective teaching behaviors and methods. Similarly, mentoring of surgical residents by teachers has benefits for performance, assessment, and career counseling. Many surgery residency programs assign a faculty mentor to each resident. This assignment should take place once it is apparent that their personalities and interests are compatible.

Incentivizing educational contributions is difficult due to increasing pressure to focus on financially rewarding activities. Mission statements of the teaching institution and surgery department should highlight commitment to education. Specific incentives often include teacher-of-the-year awards. Every teaching faculty member should receive recognition for their educational contributions at annual salary review. The residency PD should give direct input to the department chair or salary committee regarding the teaching efforts of each staff member. Some institutions factor educational activities into a salary formula, whereas others give them less formal recognition. Each year a faculty member should be informed how their educational efforts are reflected in their compensation package.

There are three levels of surgical teaching skills: basic, effective, and impactful. Basic teaching successfully transfers knowledge, experience, and technique from faculty to resident. Effective teaching is more efficient and successful by integrating teaching methods best suited to the faculty member and the needs of the resident. Impactful teaching includes mentoring and modeling behaviors and judgment. Impactful teachers achieve a degree of "surgical immortality" by strongly affecting present and future generations of surgeons and patients.

Autonomy and How to Facilitate It

Surgical training should produce graduates who can safely, skillfully, and independently care for their patients. Independence or autonomy, which is defined as freedom from external control or influence, must be progressively attained in the surgical training period in a way that protects patient safety. Residents who achieve autonomy gain confidence in clinical decision-making and performance of procedures, feel responsible for the patient, have a stronger professional identity, and are ready for independent practice.

Over the last three decades, opportunities for autonomous surgical resident experience in or outside of the OR have declined because of numerous socioeconomic factors (Table 5). One factor is increased focus on patient safety and optimization of clinical outcomes. Another is the proliferation of surgical specialty fellowships, which reduces opportunities for autonomy during residency while increasing them during postresidency fellowship.

Resident autonomy during surgical training depends on developing faculty entrustment and resident entrustability (Table 5). Faculty entrustment allows teachers to impart trust and responsibility for patient care to a trainee while providing an appropriate level of supervision. Resident entrustablity is based on the resident's knowledge, skills, behaviors, and communication that engender faculty trust. An autonomous resident experience depends on a faculty member's willingness to adapt their role in patient care, which in turn is affected by the member's teaching style and experience, the difficulty of procedure, time constraints, productivity concerns, and other factors. It also depends on how well the trainee can demonstrate their readiness for responsibility to the faculty member. Residents who lack demonstrated knowledge, technical skill, case preparation, communication skills, or team leadership skills will get fewer opportunities for autonomy.

Table 5. Barriers to resident autonomy during surgical training

1. Socioeconomic factors
   - Increased focus on patient safety and clinical outcomes
   - Health care finance regulations
   - Patient and family expectations
   - Resident duty-hour regulations
   - Medical legal considerations
   - Increased selection of postresidency surgical specialty fellowships

2. Faculty entrustment
   - Faculty teaching style and behaviors
   - Faculty experience/confidence with procedure
   - Less consistent contact with residents on service
   - Case difficulty
   - Time constraints
   - Faculty productivity pressure

3. Resident entrustability
   - Direct knowledge of resident performance
   - Indirect knowledge of resident performance (resident reputation)
   - Resident's demonstration of technical expertise
   - PGY level
   - Case preparation
   - Communication skills
   - OR team leadership

Although the socioeconomic factors listed in Table 5, are difficult to change, the PD can make some structural changes that might enhance autonomous experiences (Table 6). Surgical rotation schedules can be designed for faculty and residents to form relationships. Faculty and residents who work together frequently can more accurately assess each other's behaviors and skills, which makes autonomy more likely. Some programs have developed an autonomous experience for the chief residency year that consists of independent outpatient clinic, operating time, and hospital coverage supervised by a dedicated faculty surgeon. Finally, practice-management training during residency is essential for the independent practice of surgery.

There are several ways to improve autonomy through faculty entrustment and resident entrustablity. One is that faculty development should reinforce skills that improve procedural teaching, intraoperative communication, and resident assessment. Another is that resident education should include case preparation requirements, intraoperative communication, and operating team leadership. Finally, timely assessment of resident performance by faculty and of faculty teaching by residents is critical to developing trust.

Table 6. Potential strategies for resident autonomy during surgical training

1. Structural strategies
   - Optimize rotation schedules to foster development of relationships between faculty and residents
   - Chief resident rotation
   - Practice management curriculum

2. Faculty entrustment
   - Faculty development to improve procedural teaching, communication, and resident assessment
   - Resident assessment of faculty teaching styles and behaviors
   - Faculty compensation recognizes teaching ability

3. Resident entrustability
   - Case preparation requirements
   - Communication skills learning
   - OR leadership skills learning
   - Timely faculty assessment of resident performance

4. Faculty entrustment and resident entrustability dynamic
   - Faculty and resident discuss roles, expectations, and goals of procedure preoperatively
   - Level of autonomy monitored and modulated during procedure
   - Credentialing during residency - allowing adjustment of level of supervision
   - PASS (Procedural autonomy and supervision system) program
   - "Zwisch" four-stage model for graduated resident responsibility in the OR
   - Competency-based advancement using well-defined EPAs

Faculty entrustment and resident entrustability are inextricably intertwined; nowhere is this mutual trust more evident than in the OR. The give-and-take between faculty and resident is constant during a procedure. Well before they enter the OR, faculty and resident should discuss respective roles, expectations, and the goals of a procedure. The level of autonomy is determined during the operation as the faculty delivers entrustment in three phases: 1) monitoring resident performance, 2) assessing level of resident entrustability, and 3) granting autonomy. The level of autonomy granted may change based on this ongoing performance assessment or increasing case difficulty; these levels range from quiet assistance to verbal assistance to using an instrument to dissect and dictate "Cut here, cut there" to "Let me show you how this is done."

The faculty can assess resident performance using measures such as the Zwisch scale or PASS program. In this way, specific procedures may be credentialed during residency, which may be a component of competency-based advancement using predefined EPAs.

Competency-Based Education and Implications for Structure

Competency-based medical education (CBME) is "an outcomes-based approach to the design, implementation, and evaluation of education programs and the assessment of learners, using competencies or observable abilities," according to the Association of American Medical Colleges. It is derived from an analysis of patient and societal needs, and fosters greater accountability, flexibility, and learner-centeredness.

The fundamental principles of CBME are based upon three tenets:

1. Medical education should be based on the health needs of the population
2. The primary focus of education and training should be to achieve the desired outcomes for learners rather than to fulfill the structures or processes of the educational system
3. Physicians should be developed along a seamless continuum of education, training, and practice

CBME is being adopted in various international frameworks, including the ACGME, the Royal College of Physicians and Surgeons of Canada (CanMEDS model), the Scottish Doctor outcomes, and the Australian Curriculum Framework for Junior Doctors. Advances in cognitive educational theories, emphasis on clearly defined outcomes, greater transparency, and active learning to incorporate formative and focused feedback into the clinical setting have all catalyzed the shift to CBME. In addition, CBME is designed to produce physicians and surgeons who are competent collaborators and leaders, and able to help interprofessional teams meet the needs of 21st century complex patient care.

By adopting a systematic approach that specifies population needs and develops new and adaptive competencies based on evolving technologies and on competencies reassessed to ensure alignment, residency training can be both relevant and tailored to societal and learner priorities.

CBME proponents focus on curricular outcomes. To prepare graduates for practice, a curriculum needs to define the desired outcome capabilities and ensure they are learned, assessed, and acquired. Link each curriculum learning objective to a specific learning outcome explicitly related to the needs of the population served.

Organizing the curriculum around abilities or competencies allows the elements to build upon one another. Learners can create learning experiences that incorporate prior knowledge and skills, enabling them to progress to higher-order practice based on their observable abilities and behaviors.

The traditional residency training model was based on the learner's demonstration of knowledge acquired at preset intervals, whereas CBME shifts the focus to the learner's ability to demonstrate how to apply that knowledge. In fact, learners must show they have the necessary competency before advancing to the next stage of training. This approach standardizes learning outcomes, individualizes the learning process, sets expectations for learners, and empowers them to participate in the process.

CBME establishes a framework consistent with undergraduate medical education, GME, and continuing professional development. It helps break down the silos in traditional medical education. By determining the end goals of physicianship, this model helps learners become competent professionals and communicators.

PDs, faculty, and learners alike face many challenges to implementing CBME. Enabling learners to achieve competence requires significant time commitment and investment. Proper assessment and real-time feedback require many assessors to make many direct observations in a range of clinical settings. Faculty development is required for both teaching and assessing competency. Integrating a model to advance learners once competency is attained is inconsistent with the traditional time-based model for residency training, which creates additional challenges in program structure and design.

To teach competency efficiently and effectively to learners and faculty, the International CBME Collaborators suggests that medical educators incorporate a series of commitments to:

- *Teach, assess, and model the broad range of requisite competencies.* Beyond competencies around patient care, medical knowledge and procedural skills, competency in communication, professionalism, scholarship, leadership and practice, and system improvement also are required. These objectives need to be made explicit and weighted in the formal curriculum and applied in practice.
- *Supervision that balances safety with the professional development of learners.* Faculty must learn to be effective supervisors. They must provide the structure and support learners need to progress through residency and transition to independent and unsupervised practice.

- *Transparency with all stakeholders*. Spurred by various North American and European studies on adverse events and near-miss reporting, CBME began as an initiative to produce better physicians. Improving outcomes for desired patient populations is a basic CBME principle. CBME promotes transparent clinical and educational outcome reporting for both patients and trainees and requires learner feedback to be constructive and sourced from patients, other health care professionals, peers, and faculty.
- *Empower learners*. CBME is a learner-centered approach that includes tailored learning experiences, feedback, and reflection. Applying this principle means that practice guides training. Prioritize clinical settings that reflect the type of future practice envisioned.
- *Effective assessment strategies and tools*. Reliability improves through the diverse perspectives of broad and multisourced assessment. Because this approach requires significant resources, focus strategies on improving assessment efficiency and take advantage of mobile-based platforms and other strategies that facilitate immediate workplace-based assessment and feedback.
- *Basing transition decisions on competence rather than on time*. Learners progress at different rates, and though training may still be accomplished using a time-based model, teaching faculty can adapt and challenge learners along the training continuum based on their competence rather than seniority. Importantly, this commitment assures patients that learners advance to the next level based on demonstrating competence, not on how much time they have put in. This element also helps educators address the failure of faculty to expel failing students in traditional medical education, which has contributed to variable educational and clinical outcomes, according to certification exam performance, patient safety, and cost of care data.
- *Advancing CBME through workplace-based assessment, program evaluation, and research*. This process involves an ongoing program-level evaluation and assessment of the overall effectiveness of CBME.
- *Faculty development*. Faculty expected to teach and assess within this new framework may not have the requisite skills or knowledge. If competency-based strategies are to be sustainable as an educational model, this deficiency must be addressed through workshops, continuing professional development, and establishment of clinical productivity expectations.
- *Collaboration*. Health care delivery is a team effort that includes interprofessional colleagues and thrives on shared educational experiences in the clinical setting. Understanding the importance of teamwork will help training programs implement CBME and integrate it into the full spectrum of health care delivery.

Competency-Based Residency Education: The University of Toronto's Experience

The shift to competency-based residency education (CBRE) is a movement to transform GME to meet the changing needs of patient populations and learners by applying CBME principles to residency programs.

In July 2009, the division of orthopaedic surgery at the University of Toronto was one of the first North American residency programs to embark on a pilot program using the competency-based framework. This pioneering program has been followed by multispecialty implementation at other institutions, including Queens University in Ontario, and has informed the nationwide Competency by Design (CBD) program being implemented across all specialties under the auspices of the Royal College of Physicians and Surgeons of Canada. (The experience of the CBD program will be reviewed in some detail at the end of this chapter.)

The University of Toronto's orthopaedic training program's five guiding principles enabled successful implementation by: 1) breaking down curriculum into discrete modules reflecting progressive development of expertise, 2) altering the delivery of objectives in core surgical training, 3) ensuring a rapid ascent to technical skills competence, 4) using simulation intensely, and 5) enhancing feedback and assessment.

Curriculum Mapping

The initial steps to achieve a CBRE program involve an extensive curriculum mapping process that includes understanding the foundational competencies required for any surgical discipline and discipline-specific objectives oriented to the core training program. The mapping process specifies where learning objectives are taught and the threshold for demonstrating competence. In orthopaedics, at the University of Toronto, training was grouped into three phases. Phase 1 comprised the foundational and basic orthopaedic learning modules, including the "transition to residency" period to teach and assess basic skills. Phase 2 focused on more advanced skills that built upon phase 1. Phase 3 consolidated knowledge and skills that prepared the resident for the transition into practice. CBRE thus provides the framework for the successful application of credentialing during residency.

Need for Robust and Frequent Assessment

The CBRE paradigm requires skill acquisition and enhanced use of simulation. Deliberate practice, rehearsing technical skills in a nonclinical setting, coaching, small student-to-teacher ratios, and frequent formative feedback are some methods used to achieve competency. The most significant change in this competency-based educational model is that trainees cannot progress to the next level until they have shown that they have achieved clearly defined milestones or objectives. As a result, unlike time-based training, trainees progress through their milestones at their own pace. This requires assessment schemes to be robust and frequent.

In the Toronto experience, this approach required three to five times more assessment episodes. Determining trainee competence in CBRE also requires access to a variety of assessment tools. For residents found to have weaknesses, customized learning plans can address the deficiencies.

Eight of 14 graduates of the CBRE pilot graduated in four years of training, as opposed to five years of conventional residency training. Although the goal is not to reduce the length of the residency, efficiency was gained by refocusing on competency, according to a recent study that published eight-year outcomes evaluating all program components. Training standards and expectations were more transparent than in a traditional residency.

Challenges to CBRE include additional resources and financial costs to implement and support the training program, develop faculty development, expand simulation use, and provide enhanced teaching and frequent assessment, according to the study. Another challenge is the need for an effective technology platform. An effective mobile phone-based platform to deliver curricular maps, learning resources, and assessment tools would ease the transition to CBRE and reduce faculty time devoted to completing evaluations, according to the study.

CBRE is learner centered. The Toronto CBRE program showed that when residents understand that they are active participants in the residency, they tend to take ownership of their learning and are partners in promoting critical real-time assessment and feedback strategies.

Assessment Strategies for Trainees

Performance assessment is essential to surgical education. Assessments about each resident's progress help programs decide if the resident is ready to advance or requires supervision, remediation, or termination. This feedback is vital for trainees to learn about their strengths, weaknesses, and areas of concern. PDs can learn about global program strengths and deficiencies by reviewing normative test results and resident evaluations. Assessment must be comprehensive, encompassing all core competencies. Assessments must be timely and shared openly and honestly with the trainee. Assessment results should be reviewed with each resident at least twice a year, earlier and more frequently if there are concerns. The resident should not have to wait to hear about a concern or deficiency until they are on a performance improvement plan or receive a notice of termination. Assessment results should be summarized and well documented. Comprehensive assessment of surgeons-in-training necessarily involves objective and subjective assessment. Assessment can be more focused and structured if the performance expectations shared with faculty and residents have well-constructed goals and objectives for each educational activity and for each postgraduate year of training. Even subjective assessments can be made more "objective" by establishing clear definitions for distinct levels of performance. Finally, assessments should be completed by an array of assessors, including faculty, fellow residents, nursing staff, hospital staff, and patients.

In 2002, the ACGME introduced the six core competencies to be used by GME programs to evaluate residents in training: 1) patient care, including procedural technical skills; 2) medical knowledge; 3) practice-based learning and improvement; 4) interpersonal and communication skills; 5) professionalism; and 6) systems-based practice. Both curriculum and evaluation should be organized to include each core competency area.

In 2014, as part of the ACGME Next Accreditation System, all surgery residency programs were required to submit a milestones-based semiannual performance assessment of all residents. Clinical competency committees (CCC) were codified within each residency for formative and summative assessment. In all, 16 general surgery milestones were mapped to the six ACGME core competencies, and eight separate domains essential for surgical practice were developed by an ABS- and ACGME-led working group. Each milestone included descriptions of activities that allowed resident performance to be judged at four levels of performance. A critical deficiency level was also described for each milestone. By examining milestone results over time, a trajectory of resident performance could be used to track individual progress, identify strengths and weaknesses, and compare performance with other learners. PDs viewed the general surgery milestones favorably when compared with previous evaluation systems and noted less grade inflation and fewer "halo effects." Several groups have documented a strong correlation between resident and CCC assessments of performance using the milestones.

Effective July 2020, a second version of the surgery milestones was introduced at the Toronto program. Organized by the six ACGME core competencies, 18 new, specialty-specific milestones have been introduced—each with five levels of performance. Level 4 performance is defined as a target (not a requirement) for graduation and Level 5 performance is designated for an expert resident performing at levels higher than expected. Though a category for critical deficiency has been eliminated, two new categories have been added—one for residents who have yet to achieve Level 1 performance and another for situations in which the milestone is not yet assessable. Milestones appear best suited for broad, summative assessments of resident performance over time rather than evaluation of specific skill acquisition.

EPAs

EPAs define and evaluate essential activities before U.S. medical students enter residency. EPAs are the units of work essential to a specialty, as opposed to the competencies that refer to the ability of individuals to carry out this work. EPAs are independently executable, observable, and measurable in both process and outcome making them suitable for entrustment decisions. General surgery EPAs are designed to determine four levels of entrustability: 1) observation only, 2) performance under direct supervision, 3) performance under indirect supervision, and 4) independent practice/ ability to supervise others. The descriptors for each level are tied to discrete resident activities and behaviors that an individual can learn to perform independently. The ABS has released five surgery EPAs: gallbladder disease, trauma, surgery consult, inguinal hernia, and evaluation of right lower quadrant pain (appendicitis). EPAs provide an excellent framework for credentialing during residency and competency-based advancement toward the goals of full entrustment and autonomous practice. For EPAs to be a successful framework for competency-based credentialling, challenges related to current payment practice, medical malpractice responsibility, and adequate faculty teaching time must be resolved.

Cognitive Knowledge Assessment

Two readily available tools can be used for assessment at the start of surgical residency:

- The ACS ERRA, a psychometrically rigorous, formative assessment of PGY1 resident preparedness, was mentioned above with particular focus on how it uses intake knowledge assessments in curricular design. Focusing on 20 clinical topics that incoming surgical residents are likely to encounter, residents respond to 40 short clinical cases, each followed by questions that specifically evaluate clinical decisions. As a formative tool, the ACS ERRA is intended to assess resident decision-making upon entering surgical residency.
- The ACS Fundamentals of Surgery Curriculum® (ACS FSC), a highly interactive, case-based, online curriculum, addresses the essential content areas that all surgical residents need to master in the early years of training. In more than 109 ACS FSC simulated case scenarios, residents are asked to recognize and assess symptoms and signs, order appropriate tests and procedures, evaluate data, and initiate appropriate actions.

Assessment of cognitive knowledge once residency begins consists of the annual ABSITE and periodic topical quizzes designed and administered by each surgery residency. The ACS ATLS course also culminates in a multiple-choice examination of cognitive knowledge related to trauma care.

The ABSITE is a norm-referenced multiple-choice examination designed to measure residents' knowledge of applied science and management of clinical problems in surgery. Intended as a formative evaluation instrument, its results inform the resident and their PD of relative strengths and weaknesses in cognitive knowledge compared with colleagues in other ACGME-accredited residencies. Content of the ABSITE is aligned with the SCORE Curriculum Outline for General Surgery. In addition to annually reviewing individual resident performance, PDs also can review data regarding cumulative performance of their residents as a group to identify knowledge gaps that should be addressed. Decisions on resident advancement or termination should not be based solely upon ABSITE results.

Quizzes designed by teaching faculty are commonly used in surgery residency programs to assess specific areas of cognitive knowledge. Although these tools are not norm-referenced, they support other forms of assessment and motivate residents to participate in didactic lectures and topical reading programs.

Resident self-assessment of cognitive knowledge also is available as the SCORE Curriculum Outline for General Surgery, which includes test questions at the end of each module. Residents may also find reviewing the ACS *Surgical Education and Self-Assessment Program* (*SESAP*®) questions useful for self-assessment.

Technical and Operative Skills Assessment

Developing surgical expertise requires knowledge, judgment, decision-making, and technical skills. Although there is a long history of teaching and assessing knowledge and judgment through written and oral exams, evaluating training outcomes in the technical aspects of surgery is less developed. The traditional model of teaching the technical skills of surgery is to immerse the trainee through long hours of observation and progressive responsibility in the OR.

These skills are complex. They require application of knowledge (for example, anatomy), eye-hand coordination and visual-spatial skills, manual dexterity, strategies of exposure and retraction, the optimal use of assistants, and adaptation to the pathology of the disease.

Under constraints of work-hour restrictions, the cost of OR time, and the ethics of practicing fundamental skills on patients, interest has developed in moving the early part of the learning curve from the OR to a more controlled educational environment, such as the simulation center.

Rather than using training time or case numbers alone as surrogates for competency, there is interest in developing metrics for surgical skill that can be used for both formative and summative assessments.

Surgical skills must be developed and proven in the OR. Although case number distribution provides some measure of experience, they are insufficient to confirm competency.

The optimal verification of competence relies on multiple assessments by multiple observers under varied conditions to minimize bias and case-to-case variability. Structured assessment tools add to the validity of these assessments by focusing the learner on the goals on which they will be assessed and the evaluator on the elements of assessment. These metrics can provide structured and specific feedback and track progress.

One assessment strategy based on these principles is SIMPL, a smartphone app that allows attendings to efficiently evaluate their trainees by answering three questions based on the four-level Zwisch scale. The Zwisch scale describes the role of both the trainee and supervisor for each stage in the development of autonomy in the OR. Dictated comments can be appended to provide specific formative feedback. The approach is efficient and convenient. The supervisor provides timely feedback, and the securely stored data are aggregated and made available to the PD, who can follow a resident's progress.

The degree of guidance reported by the supervising surgeon correlates well with the blinded assessment of recorded resident performance by expert evaluators, according to the evidence. Thus, by tracking both the role of the learner and the supervisor, the Zwisch scale provides meaningful information. Likewise, the Global Operative Assessment of Laparoscopic Skills (GOALS) provides another convenient global rating scale, with published evidence of reliability and validity in assessing laparoscopic surgery skills.

Simulation lends itself well to training and assessment of surgical technical skills. This highly controlled environment places the learner, rather than the patient, at the center of the experience, eliminating patient and pathology variables and allowing for reliable and valid assessment. By developing and confirming acquisition of fundamental skills at the simulation center, the learner can build a strong foundation and accelerate the learning curve in the clinical setting. FLS has been incorporated into all general surgery and obstetrics/gynecology programs in the U.S. and this laparoscopic skills training is a prerequisite for eligibility for the ABS Qualifying Exam (ABS QE). The effectiveness of FLS in enabling residents to acquire laparoscopic skills has been demonstrated in a randomized controlled trial.

The FLS approach of defining a foundational set of skills, modeling them in a structured, standardized simulation environment, and embedding reliable and validated metrics to verify acquisition of these skills has been applied to flexible endoscopy training. The Fundamentals of Endoscopic Surgery Program (FES) was developed by SAGES and distributed to all general surgery residency programs in the U.S.; it is a prerequisite for entry into the ABS QE.

Because general surgery graduates are expected to be competent in flexible gastrointestinal (GI) endoscopy, and because clinical training opportunities vary between programs, the ABS, working with SAGES and other leading GI surgical specialty societies, defined a curriculum for endoscopy training, They mandated completion of FES to demonstrate the knowledge and skills of flexible endoscopy required for graduates of general surgery training programs.

OSATS, developed at University of Toronto, is a widely used and well-validated assessment of a range of surgical skills in the simulation setting. Another assessment, for first-year residents, is Verification of Proficiency.

ATLS and ACLS are mature programs that provide a structured approach to trauma care and cardiac resuscitation, respectively. They have been universally incorporated because of their proven impact on patient outcomes. To expand the capabilities of surgeons to operate in rare and complex trauma situations, the ACS developed the Advanced Surgical Skills for Exposure in Trauma (ASSET) course. This is a cadaver-based one-day course to demonstrate optimal surgical exposure in five key anatomic areas: neck, chest, abdomen and pelvis, and upper and lower extremities. The ACS Advanced Trauma Operative Management (ATOM®) course teaches operative techniques for managing penetrating injuries of the chest and abdomen to senior surgical residents, trauma fellows, military surgeons, and general surgeons who infrequently treat these types of injuries.

An established way to evaluate surgical competence is the objective structured clinical examination (OSCE), a standardized method to assess a variety of clinical skills, such as technical, diagnostic, and professional skills, using a standardized scoring system. OSCEs use standardized clinical scenarios involving stations with task trainers, models and standardized patients.

Leadership and Team Skills

Surgical education goes beyond the acquisition of knowledge and technical skills and demands training in a variety of competencies. The Royal Australasian College of Surgeons defines nine competencies:

- Collaboration and teamwork
- Communication
- Health advocacy
- Judgment: decision-making
- Management and leadership
- Medical expertise
- Professionalism
- Scholarship and teaching
- Technical expertise

An effective surgical training program educates its trainees in each of these areas and incorporates these competencies in regular formative evaluations.

Originally used to assess the non-technical (social and cognitive) skills of crew members in the aviation industry, the non-technical skills (NOTECHS) scale assessed cooperation, leadership and managerial skills, situation awareness and vigilance, and decision-making. This system has been applied to surgical training by Sevdalis and colleagues, who added a "communication and interaction dimension" and adapted all subscales for use in the surgical context.

Another effort to train and evaluate non-technical skills in surgery and to improve behaviors in the OR that affect performance and patient safety is Non-Technical Skills for Surgeons (NOTSS), which was developed at the University of Aberdeen with funding from the Royal College of Surgeons of Edinburgh and National Health Services Education for Scotland. NOTSS establishes an educational system for assessment and training based on observable behavior in the intraoperative phase of surgery.

A group from Imperial College in London also described and refined the Observational Teamwork Assessment for Surgery (OTAS) and provided evidence for content and construct validation. Their data demonstrate that OTAS' psychometric properties are sound when used to evaluate teamwork in the OR.

Quality

Because surgical education should ensure that surgeons deliver competent and safe clinical care, it should strive to demonstrate that an educational intervention enhances patient safety. In practice, this ability is difficult to measure because residents primarily perform clinical tasks in a supervised setting. Supervising faculty members are responsible for protecting the patient and are mandated to intervene if a trainee may put the patient's safety at risk. Although training has been shown to transfer from simulation to the OR with respect to performance, limited quality evidence is available regarding clinical outcomes or safety.

Benchmarking and Autonomy: The CBD Program in Canada

The transition from time-based surgical education to competency-based training requires the establishment of benchmarks which must be achieved for promotion and for graduation. Measures that can be used for benchmarks, described previously, should be governed by the principles of reliability and validity, multiple assessments by multiple faculty, and efforts to minimize bias, whether explicit or implicit. The Royal College of Physicians and Surgeons of Canada transitioned in recent years to CBD, based on evidence that showed learners advanced at different rates and that years of training or case volume alone were insufficient measures of competency.

CBD is underpinned by assessment after almost every operation or clinical encounter that is based on a smartphone app to provide continuous feedback to the learner and the PD. A promotions committee independently reviews these data to determine whether the learner has met the performance standards and achieved the requisite benchmarks, which allows the PD to identify and remediate struggling residents more easily.

CBD divides each program into four stages of training with clear learning objectives for each stage. Trainees receive a list of EPAs and milestones based on the CanMEDS competency framework, which are embedded in their normal clinical workflow. Faculty are required to directly observe residents as they perform the EPAs, which encourages coaching and constructive feedback. These EPA evaluations then populate an electronic portfolio, which can be reviewed by the resident as well as a competency committee, which determines if the resident is ready to progress to the next stage of training.

Remediation Strategies

Prior single-program studies suggest that about one out of five trainees in GME programs will demonstrate a significant problem during training. These challenges are often multifactorial, bridging the areas of clinical function, academic progress, and the most common challenge, professionalism. Such challenges often present in the junior residency years but may not be successfully addressed over the course of training. Hence, remediation frequently requires evaluation across multiple domains, including assessments of personal and workplace pressures that may affect the trainee; sometimes it involves managing, rather than solving, a challenge. In general, character-based challenges, such as honesty, integrity, work ethic, altruism, humility, and perseverance, are difficult to address. Research among business executives shows character issues can be addressed by pointing the learner to prior role models and teachers who demonstrated these qualities, coupled with deeper self-reflection exercises, such as those that might accompany a life-altering illness or spiritual experience. More readily addressed may be issues such as time management, study patterns, academic development behaviors, technical deficiencies, and communication competencies. Determining the nature and source of the challenge, including causes outside of the workplace, is important to the remediation process.

Establishing a culture of evaluation in training and incorporating multiple measures and validated assessment instruments offers a PD an accurate and unbiased profile of each resident's progress, including identifying individuals who are unready to advance and where they need remediation. Objective and valid assessments remove bias and provide opportunity for specific action. Remediation should be goal-directed, specific to each trainee, and have an objective endpoint, wherever possible. Ideally, remediation should use simulation, if feasible and appropriate. The simulation center is a safe space where the learner is central and an educational scenario can be developed to meet the learner's specific need. Progress can be monitored with specific metrics and a performance improvement goal should be established.

Once remediation targets have been achieved, the learner can return to the clinical environment. For technical skill deficiencies, video assessment of performance with feedback is valuable during remediation. Emerging technology using computer vision-powered algorithms allow the coach to focus on the specific aspects of the procedure requiring improvement and to efficiently embed feedback, comments, and assessment into the video.

Remediation strategies should be developed with broad-based, corroborative faculty input using collective wisdom and experience to diagnose the challenge. The nature of the problem should be documented with clarity and presented to the trainee in a structured and constructive fashion along with an agreed-upon improvement plan. Developed in partnership with the faculty, this plan should establish mutual accountability through a series of check-ins and progress updates, which can document the resolution of the challenges or the need for remediation to progress to more significant interventions, such as extended training or dismissal. Diligent documentation of the case for remediation, plan, progress monitoring, and outcome of the intervention is critical to a fair and successful process and serves the interests of both the trainee and the program.

Institutional GME overseers and external resources, such as individuals who can assist with learning diagnostics or psychological and/or psychiatric support, should be included in the process, especially in more complex cases, such as those that may to lead to termination. Strategies such as coaching and mentorship, when applied to all learners and faculty, provide an environment that acknowledges personal growth and a culture of lifelong learning that make constructive feedback and interventions a normal part of ongoing development and sustainability. Finally, if all else fails, adherence to institutional policy and legal consultation form the foundation for an effective, albeit painful, termination process. A useful approach to these challenges honors the program's commitment to the trainee as well as high standards of care commensurate with the public trust.

Assessment Strategies

This chapter, which has focused on the assessment of people and evaluation of program elements, now turns to overall program evaluation. The Association of American Medical Colleges (AAMC) and ACGME outline various types of evaluations for both specific programs and for medical schools and residencies. Those involved in medical education should become familiar with these required evaluations as well as any internal requirements.

With regard to residences and fellowships, the ACGME has separate sections to evaluate residents, faculty, and program, along with a section on the learning and working environment. Programs must report on these areas in their annual program report.

As part of these processes, programs are required to establish a Program Evaluation Committee (PEC) that advises the PD and conducts the Annual Program Evaluation (APE). The APE evaluates program changes from the prior year and plans for upcoming changes, whereas the PEC evaluates overall resident/fellow performance, faculty development activities, results of graduate performance (such as board examination performance), and program quality, including the clinical learning environment. The PEC outlines program strengths, areas for improvement, and establish timelines for any planned changes.

The APE is more than a requirement; it is a tool to ensure that the program participates in continuous quality improvement and uses reasonable metrics to ensure timely progress. This evaluation process must involve core educators and requires acceptance of the proposed changes by all who interact with learners. Establishment of the PEC and implementation of an APE is a commitment to quality education.

The APE may be used as a starting point for outside evaluation of a struggling program. Consultation with a historically successful program can initiate program change aligned with established best practices.

Programs also must evaluate faculty in a report that should be written, anonymous, and provided to the PD for review. Faculty members must receive evaluation feedback at least once a year. In addition, faculty evaluations identify topics for a faculty development program. In institutions where education and teaching are part of the promotion and retention process, these evaluations can support the faculty member's academic promotion credentials.

Faculty evaluations also should address negative behavior. It is not enough to provide a faculty member with a group of poor evaluations; a remediation program should also be designed, including defining support needed for improvement. This process should be documented in the APE and the annual program report to the ACGME.

Evaluation of the clinical learning and working environment is critical. Education is best achieved in an environment free of perceived threat. The ACGME outlines what is needed for a safe working environment, including patient safety, quality, supervision, well-being, and professionalism. The ACGME also monitors the learning environment through a site visit process known as the Clinical Learning Environment Review (CLER), which each sponsoring institution must undergo every two years or so. The ACGME publishes summaries of expectations for best-practice learning environments and for applying CLER principles to unique training settings, such as those programs with few trainees or faculty or unique content focus, such as aerospace medicine. The clinical learning environment, assessed at an institutional level, is still a required focus for each program, which must have tools to evaluate the environment. An area deemed noncompliant can become part of the APE delineation of areas for improvement.

Areas difficult to evaluate include fatigue and fatigue mitigation, resident well-being, toxic work environment, and professional responsibilities and their execution. Several well-designed tools to evaluate each of these areas are available online.

Programs not meeting these standards must identify the root cause of the issue and design a remediation program with measurable outcomes to ensure improvement.

Conclusion

Surgical residency training has evolved dramatically in the past 30 years, with the advent of duty-hour restrictions, Internet-based content delivery, competency-founded and outcome-oriented strategies, simulation, quality and cost priorities, technologic advances affecting both practice and assessment, benchmarking capabilities, awareness of the role and importance of non-technical skills, and the growth of assessment science in general. All of these elements, among others, have created an environment in which curricular development and assessment are more challenging yet more meaningful. The surgical educator of the future will need to develop adaptive educational competencies that include levels of accountability and specificity that can be measured and documented rather than simply governed by personal observation and inference. Critical to this process will be public and professional accountability for the educational process and product, navigation of an increasingly complex regulatory and fiscal environment, and reorientation processes to match outcomes. Evolving technologies that create the opportunity for frequent and scalable workplace-based assessments, skill analysis, and benchmarking to external standards are needed for implementation. In addition, progress in cognitive science and understanding how foundational knowledge and skills are formed and maintained will inform these processes and lead to the more efficient program designs that contemporary health care and education require.

The future is bright, dynamic, and offers promise for a more standardized and qualifiable product that could affect global health. By operationalizing these strategies, surgical learners, educators, professionals, and most importantly, patients will be better served.

Suggested Readings

Allen M, Gawad N, Park L, Raîche I. The educational role of autonomy in medical training: a scoping review. *J Surg Res.* 2019;240:1-16.

Carraccio C, Englander R, Van Melle, E, et al. Advancing competency-based medical education: a charter for clinician-educators. *Acad Med.* 2016;91(5):645-649.

Carraccio CL, Englander R. From Flexner to competencies: reflections on a decade and the journey ahead. *Acad Med.* 2013;88(8):1067-1073.

Chen XP, Sullivan AM, Smink DS, Alseidi A, Bengtson JM, Kwakye G, Dalrymple JL. Resident autonomy in the OR: how faculty assess real-time entrustability. *Ann Surg.* 2019;269(6):1080-1086.

Englander R, Frank JR, Carraccio C, Sherbino J, Ross S, Snell L, on behalf of the ICBME Collaborators. Toward a shared language for competency-based medical education. *Med Teach.* 2017;39(6):582-587.

Frank JR, Snell LS, Cate OT, et al. Competency-based medical education: theory to practice. *Med Teach.* 2010; 32(8):638-645.

George BC, Teitelbaum EN, Meyerson SL, et al. Reliability, validity, and feasibility of the Zwisch scale for the assessment of intraoperative performance. *J Surg Educ.* 2014;71(6):e90-96.

Hull L, Arora S, Kassab E, Kneebone R, Sevdalis N. Observational teamwork assessment for surgery: content validation and tool refinement. *J Am Coll Surg.* 2011;212:234-243.

Jarman BT, O'Heron CT, Kallies KJ, Cogbill TH. Enhancing confidence in graduating general surgery residents: establishing a chief surgery resident service at an independent academic medical center. *J Surg Educ.* 2018;75(4):888-894.

Karpicke JD, Roediger HL III. The critical importance of retrieval for learning. *Science.* 2008;319:966-968.

Klingensmith ME, Cogbill TH, Samonte K, Jones A, Malangoni MA. Practice administration training needs of recent general surgery graduates. *Surgery*. 2015;158(3):773-776.

Kneebone R, Nestel D, Wetzel C, Black S, et al. The human face of simulation: patient-focused simulation training. *Acad Med*. 2006;81(10):919-924.

Leppink J, Duvivier R. Twelve tips for medical curriculum design from a cognitive load theory perspective. *Med Teach*. 2016;38(7):669-674.

McSparron JI, Vanka A, Smith CC. Cognitive learning theory for clinical teaching. *Clin Teach*. 2019;16(2):96-100.

Mohammad A, Branicki F, Abu-Zidan FM. Educational and clinical impact of Advanced Trauma Life Support (ATLS) courses: a systematic review. *World J Surg*. 2014;38(2):322-329.

Nousiainen MT, Mironova P, Hynes M, et al. Eight-year outcomes of a competency-based residency training program in orthopedic surgery. *Med Teach*. 2018;40(10):1042-1054.

Sanfey H, Ketchum J, Bartlett J, Markwell S, Meier AH, Williams, Dunnington G. Verification of proficiency in basic skills for postgraduate year 1 residents. *Surgery*. 2010;148:759-767.

Sedvalis N, Davis R, Koutantji M, Undre S, Darzi A, Vincent CA. Reliability of a revised NOTECHS scale for use in surgical teams. *Am J Surg*. 2008;196(2):184-190.

Soper NJ, DaRosa DA. Presidential address: engendering operative autonomy in surgical training. *Surgery*. 2014;156(4):745-751.

Sroka G, Feldman LS, Vassiliou MC, Kaneva PA, Fayez R, Fried GM. Fundamentals of laparoscopic surgery simulator training to proficiency improves laparoscopic performance in the OR-a randomized controlled trial. *Am J Surg*. 2010; 199(1):115-120.

Sturm LP, Windsor JA, Cosman PH, Cregan P, Hewett PJ, Maddern GJ. A systematic review of skills transfer after surgical simulation training. *Ann Surg*. 2008;248(2):166-179.

Swendiman RA, Hoffman DI, Bruce AN , Blinman TA, Nance, Chou CM. Qualities and methods of highly effective surgical educators: a grounded theory model. *J Surg Ed*. 2019;76(5):1293-1302.

Taylor DCM, Hamdy H. Adult learning theories: implications for learning and teaching in medical education: AMEE Guide No. 83. *Med Teach*. 2013;35(11):e1561-e157.

Teman NR, Gauger PG, Mullan PB, Tarpley JL, Minter RM. Entrustment of general surgery residents in the OR: factors contributing to provision of resident autonomy. *J Am Coll Surg*. 2014;219(4):778-787.

Torbeck L, Wilson A, Choi J, Dunnington GL. Identification of behaviors and techniques for promoting autonomy in the OR. *Surgery*. 2015;158(4):1102-1110.

Undre S, Healy AN, Darzi A, Vincent CA. Observational assessment of surgical teamwork: a feasibility study. *World J Surg*. 2006;30:1774-1783.

Vassiliou MC, Feldman LS, Andrew CG, Bergman S, Leffondré K, Stanbridge D, Fried GM. A global assessment tool for evaluation of intraoperative laparoscopic skills. *Am J Surg*. 2005;190:107–113.

Williams RG, Roberts NK, Schwind CJ, et al. The nature of general surgery resident performance problems. *Surgery*. 2009;145(6):651–658.

Winn W. Some implications of cognitive theory for instructional design. *Instr Sci*. 1990;19:53-69.

AMERICAN
SURGEONS
OF SURGEONS
COLLEGE OF
AMERICAN
SURGEONS
OF SURGEONS
COLLEGE OF
AMERICAN
SURGEONS

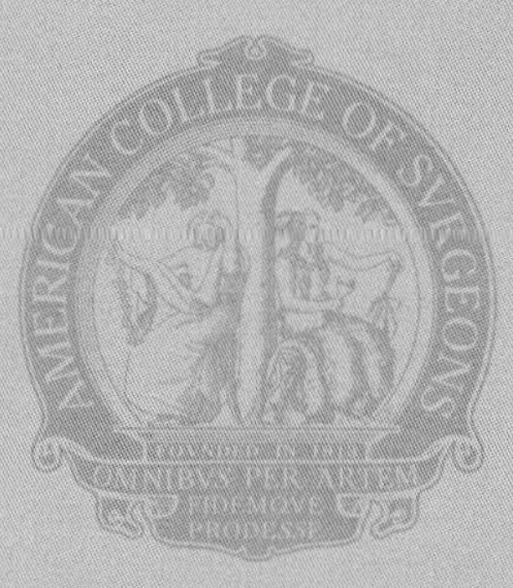

CHAPTER 13
Resources

Lead Author

Ronald J. Weigel, MD, PhD, MBA, FACS

Co-Authors

Karen J. Brasel, MD, MPH, FACS, MAMSE

Christian Miguel de Virgilio, MD, FACS

Taylor S. Riall, MD, PhD, FACS

Patricia L. Turner, MD, MBA, FACS

CHAPTER 13

Resources

Executive Summary

- Who are the key players involved in running a training program?
- What are their responsibilities to the resident?
- What system resources should be available to trainees?
- What physical resources should be available to residents?
- How can we promote well-being to help residents avoid burnout?

The optimal training environment for surgery residents requires the commitment and coordinated effort of many individuals across the spectrum of the health care system. Health system structure, including the integration of different educational programs and access to adequate patient volume, is critical for success. Physical resources, such as hospital and training facilities, must meet standards appropriate for resident education. Additional resources that support the wellness of residents during training are needed to maintain a strong working environment conducive to learning. These resources need to be integrated and coordinated to achieve an optimal training environment.

People Resources

A successful surgical training program depends on committed individuals within the department of surgery as well as individuals in other departments, college of medicine, and hospital.

Department of Surgery Chair

The department chair has ultimate oversight for recruiting and maintaining the faculty and staff required for optimal resident education. The chair is responsible for ensuring resources are available for the residency training program and needs to develop productive relationships with the dean, associate deans for graduate medical education (GME), chief executive officer (CEO) of the hospital, and chief financial officer (CFO) of the health care system. For independent programs that are not university-based, affiliating with a medical school engages medical students and research faculty and enhances the academic opportunities for surgery residents. The chair should recognize the need to engage other faculty and enable them to successfully perform their duties within the residency education system. A culture of professionalism requires maintaining and expanding diversity among faculty, staff, and residents. Establishing and maintaining diversity among the faculty helps ensure that the department's learning environment is free of bias and harassment. A recent American Surgical Association white paper offers a valuable resource to develop diversity, equity, and inclusion in academic surgical departments.[1]

A program must have a team dedicated to resident education that includes a vice-chair for education, a residency program director (PD), associate PDs, and nonsurgical faculty educators, particularly surgeons with professional educational experience, as well as program support staff and administrative assistants. This team needs to coordinate efforts to create a "culture of education" within the department of surgery. The department chair needs to advocate for appropriate institutional resources to provide financial support, space, training facilities, and a safe working environment within the hospital, operating rooms (ORs), and clinics. The chair should enforce policies that support a conducive educational environment, such as resident work-hour regulations. The chair also must maintain the appropriate balance between competing priorities, such as education and service, as well as the balance between the residency training program, fellowship training programs, and medical student education programs.

Department of Surgery Vice-Chair for Education

Some departments will have a specific vice-chair role for education much like they might have for research. The role of the vice-chair may be responsible for integrating educational programs within the department, across departments, and within service lines. The vice-chair, along with the PD, supports an appropriate educational structure within the department. A key role for a vice-chair could include overseeing educational programs, educational priorities, and educational budgets. Educational resources need to be balanced between medical student, resident, and fellowship needs. Increasing specialization in surgical practice has led trainees to pursue fellowship training. The vice-chair, the office of the designed institutional office (DIO), and the PDs must ensure that fellowship training programs do not interfere with the general surgery residency training program. The vice-chair for education also can mentor leaders in the various educational programs within the department.

Residency PD

The residency PD is responsible for all aspects of a specific surgery residency training program. PDs need to be able to devote at least 30 percent of their time to the residency program. Individuals chosen for this role need to be well regarded and respected among peer faculty and the surgery residents. Although junior faculty members could do this job, more seasoned surgeons may be better suited to it. If junior faculty members are appointed PDs, they may need structured mentoring. PDs should have a strong history of interest in, and dedication to, education and would benefit from formal training in education, such as a masters degree in education or intense courses in education. PDs should have a passion for resident education, familiarity with the department's culture, and knowledge of the necessary oversight and regulations required to run a surgery residency program. A PD needs to be unbiased, emotionally intelligent, and politically astute to work successfully with division chiefs, chairs of other departments, and institutional leaders. This individual must be able to engage faculty and residents in necessary and required training priorities.

Within the educational structure, the PD has authority and accountability for administering the residency program. Ideally, the PD will coordinate and help develop scholarly activity centered on resident education. A PD is accountable for establishing an appropriate resident recruitment plan, a system to evaluate current residents, clear criteria for promotion of residents, and action plans for residents who fall short of program expectations. The PD oversees all training sites within the program and must have the authority to approve or separate faculty members from teaching and assessment responsibilities within the residency program.

Associate PD

Associate PDs can assist the PD in the complex task of resident education; the number of associate PDs will vary depending on the size of the residency program. Associate PDs provide leadership over various aspects of the residency program, including fundamental knowledge areas encompassed by the American Board of Surgery In-Training Examination (ABSITE). In addition, associate PDs share responsibilities with the PD, which may include monitoring and confirming operative experience and technical skills, providing opportunities for resident assessment and feedback, and maintaining an appropriate skills laboratory. Other shared tasks may include developing didactic lectures for the residents; mock oral examinations; a system for up-to-date and accurate records and logs of resident activities; research opportunities that include both clinical and basic science; quality improvement and system-based learning projects; training for the residents to be effective teachers in the clinical services; and disciplinary structures and remediation. These leadership duties provide excellent faculty development opportunities. Serving as associate PD can serve as a training opportunity for a future PD role.

Primary Clinical Faculty

Primary clinical faculty within a general surgery residency training program must be certified by the American Board of Surgery. Accreditation Council for Graduate Medical Education (ACGME) requirements for core versus noncore faculty ensure appropriate teachers are available for the surgical residents. The size and scope of practice to maintain the required educational opportunities for surgery residents should be commensurate with the size of the residency program. Residents need adequate exposure to surgical volume to train in the required aspects of surgical practice. Faculty need to understand that the principal responsibility of residents on a surgical service is to address their educational needs, not just to provide service. As a result, to meet the needs for education, certain services within the health care system may not be assigned residents. Appropriate scope of resident experience includes adequate time and surgical volume on various clinical services, including acute care, gastrointestinal and colorectal, oncology, endocrine and vascular; thus, the primary clinical faculty need to have an adequate breadth of clinical expertise. Other clinical experiences can enhance and contribute to the general surgery training experience, such as organ transplantation, cardiac surgery, plastic and reconstructive surgery, and pediatric surgery. Clinical faculty both at academic and community-based practices can provide an important diversity of practice type for the residency training program.

Research Faculty

Academic faculty who are involved in research are the ideal educators to train residents in research. They enhance the research opportunities necessary to develop future faculty for academic training programs, which require research experience and improve resident preparation for future fellowship training. Faculty and staff involved in grant management, institutional review board (IRB) management, and biostatistical support also help train surgery residents in research. Faculty significantly devoted to research can help mentor residents in developing their role as surgeon-scientists. Other research areas, such as health services, can be developed by engaging faculty in other colleges, such as the college of public health. Performing clinical research provides additional opportunities for residents to understand the role of the IRB and other mechanisms that may relate to clinical trials and studies that optimize patient care. Formal mechanisms for teaching the conduct of ethical research or examining global medicine projects are important for future academic development of residents as faculty members. Even for those individuals who eventually develop a career in a community practice, interpreting the literature and helping conduct clinical studies prepares them to objectively evaluate the literature. Opportunities for surgery residents to obtain advanced degrees, including a master of public health (MPH), doctor of philosophy (PhD), or master of business administration (MBA), enhance the development of future academic surgical faculty and are strongly recommended for academic surgical training programs.

Program Administrators

Administrative support for the residency program is a critical resource necessary to coordinate the various aspects of the program. At least one full-time equivalent program coordinator should be on staff, along with administrative support for every 20 residents in the program. Program coordinators would benefit from formal educational training such as a masters degree in education or other experience that prepare them to understand the necessities of educational programs.

Additional Educational Personnel

Additional faculty with a breadth of expertise may enhance residency training, such as a doctorate-prepared professional educator who can contribute to curriculum design and implementation, faculty development, and research. These faculty can develop specific programs focused on quality improvement, approaches to enhance communication, and the development of surgical faculty as educators. They may also serve on other committees related to education and be an important liaison to the department's educational programs. Other educational personnel can include physician assistants, advanced registered nurse practitioners, and bedside nurses, who can teach residents at the point of care. Programs with medical students on surgical service require coordination with the student clerkship director, associate directors, and the student clerkship coordinator. Residents provide a key educational opportunity for medical students rotating on the surgical service; in fact, resident teaching is a requirement of the Liaison Committee on Medical Education. The better the educational experiences offered by surgical residents, the more likely medical students will choose a career in surgery. Programs that develop surgery residents as educators enhance the education of both residents and medical students.

Health System Faculty and Staff

Many other institutional individuals need to be engaged and committed to training surgical residents. The dean of the college of medicine serves as the chief academic medical officer and is responsible for supervising the associate dean for GME. The associate dean for GME oversees all residency programs at the institution and ensures that they have appropriate institutional resources.

General surgery residents are hospital employees; in most organizations the number of residents in the various training programs exceeds the Centers for Medicare & Medicaid Services (CMS) cap established decades ago. For this reason, the hospital's financial commitment is to ensure adequate support for residents and their well-being. The hospital CEO must commit to providing adequate health care benefits, essential needs (such as library access, meals, parking, uniform services, and so on), and a safe working environment. There needs to be a strong working relationship between the various departments that have residency training programs.

For example, the surgical skills lab/simulation center should be developed as an institutional resource and requires a productive working interaction between the PDs of various surgical programs, all of whom benefit from this center. The center's director should work with or be part of the department of surgery to implement the American College of Surgeons/Association of Program Directors in Surgery (ACS/APDS) Surgery Resident Skills Curriculum and other essential surgical skills curricula. The resources of a surgical skills lab/simulation center are increasingly important to residency training, and it's important to have someone who understands these evolving requirements and establishes appropriate training modules. A skills lab director and coordinator with additional faculty dedicated to teaching surgical techniques provide an invaluable educational opportunity for surgical residents.

In addition, recognizing that residents work on many different clinical services, the chief nursing executive must establish a strong educational environment for the surgery residents. This responsibility includes ensuring that nursing staff in the OR, clinic, and hospital inpatient services recognize and interact well with surgical residents who manage patients on the surgical services.

System Resources (for General Surgery)

In addition to the right people, a successful general surgery residency program requires system resources to make sure residents become independent surgeons capable of operating autonomously across a range of general surgical procedures. Importantly, these system resources must provide residents with the technical skills, knowledge, and experience to effectively manage both the pre- and post-operative aspects of general surgical care, including knowing when—and when not—to operate.

In acquiring system resources, it is important to understand that the goal of training an independent general surgeon is more challenging today than it was in previous eras. Since July 2003, the 80-hour resident duty-hour restrictions have limited the number of hours that residents can spend at the hospital. This workweek limit has forced programs and PDs to streamline education.

A less discussed, but perhaps more influential, change to resident and fellowship training occurred in November 2002, when Medicare announced it would no longer pay for any service provided by a student. Consequently, clinic and inpatient notes, formerly assigned to medical students, had to be completed by residents. The increasing demand for residents to write notes puts more emphasis on service than on education. In addition, Medicare required that the teaching surgeon be present in the OR for the critical portion of the procedure to qualify for reimbursement. For concurrent surgeries, the teaching surgeon should be present for the critical portions of both operations. Furthermore, trainees in ACGME-approved fellowships cannot bill even if they have a faculty appointment.

Collectively, the duty-hour restrictions, combined with these changes in Medicare reimbursement, have allowed less flexibility in supervision if billing is to occur, creating an environment in which, without adjustments, general surgery residents will have less opportunity to achieve autonomy. Although important for patient safety and accuracy of documentation, these changes have led to more regulatory oversight, more paperwork, and less opportunity to focus directly on patient care; they have also contributed to burnout. The solution is not simply shifting the burden to trainees, but providing adequate resources to achieve patient safety, including progressive solutions that ensure effective, beneficial, and lasting change. Unfortunately, the provider of the necessary resources (in general, the hospital administrative leadership) may not be directly aware of these unintended consequences. The Coronavirus Disease 2019 (COVID-19) pandemic has taught us that solving a problem by assigning additional work to health care professionals requires sensitivity to overwork and stress. These stresses can be relieved, at least partially, through protected time off, support services for physical and psychological health, and a healthy work-life balance. Top leadership needs to recognize these needs and obtain the necessary remedial resources.

General surgery procedure skills, technological improvements, and disease epidemiology also have changed. For example, trainees today may need to learn three different approaches to performing an inguinal hernia (open, laparoscopic, and robotic) or four ways to perform an esophageal myotomy (open, laparoscopic, robotic, and endoscopic); in addition, they may not encounter severe ulcer disease due to acid-reducing drugs and improved treatment of helicobacter pylori. In many centers, open vascular surgery comprises less than one in five cases, so they must learn endovascular and open vascular approaches.

Along with this explosion of technology, public reporting is bringing surgeons under greater scrutiny regarding surgical outcomes. Some complex operations should be performed at centers with optimal resources and experience.[2,3] The modern general surgery training program must meet the expanding needs of volume and hospital quality while offering residents sufficient case volume, variety, and complexity in an array of surgical areas.

The modern surgical training experience can be divided into three domains:

- The first domain includes the core components, such as the surgical disorders of the abdomen and its contents, the alimentary tract, skin, soft tissues, breast, endocrine organs, and trauma. For these disciplines, the resident must graduate with the ability to provide independent and comprehensive care.
- The second domain comprises oncologic, vascular, pediatric, and intensive care disorders. The program needs to encompass the surgical evaluation and management of these conditions.
- For the third domain, which includes cardiothoracic, urologic, gynecologic, neurologic, and otolaryngologic diseases, the training program must ensure the resident has adequate knowledge and experience for the assessment and requisite emergency surgical stabilization of these patients with these conditions. It should provide adequate equipment for open, laparoscopic, robotic, endoscopic, and endovascular procedures.

Given the complexity of training requirements, it is unlikely that a single hospital, university-based or independent, can meet all these demands; as a result, they will likely need to affiliate with other hospitals to achieve the requisite training.

Documentation Expectations and Resources

In 2014, a federal mandate to require use of the electronic health record (EHR) was enacted to improve the quality of patient care by making patients' medical histories available to the physicians treating them. The EHR was expected to improve the efficiency of physician's offices by eliminating patient charts and illegible handwriting. Unfortunately, most studies suggest that physician time spent charting has increased, and the EHR frequently has been cited as a major factor contributor to physician burnout.[4]

The EHR must be considered within the context of balancing resident service versus education, which the ACGME monitors. Anonymous annual ACGME surveys sent to residents may influence the accreditation status of a residency program. The morale of the residents may be negatively impacted in situations where provision of service is prioritized over the educational needs of residents and this may result in negative resident responses on the survey. There may be perceptual differences about what constitutes service. For example, most residents feel that EHR documentation and writing notes is service, whereas faculty often view it as education; likewise, many surgical interns see talking to patients as service, while senior residents see it as education. Thus, it is important that programs define and come to a mutual agreement on what constitutes service and what is education.

Coexisting Training Programs

The coexistence of a general surgery program with one or more fellowship programs may either enhance or harm the educational experience of both sets of trainees. A fellowship program may stimulate an increase in the referral of complex cases. When logging cases, e-codes can be used to allow more than one resident to take credit for different parts of the operation. For instance, the general surgery resident can take credit for a femoral arterial exposure and repair, and the fellow can take credit for the endovascular intervention. The fellow adds another, more experienced surgeon to the program, who can therefore teach more junior general surgery residents. Thus, the fellowship has the potential to enhance general surgery resident training.

However, the training and education of the core general surgery training program must take priority. In considering new fellowships in a general surgery subspecialty, the operative experiences of the general surgery residents in those domains need to be evaluated; if the experiences of residents are found to be deficient or marginal, the fellowships should not be approved. This policy applies to both ACGME-accredited and nonaccredited fellowships. In determining whether to start a new fellowship (ACGME-accredited or not), the program must ensure that the chief resident and a fellow have primary responsibility for different patients, although a general surgery resident and surgical critical care fellows may co-manage the nonoperative care of the same patient. Ultimately, programs must determine if they have sufficient case volume and resources to create separate experiences for residents and prospective fellows.

Models for Resident Autonomy

General surgery resident autonomy in the OR must be meaningful in that the resident operates with either passive help from the supervising (attending) surgeon or supervision only for the key portions of the case. Independent operative experience is vital, especially for the critical parts of the operation during which the resident will have the opportunity to direct the flow of the operation.

Meaningful autonomy can be achieved in several ways. In the OR, the supervising surgeon can scrub in on the case and observe silently or, alternatively, can be physically present in the OR without scrubbing in. Another approach is a designated chief resident service in which carefully selected patients are assigned to be cared for by a chief resident, including operative care. The designated chief resident service should be designed so that there is still an attending of record, and sufficient evidence of supervision so that Medicare billing is done appropriately. Another valuable way to gain autonomy is for a resident to serve as a teaching assistant; the ACGME permits teaching assistant cases to count toward the 850 major cases required for graduation.

Regardless of the approach used, programs must provide progressive independence with appropriate supervision and mentored autonomy, as it is a requirement for graduation. To achieve the goals of autonomy, periodic assessment of the progress of each resident in achieving the mutually agreed upon technical milestones is necessary. For example, experience monitoring or gap analysis might reveal that a resident has had insufficient experience in breast surgical procedures. These experiences typically occur in years two and three of residency. Through careful monitoring of experience, the resident's remaining clinical rotations can be adjusted to fill the experience gap. Ongoing gap analysis can prevent residents who are unsure of themselves or who lack the necessary confidence from going directly into practice. Residency programs must assess skill acquisition progress to ensure residents are practice-ready.

Patients must be informed about surgical residents' involvement in their care. Most patients welcome resident participation,[5] but the approval percentage drops when they are asked if they are willing to have residents involved in their intraoperative care, and decreases further (though still a majority) for resident involvement in complex operations.[6] Yet, patients overwhelmingly want residents who graduate from general surgery training able to operate independently. Studies examining surgical outcomes when residents participate have not demonstrated a higher morbidity or mortality.[7] Most surgeons believe that resident involvement improves overall quality of care. However, most studies indicate that resident involvement does lengthen operative times.[7] Thus, it is essential that there is good communication between surgeons and patients in advance, so that they understand the residents' roles as well as potential risks and benefits.

Programs must seek ways to develop resident autonomy in the OR. The faculty must build trust with residents and be committed to increasing their independent experience. This can be achieved by rotations that are long enough for faculty and residents to work together to develop trust. For example, a one-month rotation in which a faculty member operates only once with a resident is unlikely to offer experiences that support autonomy. In addition, faculty must not allow external pressures to compromise the patience and extra time it takes for trainees to perform procedures with adequate independence. Faculty behavior, such as their teaching style, may affect the development of entrustment. For example, autonomy and entrustment may be subject to unconscious bias on the part of faculty, as some studies suggest that women surgery residents are less likely to receive meaningful autonomy than their male counterparts.[8]

Resources for Developing Inquiry and Innovation

Finally, rapid growth in surgical technology requires that general surgery residents learn about surgical innovation. Residents also must learn, ideally through direct involvement in scholarly projects, the basic principles of research, including how to conduct research and apply this knowledge to patient care. The institution should offer resources to facilitate resident research, including access to databases, statistical support, administrative support, and access to an IRB. Residents need adequate access to experienced faculty mentors in study design, data interpretation, and in writing.

Physical Resources

Hospital Type

Determining the optimal physical resources for surgical training depends on how much benefit those resources bring to the trainee. For instance, a children's hospital should ensure that the trainee will have access to the required number of pediatric surgical cases. Similarly, a university hospital or an independent quaternary care hospital could provide training experience that exposes residents to advanced technology and its possibilities and limitations, as well as resources for intensive care and how that care can benefit patients. A university hospital also offers exposure to complex cases but may offer too few routine cases. Other hospitals provide exposure not only to common and complex cases, but also to other types of surgical training benefits. For example, in the community or independent hospital, trainees may see the advantages and disadvantages of private and hospital-based practice. They expose residents to different practice models, helping them better prepare for making career decisions. The integrated hospital and closed medical group system (such as Kaiser) offers an experience that teaches the importance of decisions both large and small; for example, they learn what type of cases get referred to another hospital or how centralized decision-making about supplies (sutures) can help maximize efficiency and minimize cost. Finally, both Veterans Administration (VA) hospitals and public safety-net hospitals provide experiences with different patient populations, including those who face barriers to accessing care. The VA hospital system, as well as affiliated hospitals, offer trainees experience in caring for the geriatric patient. Public safety-net hospitals also show the impact on health outcomes of inadequate access to preventive care and, ideally, how to improve this access.

A good residency program recognizes and takes advantage of the opportunities each of these hospital types affords. Nevertheless, many training programs do not offer rotations or experiences at a wide variety of hospital types. Table 1 outlines the nonexclusive educational opportunities that each hospital type brings to the trainee. Training programs that cannot offer exposure to a range of settings should find another way to deliver these additional experiences.

Ambulatory Surgery Center

Experience in an ambulatory surgery center also is optimal for resident training in that it allows residents to do many cases in a day with a single attending surgeon and shows them what cases can be done in this venue and how to maximize the patient experience. Also, because more and more routine operations are done in the outpatient environment, residents learn how to adequately prepare a patient before surgery and anticipate and address their postoperative needs.

Clinic

Given the constraints of faculty practice and resident education, it is difficult to offer residents a longitudinal clinic experience, in which they see the same patients throughout their course of care, from the initial clinic visit as a new patient, to the procedure, to the postoperative visit. Since clinic is an ACGME-required component of resident education, the challenge is to make the experience an optimal one. One strategy is to preview clinic lists to have residents see new patients, first-time postop visits, and patients they have seen previously.

Table 1. Hospital type and training benefits

Hospital type	Cases	Additional education
Children's	Pediatric; common and complex	Pediatric index cases
University	Complex	Innovative, high-technology approaches; resource-intensive care
Independent hospital (community)	Common and complex	High volume, mix of private and hospital-based practice
Integrated not-for-profit (e.g., Kaiser)	Common and complex	High volume, drive for efficiency
VA or DoD	Common and complex	Care for patients with access to care issues; care of geriatric patients
Safety net	Common and complex	Care for patients without equal access to care, with disparate health outcomes

Before COVID-19, telehealth was an aspect of surgical care delivered in the clinic that received little attention. The exponential growth of virtual visits, both phone and video, and the satisfaction of both patients and providers with this medium, ensure that virtual visits are here to stay. Surgical residents want and need to be trained in its use.

Coordinated Care Teams

Medical and surgical care are practiced in teams, and surgeons often serve as team leaders. Leading a trauma resuscitation is an ACGME requirement – the optimal educational experience requires feedback about the ultimate patient care delivered and the leadership characteristics and behaviors displayed. Participating in a cancer care team, which often occurs over a longer period, allows the trainee to see surgical leadership and team membership in a different and equally important light. Working with an interdisciplinary team also offers a tremendous opportunity to learn about team leadership, emotional intelligence, the value of multidisciplinary input, and patient-centered care. These are important assets for a modern surgeon and can help secure their leadership in health care delivery in the future.

Simulation Center

The simulation center is an invaluable resource for any surgery residency program. A centralized simulation facility can serve the needs of many surgical and medical specialties with effective utilization of scarce resources. Such institutional resources can be vital in training residents in cognitive, technical, and non-technical skills. A variety of simulations, including bench models, simulators, virtual reality tools, endoscopic trainers, consoles for robotic-assisted surgery, and simulated patients may all be used effectively to address specific skills. In addition, human patient simulators can be very useful in addressing effective teamwork. Simulated patients are especially helpful in addressing interpersonal and communication skills focusing on a variety of critical tasks, including obtaining an informed consent, sharing bad news, conducting a family meeting, or other tasks that involve effective communication to promote optimal patient care. The aforementioned simulation-based training and assessment activities can be very important in promoting patient safety. Simulation-based education and training remain vital in the acquisition, verification, and maintenance of critical skills. They also play an important role in remediation to address gaps in performance.

The ACS Division of Education has established a program for accreditation of simulation centers based on specific standards and criteria. These accredited simulation centers are called American College of Surgeons Accredited Education Institutes (ACS-AEIs) and a Consortium of ACS-AEIs has been created to advance simulation-based teaching and assessment, develop innovative training models that involve the use of simulation, share educational materials and best practices, and conduct collaborative research and development. Also, the ACS Division of Education has implemented a 5-step Verification Model that includes Verification of Attendance; Verification of Satisfactory Completion of Course Objectives; Verification of Knowledge and Skills; Verification of Preceptorial Experience; and Demonstration of Satisfactory Patient Outcomes. This Model is used to provide learners specific Certificates of Verification that may be useful in credentialing and privileging.

Information Technology and Library Access

Digital transformation of knowledge is rapidly making traditional content delivered through textbooks and paper-based journals obsolete; residency programs must adapt accordingly. Many residents will not visit a physical library; instead, they will depend upon electronic and personnel resources that include easy onsite and offsite access to surgical textbooks, journals, web-based resources, video libraries, and the services of a resource and reference librarian. As such, a modern program must invest in these resources, offering residents access to them every hour of every day throughout the year, just as was traditionally done with a hospital's physical library.

Personal Workspace

Given the demands of training and work and the need to promote personal well-being, personal workspace should be provided as a retreat for learning, secure computer access, and storage of personal items, such as jackets, backpacks, and food. Protected space needs to be quiet and nearby, free from interruption, accompanied by appropriate lactation resources, showers, changing facilities, lockers, and exercise facilities. Active, deliberate planning for this kind of protected environment is the responsibility of the hospital, PD, and department.

Well-Being Resources

Physician well-being is the foundation of high-quality patient care and is essential to the success of our health care system. In contrast, physician burnout presents a threat to the surgical workforce. National data suggest that 50 percent of general surgeons experience symptoms of burnout. Likewise, a 2015 study reported that 69 percent of surgical residents met criteria for burnout on at least one subscale of the Maslach Burnout Inventory (MBI) and 44 percent considered leaving residency.[9] Even more concerning, nearly one-third of medical students experience symptoms of burnout before even starting their residency. Residency training is an intense experience requiring long work hours and is associated with loss of perceived autonomy; the frequency of burnout symptoms rise during surgical training.[10]

Burnout harms physicians' personal well-being and can lead to career dissatisfaction, divorce, disruptive behavior, home or workplace violence, depression, substance abuse, and increased risk for suicide. Burnout among surgical residents contributes to attrition. Faculty and resident burnout is costly not only to individuals, but also to departments and institutions. Burnout contributes to increased health care costs through physician turnover, reduced clinical effort, and early retirement. Physician burnout has been shown to decrease patient safety, quality of care, professionalism, and patient satisfaction, as well as increase medical errors and legal risk.[11-14]

Resident well-being is more than the absence of burnout; it accounts for all aspects of well-being, including the trainee's physical health, psychological health, and social support system. Although academic surgeons, leaders, and educators must do more than teach surgeons how to operate and take care of patients, it is equally important that they also model, develop, and teach the noncognitive aspects of surgery that are essential to well-being and success. These include self-awareness, effective communication, mindfulness, motivation, emotional intelligence, drive, perseverance, and resilience. Most importantly, the departmental culture must support these behaviors.[15]

ACGME Expectations for Faculty and Resident Well-Being

Wellness and the factors that threaten it have become a recent concern for several reasons. First and foremost are the challenges of the complexity of training, the acquisition of knowledge, the constantly changing learning environment, and the digital/technological transformation. Next is the ethos that surgeons can take on anything—that they thrive when given more work, more responsibility, more tests, and more challenges. In some respects, this work ethic, high self-expectation, and desire for self-discipline is in the best interest of excellent patient care. Yet everyone has limits, and surgeons and residents must accept that limitations, sickness, fatigue, depression, and frustration are important human attributes and should not be considered signs of weakness.

In 2015, the ACGME launched a campaign to foster physician well-being. Similar to a commitment to ensure all aspects of clinical competence, the ACGME highlights the program's/sponsoring institution's responsibility to address resident and faculty well-being.[16] In 2017, the ACGME introduced specific requirements to promote resident well-being, including developing and implementing programs that prioritize resident well-being[17] to focus on: creating an environment that encourages self-care, helping residents find meaning in work, enhancing communication and professional relationships, evaluating and promoting safety in the working and learning environment, and providing education and resources to identify and treat burnout, depression, substance abuse, and other challenges that arise. Although the mandate is clear, the format and effectiveness of such programs are not yet well-defined or addressed in residency curricula.

Measuring Burnout and Well-Being

Implementing change and measuring the impact requires understanding the current state. By regularly measuring well-being and burnout, programs can determine how to develop and implement initiatives to improve well-being, decrease burnout, and assess the impact of these initiatives. Multiple individual surveys measure burnout, well-being, resilience, self-efficacy, grit, and other factors essential to success. Table 2 has a list of assessments with a description of what they measure and where they are available. By no means comprehensive, this list includes the most commonly used tools, including the Maslach Burnout Inventory, the Physician Well-Being Index (PWBI), and the Perceived Stress Scale.

Table 2. Individual assessments of physician well-being, burnout, self-efficacy, resilience, grit, and other measures

Assessment	Description	Availability
Maslach Burnout Inventory - Human Services Survey Medical Personnel	22-item scale that measures: *Emotional Exhaustion* (feelings of being emotionally overextended and exhausted by one's work) *Depersonalization* (unfeeling and impersonal responses toward patients) *Personal Accomplishment* (feelings of competence and successful achievement in one's work)	Purchased for individual or can purchase licenses for group use (*https://www.mindgarden.com/315-mbi-human-services-survey-medical-personnel*)
Physician Well-Being Index (PWBI)	7-item scale designed as a brief screening tool to identify physicians at risk for burnout	Available free online to any member of the American College of Surgeons (*www.facs.org/member-services/surgeon-wellbeing*)
Response to Stressful Experiences Scale (RSES)	22-item and abbreviated 4-item scales; measures individual differences in cognitive, emotional, and behavioral responses to life's most stressful events	*https://www.reginfo.gov/public/do/DownloadDocument?objectID=39162801*
Connor-Davidson Resilience Scale	10-item abbreviated scale that measures resilience	Obtained by submitting online form (*http://www.connordavidson-resiliencescale.com/submit-ofr.php*)
Short Grit Scale	8-item scale to assess the personality trait of grit, defined as perseverance and passion for long-term goals; characterized by strenuously working toward challenges, and maintaining effort despite failure, adversity, and plateaus	*http://www.sjdm.org/dmidi/files/Grit-8-item.pdf*
Perceived Stress Scale	10-item scale designed to measure individual stress levels	Available through MindGarden; no charge (*http://www.mindgarden.com/documents/PerceivedStressScale.pdf*)

Optimal Resources to Enhance and Encourage Resident Well-Being

The commitment to adequate wellness resources must start at the top. DIOs, department chairs, hospital administrators, and PDs must articulate their commitment and prioritize developing resources to address these issues. Too often, there is more discussion than action about these concerns. For example, it's fine to hold an ice cream social to promote positive feelings, but it doesn't count for much if a program avoids addressing significant well-being issues, such as sleep deprivation among residents.

Bohman and colleagues from Stanford describe three reciprocal domains of resident well-being: personal resilience, culture of wellness, and efficiency of practice. While individual-level interventions are critical, such interventions are more likely to be effective when supported by organizational approaches.[18]

American College of Surgeons Well-Being Resources for Resident Surgeons

ACS offers many well-being resources for residents.

From the Surgeon Well-Being Workgroup

- Creating Well-Being
- Identification of Burnout
- Prevention of Burnout
- Experiencing Burnout
- Maintaining Well-Being

Resources on the above can be found at: *www.facs.org/member-services/surgeon-wellbeing/resources*

- Mental Health Awareness

Resources can be found at: *www.facs.org/publications/bulletin-brief/052521/wellbeing* and *www.facs.org/publications/ bulletin-brief/051821/wellbeing*

From Resources in Surgical Education (RISE)

- How the Personal Characteristics of Grit and Resilience Relate to Surgeon Well-Being: *www.facs.org/education/division-of-education/publications/rise/articles/grit-resilience*
- Enhancing Surgeon Wellness: Integrating a Multidimensional Behavioral Medicine Approach into a General Surgery Residency Program: *www.facs.org/education/division-of-education/publications/rise/articles/multidimensional*
- Making Average Performance Excellent: Mental Skills for Performance Enhancement: *www.facs.org/education/division-of-education/publications/rise/articles/performance*
- Work-Life Integration: Being Whole at Work and at Home: *www.facs.org/education/division-of-education/publications/rise/articles/work-life*
- Burnout in Surgery: *www.facs.org/education/division-of-education/publications/rise/articles/burnout*

Webinars

- From the Surgeon Well-Being Workgroup
  - Reframing Surgeon Well-Being: *https://www.facs.org/member-services/surgeon-wellbeing/reframing-wellness*
  - Managing Microaggressions: What to Do When It Gets Personal, Part 1 & Part 2: *www.facs.org/member-services/surgeon-wellbeing/microaggressions-series*

- From the Resident and Associate Society of the American College of Surgeons (RAS-ACS) Grand Rounds Webinar Series
  - PTSD/Burnout in General Surgery Residents and Attendings versus Other Specialties
  - A Juggling Act: Work Life Integration and Avoiding Burnout in Surgery
  - Navigating the Balance of Life as a Surgeon
  - Mindfulness and Work-Life Balance for the Busy Surgeon
  - The Impact of Diversity on Physician Resiliency
  - Physician Heal Thyself? A Reflection on Resident Psychological Wellness
  - There's No Crying in Surgery

The above can be found at: *www.facs.org/member-services/ras/webinars*

Addressing Personal Resilience

Resident well-being programs should be holistic, addressing the psychological, physical, and social aspects of well-being. Programs should also address the noncognitive aspects of surgery that are essential to long-term success, including emotional intelligence, mindfulness, resilience, and effective communication.

Emotional intelligence, a strong predictor of success, is defined as the ability to recognize one's own and other people's emotions, to discriminate between feelings and appropriately label them, and to use emotional information to guide thinking and behavior. Emotional intelligence comprises an array of noncognitive skills, capabilities, and competencies that influence a person's ability to cope with environmental demands and pressures; it includes self-awareness, self-management, social awareness, and relationship management.

The emotionally intelligent surgeon takes a broad view of situations, acknowledges others' feelings and struggles, and develops collaborative interactions. Teaching skills to enhance faculty and resident emotional intelligence can prevent disruptive behavior and support the collaboration necessary for complex systems to function. By prioritizing and modeling the principles of emotional intelligence, leaders can establish the cultural underpinnings needed to achieve a high state of emotional intelligence.

Mindfulness, which is defined as nonjudgmental awareness of the present moment, can reduce an individual's stress levels and burnout. It is the ability to observe one's own thoughts, emotions, and experiences in a nonreactive way.[19] Many obstacles block the surgeon's ability to be mindful, especially during training, where there is little autonomy and many competing demands are placed on the surgeon's time. Fortunately, mindfulness can be learned through guided reflection and meditation practices that take only minutes per day. To reduce stress and burnout in surgical residents,[19,20] training programs should offer guidance in mindfulness techniques. Emotional intelligence and mindfulness improve communication, allowing individuals to decide how they want to respond to situations that inevitably arise. Residents and faculty can be taught to recognize their tendency to become emotional and anticipate the associated unintended consequences. Abraham Lincoln wrote that when he was stressed and aware that he may become emotional or angry with his colleagues, he made it a practice to cool off by going "to the balcony;" once the emotion had passed, he could address the issue with clarity and even disagreement without escalating the conflict. Learning to identify and control the tendency to overreact before it happens is an important emotional intelligence skill. The emotional intelligence skill set, which can be practiced, is perhaps the most important non-technical capability to which surgeons aspire.

The concept of resilience, which is less well-characterized, refers to an individual's ability to recover from distress. High individual resilience is thought to be inversely correlated with burnout.[21] Surgeons, by nature, are resilient; on the other hand, for many surgeons, the concept of burnout suggests a failure of resourcefulness and resilience. The surgical environment poses many challenges to the surgeon's ability and mission to provide high-quality care. Surgeons and residents must simultaneously address these issues and normalize the intense feelings associated with their career choice. Resilience can be difficult to define, but for surgeons resilience is the ability to succeed despite challenges and perceived failures. As important as resilience is, it cannot be oversimplified. It must be authentic, developed, and internalized into the personality of the individual surgeon.

A formal resident curriculum to improve overall well-being and resilience should include modules on stress reduction, mindfulness, meditation, resilience, normalization of experiences, effective communication, and team building. Such curricula have been implemented at various programs with success and can be exported and adapted to other programs.[20,22-24]

The resident curriculum should also include education that optimizes physical wellness. This includes strategic diet and exercise that can be incorporated into the surgeon's busy schedule and ergonomics to prevent long-term injury and disability. Sessions on work-life integration can help residents balance the many competing demands on their time and help them prioritize how they spend their time and energy.

Addressing the Culture of Well-Being

As stated previously, these interventions are more effective in a culture and organizational approach that supports and encourages them. A department must have a well-being champion to lead well-being efforts for the faculty, residents, and staff. Ideally, the leader of these initiatives is the chairman or the PD, but in either case, the chairman should publicly endorse its importance, model the behavior, and empower the champion to accomplish the task. The efforts should focus on all surgeons; after all, the well-being of residents is negatively affected when faculty and staff are unhappy. The champion should be trusted by the residents and faculty.

The faculty and department leaders must model the individual behaviors being taught to the residents. This includes supporting healthy behaviors, acknowledging the many aspects of residents' lives that make them well-rounded individuals, and creating a social-support structure in which struggling residents know where to go to get helpful resources. In addition, it is critical to destigmatize requests for help and model this behavior amongst the faculty.

Cultural and organizational interventions that support resident well-being and the behaviors that promote individual resilience should include: clear and equitable parental leave policies and lactation facilities for lactating mothers; appropriate spaces for families and residents to meet at the hospital; resident lounges with healthy food, games, and resting space; appropriate sleeping arrangements on call; protected time for education, including the formal well-being curriculum; and interactive sessions addressing real-life situations to teach noncognitive skills, which help build camaraderie and a culture of support.

Programs also should provide access to exercise facilities for residents on call and reduced fees to campus fitness facilities so that residents can work out during downtime. They should offer opportunities for physical activity and meditation in the department or organization. Group races, hikes, softball games, or competitions with activity trackers promote well-being and increase the sense of community support. Other possible group activities may include book clubs, cooking, gardening, and so on. A well-being champion can collect these ideas and coordinate events throughout the year.

An example of an organizational intervention is Banner Health's Cultivating Happiness in Medicine (CHIM), a comprehensive model that tackles physician well-being from the operational, leadership, organization, individual, community, and second-victim perspectives.[25] CHIM has multiple components including measuring physician burnout on an annual basis using the Maslach Burnout Inventory survey, monitoring performance, and planning/evaluating interventions; integration with the Banner Health My Well-Being Strategy and health plan; and partnership with the physician human resources department to engage, equip, and enable physicians and advanced practice providers (APPs) to deliver optimal care and achieve their career aspirations. As part of CHIM, Banner Health also offers funds to support social events.

As most residents (and faculty) will experience an adverse event during their careers, they must be able to talk about these experiences and get the help they need to move forward, restore their confidence, and heal emotionally. Formal second-victim programs with peer-supporters have been shown to be effective.[26]

Residents and faculty should have access to coaching and psychological support as necessary to improve resident well-being. While resource intensive, these individuals offer an objective perspective and allow residents access to a safe space to share their concerns and challenges – especially topics about which they may feel uncomfortable in discussing with faculty. Residents can meet with coaches or psychologists in groups to address these challenges in real time. In addition to these resources, safe space interest groups enable residents to express themselves and discover solutions.

Finally, appropriate support systems must be available to help a resident who is struggling in any aspect of their life. The Surgical Education Culture Optimization through targeted interventions based on National comparative Data (SECOND) trial is a national prospective, pragmatic cluster-randomized trial examining the learning environment and well-being of residents.[27] Participating programs will receive a program-specific report on their residents' well-being metrics. Programs will be randomized to intervention versus control and intervention programs will receive a learning environment report, a wellness toolkit, and implementation support. After the trial is complete, all programs will have access to the wellness toolkit, which contains many interventions that can improve individual resilience, the culture of wellness, and organizational factors that promote well-being.

Addressing Efficiency of Practice

Residents should have schedules that promote adherence to work-hour regulations, while optimizing their education. Appropriate ancillary support with APPs who assist with case management, administrative burden, and continuity of care can increase resident satisfaction and optimize educational opportunities. By working with EHR "super users" to increase their efficiency in documentation, residents can significantly decrease their workload. Finally, education on coding and documentation should demonstrate the value of developing skills for their use in future practice.

Summary

Physician well-being is essential to high-quality patient care. Programs are responsible to address resident and faculty well-being just as they are to ensure clinical competence. Formal education on well-being should focus on creating an environment that encourages self-care, helping residents find meaning in work, enhancing communication, developing professional relationships, evaluating and promoting safety in the working and learning environment, and providing a sufficient support system to assist residents as struggles arise. While programs can provide education to improve emotional intelligence, mindfulness, resilience, and personal wellness, they must also create a culture and environment that support these behaviors. Programs should share best practices in this emerging area of surgical training as our profession explores the optimal format of such programs. Finally, well-being must be addressed in residents, faculty and staff, and organizational support for well-being makes residency program interventions more effective. Future department leadership will be assessed on the metrics of clinical service excellence, scholarly productivity and innovation, and creating a culture conducive to training the next generation of surgeons and surgical leaders.

Conclusion

In conclusion, a successful training program has to be well-planned, well-led, and well-administrated, taking into account the resources needed. These include physical resources, systems resources, coexisting training programs, people resources, cognizance, and deliberate attention to resources that support resident well-being. Training the next generation of surgeons is a major professional responsibility and the acquisition of these resources is essential.

References

1. West MA, Hwang S, Maier RV, Ahuja N, Angelos P, Bass BL, Brasel KJ, Chen H, Davis KA, Eberlein TJ, Fong Y, Greenberg CC, Lillemoe KD, McCarthy MC, Michelassi F, Numann PJ, Parangi S, Reyes JD, Sanfey HA, Stain SC, Weigel RJ, Wren SM. Ensuring equity, diversity, and inclusion in academic surgery: an American Surgical Association white paper. *Ann Surg.* 2018;268(3):403-407.
2. Birkmeyer JD, Dimick JB, Staiger DO. Operative mortality and procedure volume as predictors of subsequent hospital performance. *Ann Surg.* 2006;243(3):411-417.
3. Hunger R, Mantke R. Outcome quality beyond the mean - an analysis of 43,231 pancreatic surgical procedures related to hospital volume. [published online ahead of print, November 2020]. *Ann Surg.* 2020. DOI: 10.1097/SLA.0000000000004315.
4. Kroth PJ, Morioka-Douglas N, Veres S, Babbott S, Poplau S, Qeadan F, Parshall C, Corrigan K, Linzer M. Association of electronic health record design and use factors with clinician stress and burnout. *JAMA Netw Open.* 2019;2(8):e199609.
5. Kempenich JW, Willis RE, Blue RJ, Al Fayyadh MJ, Cromer RM, Schenarts PJ, Van Sickle KR, Dent DL. The effect of patient education on the perceptions of resident participation in surgical care. *J Surg Educ.* 2016;73(6):e111-e117.
6. Kempenich JW, Willis RE, Rakosi R, Wiersch J, Schenarts PJ. How do perceptions of autonomy differ in general surgery training between faculty, senior residents, hospital administrators, and the general public? A multi-institutional study. *J Surg Educ.* 2015;72(6):e193-201.
7. Whealon MD, Young MT, Phelan MJ, Nguyen NT. Effect of resident involvement on patient outcomes in complex laparoscopic gastrointestinal operations. *J Am Coll Surg.* 2016;223(1):186-192.
8. Meyerson SL, Odell DD, Zwischenberger JB, Schuller M, Williams RG, Bohnen JD, Dunnington GL, Torbeck L, Mullen JT, Mandell SP, Choti MA, Foley E, Are C, Auyang E, Chipman J, Choi J, Meier AH, Smink DS, Terhune KP, Wise PE, Soper N, Lillemoe K, Fryer JP, George BC, Procedural Learning and Safety Collaborative. The effect of gender on operative autonomy in general surgery residents. *Surgery.* 2019;166(5):738-743.
9. Elmore LC, Jeffe DB, Jin L, Awad MM, Turnbull IR. National survey of burnout among US general surgery residents. *J Am Coll Surg.* 2016;223(3):440-451.
10. Dyrbye LN, West CP, Satele D, Boone S, Tan L, Sloan J, Shanafelt TD. Burnout among U.S. medical students, residents, and early career physicians relative to the general U.S. population. *Acad Med.* 2014;89(3):443-451.

11. Misra-Hebert AD, Kay R, Stoller JK. A review of physician turnover: rates, causes, and consequences. *Am J Med Qual*. 2004;19(2):56-66.
12. Shanafelt T, Goh J, Sinsky C. The business case for investing in physician well-being. *JAMA Intern Med*. 2017;177(12):1826-1832.
13. West CP, Dyrbye LN, Erwin PJ, Shanafelt TD. Interventions to prevent and reduce physician burnout: a systematic review and meta-analysis. *Lancet*. 2016;388(10057):2272-2281.
14. Panagioti M, Geraghty K, Johnson J, Zhou A, Panagopoulou E, Chew-Graham C, Peters D, Hodkinson A, Riley R, Esmail A. Association between physician burnout and patient safety, professionalism, and patient satisfaction: a systematic review and meta-analysis. *JAMA Intern Med*. 2018;178(10):1317-1330.
15. Riall TS. Enjoy the journey. *Surgery*. 2018;164(6):1382-1387.
16. Accreditation Council for Graduate Medical Education. Symposium on Physician Well-Being Summary and Proposal to the ACGME Board of Directors. Available at: https://www.acgme.org/globalassets/PDFs/Symposium/Symposium_on_Physician_Well-Being_Summary_and_Proposal_Feb_2016_BOD.pdf. Accessed October 11, 2021.
17. Accreditation Council for Graduate Medical Education. Common Program Requirements (Residency). Available at: https://www.acgme.org/globalassets/PFAssets/ProgramRequirements/CPRResidency2021.pdf. Accessed October 11, 2021.
18. Shanafelt TD, Noseworthy JH. Executive leadership and physician well-being: nine organizational strategies to promote engagement and reduce burnout. *Mayo Clin Proc*. 2017;92(1):129-146.
19. Lebares CC, Guvva EV, Ascher NL, O'Sullivan PS, Harris HW, Epel ES. Burnout and stress among US surgery residents: psychological distress and resilience. *J Am Coll Surg*. 2018;226(1):80-90.
20. Lebares CC, Hershberger AO, Guvva EV, et al. Feasibility of formal mindfulness-based stress-resilience training among surgery interns: a randomized clinical trial. *JAMA Surg*. 2018 Oct 1;153(10):e182734.
21. Dyrbye LN, Power DV, Massie FS, Eacker A, Harper W, Thomas MR, Szydlo DW, Sloan JA, Shanafelt TD. Factors associated with resilience to and recovery from burnout: a prospective, multi-institutional study of US medical students. *Med Educ*. 2010;44(10):1016-1026.
22. University of Rochester. Better health, better you. Available at: https://www.urmc.rochester.edu/education/graduate-medical-education/prospective-residents/surgery/about-the-program/wellness-program.aspx. Accessed August 24, 2021.
23. Stanford balance in life program. Available at: http://med.stanford.edu/content/dam/sm/scalpel/documents/InternOrientation/2017Orientation/-R-A-Program-to-Create-Balance-in-the-Lives-of-our-Residents.2015.pdf. Accessed August 24, 2021.
24. Riall TS, Teiman J, Chang M, Cole D, Leighn T, McClafferty H, Nfonsam VN. Maintaining the fire but avoiding burnout: implementation and evaluation of a resident well-being program. *J Am Coll Surg*. 2018;226(4):369-379.
25. Banner Health. Cultivating happiness in medicine. Available at: http://bycell.mobi/wap/default/item jsp?entryid=ECMTAyNA==&itemid=87407#m. Accessed August 24, 2021.
26. El Hechi MW, Bohnen JD, Westfal M, Han K, Cauley C, Wright C, Schulz J, Mort E, Ferris T, Lillemoe KD, Kaafarani HM. Design and impact of a novel surgery-specific second victim peer support program. *J Am Coll Surg*. 2020;230(6):926-933.
27. U.S. National Library of Medicine. The Surgical Education Culture Optimization Through Targeted Interventions Based on National Comparative Data - "The SECOND Trial" (SECOND). Available at: https://clinicaltrials.gov/ct2/show/NCT03739723. Accessed October 11, 2021.

AMERICAN C
SURGEONS A
OF SURGEONS
COLLEGE OF
AMERICAN C
SURGEONS A
OF SURGEONS
COLLEGE OF
AMERICAN C
SURGEONS A

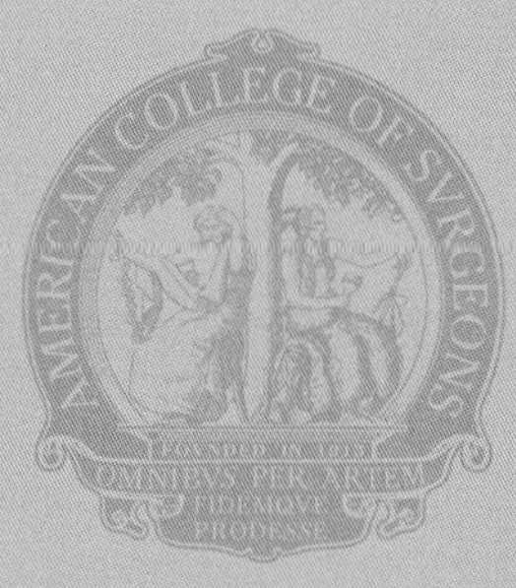

CHAPTER 14
Faculty and Trainee Expectations

Lead Author

Melina R. Kibbe, MD, FACS, FAHA

Co-Authors

Barbara L. Bass, MD, FACS, MAMSE

Muneera R. Kapadia, MD, MME, FACS, FASCRS

CHAPTER 14
Faculty and Trainee Expectations

Executive Summary

- What are the educational expectations of residents and faculty?
- How do faculty and residents work together?
- How can we provide residents with wellness, quality of life, and a secure learning environment?
- What is the role of professional oversight, including the following?
  - American College of Surgeons (ACS)
  - Accreditation Council for Graduate Medical Education (ACGME)
  - American Board of Surgery (ABS)
  - Association of American Medical Colleges (AAMC)
- What resources are available to leadership and faculty?
- What are some common case scenarios?

Introduction

Common to all the chapters in this book is the underlying assumption that faculty and trainees have certain expectations. These expectations span many domains that are critical to the mission and vision of any college or school of medicine and affiliated health care institutions that have accepted the responsibility of educating and training medical and allied health students, residents, and fellows. With respect to the educational mission, it is commonly expected that faculty will educate the next generation of surgeons as well as participate in their own continuing medical education, a fundamental element of professionalism. Upon entering a residency training program, all trainees commit to participating in their own education as well as the education of the junior residents and medical students who follow them. Faculty have a commitment to train residents and medical students in the art and science of surgical craft. However, the commitment goes much further than that. To meet the needs of the current generation of learners, trainees and faculty must commit to be open to new educational teaching methods, receive continual feedback, and serve as role models in the pursuit of lifelong learning.

Education not only spans the diagnosis and treatment of patients with surgical disease, but also extends into professionalism and accountability, both of which are foundational to the vocation. A positive learning environment that supports trainee and faculty wellness is essential for the current generation of surgeons and draws the next generation to our field. Fundamentally, education prepares the next generation of our surgical workforce. Thus, a commitment to educating the next generation of surgeons is closely aligned with our commitment to patients, to the community we serve, and to upholding the Hippocratic Oath. Part of fulfilling our commitment to patients is to impart our knowledge to the next generation of surgeons. This chapter will explore the expectations of both trainees and faculty toward the educational mission and will provide resources for further development of surgical residency programs.

Educational Expectations

Three organizations set the bulk of the educational expectations for surgeons, residents, and surgical residency programs: the American College of Surgeons (ACS), the Accreditation Council for Graduate Medical Education (ACGME), and the American Board of Surgery (ABS). Following is a summary of their educational expectations.

American College of Surgeons

The ACS "Statements on Principles," updated in April 2016, clarify that the ACS expects its Fellows to "meet the obligation for continuous education and development" through several routes.[1] The goal of continuous education and self-assessment is to "ensure a high level of skill in the domains of medical knowledge, technical proficiency, professionalism, interpersonal communications, and systems-based practice." Surgeons can meet these goals by attending national conferences, hands-on programs, and ACS educational programs; by reading peer-reviewed journals and textbooks; and through participation in Continuing Medical Education (CME) events. The ACS also expects surgeons to be "teachers of patients, medical students, residents, and other health care professionals." The ACS further states that "surgeons have a special responsibility to supervise resident training because of the unique characteristics of surgical conditions and operations."

Accreditation Council for Graduate Medical Education
Defining and understanding educational expectations is critical for all surgical programs. The ACGME has very clear and well-defined requirements for faculty and trainees alike.[2] First and foremost, the ACGME expects faculty members to serve as "role models of professionalism." Without modeling professional behavior, all efforts toward education will be futile. The ACGME expects faculty to demonstrate a "strong interest in the education of residents." This involves devoting "time to the educational program to fulfill their supervisory and teaching responsibilities," maintaining "an environment conducive to educating residents," and participating in "organized clinical discussions, rounds, journal clubs, and conferences." Furthermore, the ACGME expects that faculty will commit to their own development on an annual basis with respect to "enhancing the transference of knowledge, skill, and behavior from educator to learner." Achieving this objective may involve such activities as attending lectures or external courses or participating in workshops or well-being initiatives. Surgeon educators need ongoing professional development to remain effective; this endeavor includes learning how to apply multiple teaching styles and tools to meet individual needs.[3]

The ACGME expects all residents to successfully develop its core competencies, which describe the required domains for a "trusted physician to enter autonomous practice." The ACGME core competencies include professionalism, patient care and procedural skills, medical knowledge, practice-based learning and improvement, interpersonal and communication skills, and systems-based practice. These core competencies were developed to broadly shape the education of residents and serve as the foundation for resident evaluation.

American Board of Surgery
The mission of the ABS is to serve the "public and the specialty of surgery by providing leadership in surgical education and practice, by promoting excellence through rigorous evaluation and examination, and by promoting the highest standards for professionalism, lifelong learning, and the continuous certification of surgeons in practice."[4] Hence, it is critical for both trainees and faculty to commit to education. In fact, one of the stated purposes of the ABS is to "improve and broaden the opportunities for the graduate education and training of surgeons," and a principal objective of the ABS is to "pass judgment on the education, training and knowledge of broadly qualified and responsible surgeons and not to designate who shall or shall not perform surgical operations." To become board-certified in surgery, the ABS expects trainees to meet educational, professional, and ethical standards. Trainees must acquire a broad understanding of surgical diseases and technical skills to care for surgical patients, and they must be afforded opportunities to progressively take on responsibility and independently make decisions.

Perspective of Chairs for the Faculty

Many of the authors of this manual have served as chairs of departments of surgery. Chairs of surgery believe that all faculty in a department of surgery must consider their commitment to educating the next generation of surgeons as an essential core responsibility. To provide residents direct education from shared experiences, faculty must closely interact with residents in the clinic, operating room (OR), and at the bedside. Through such interactions, the knowledge, wisdom, decision-making, and technical skills of the faculty can foster true comprehension and retention in the learner. This must be a two-way dialogue and exchange, and this education must be performed in a graded, experiential fashion, taking into account the stage of the trainee, subject matter complexity, and mutual expectations. In addition, faculty should commit to their own development and lifelong learning, including professionalism, communication, personal wellness, knowledge, decision-making, and technical skills. All of these attributes are necessary to practice the art and craft of surgery. Persistent dedication to improving education can help create an optimal learning environment that is current, evidence-based, and rich with opportunity.

Perspective of Chairs for the Residents

All trainees must be willing and eager to learn all aspects of the surgical discipline; they must be open to new ideas, approaches, or concepts. Trainees must be committed to active learning; education is a two-way experience of mutual give and take. A basic expectation is that trainees will read and learn on their own time, practice fundamental skills, and develop interpersonal behaviors—all of which are essential to becoming an independent surgeon. This self-preparation will enhance their ability to absorb the educational opportunities of the experiential patient care environment and the didactic learning sessions. Trainees must also possess a certain level of self-awareness regarding their own knowledge, skill, and professional maturity; they must know or learn very quickly when to ask for help with the expectation that the request will be met without penalty. Without this level of understanding and a mature learning environment, patient care can be jeopardized and the trust established between learner and teacher will be lost, resulting in many undesirable consequences.

The Changing Paradigms of Surgical Education

Increasingly, often to the frustration of faculty, learners rely on point-of-care sources for clinical decision-making. This reliance cannot replace the need for trainees to develop a body of internally accessible knowledge, such as patterns of disease, fundamentals of human physiology and anatomy, concepts of treatment, and interventions that are needed to become a knowledgeable and skilled surgeon. However, at the same time, surgeon educators must recognize that learners today gain knowledge through different means than they did when they trained. Textbooks provide comprehensive reviews but no longer serve as the primary learning tools. Now trainees (and surgeons engaged in lifelong learning) often acquire information from Internet websites—some exceptionally rich in good content, others much less so. There needs to be better editorial oversight for Internet-based content, comparable to that for textbooks or peer review. Until content oversight develops, social media needs to be used cautiously. Knowing that residents will access content on the Internet, faculty should regularly address its limitations. This itself can be a useful learning experience because anecdotal reports with unedited content may be an impediment to young learners.

Surgical skill labs or surgical simulation labs, now part of most training curricula, have demonstrated that "part task" training can create more technically savvy surgeons in the OR as trainees progress to increasingly complex cases. However, these scenarios do not replace the need to understand the entire procedure. Many lectures are now viewed from prerecorded and populated databases. So, although these tools can serve as useful reminders about how procedures are done, they should not be the trainee's only learning experience.

The Importance of Professionalism and Respect in Faculty and Resident Interactions

Professionalism and mutual respect between the faculty and trainees are critical to the success of a training program. Professionalism must be extended toward colleagues, learners, patients, and other members of the health care team. This includes respectful communication, promptness, and thoughtfulness. Faculty and trainees must develop a high level of emotional intelligence to detect and manage breaches of professionalism. Dishonest behavior, such as cheating, lying, or failure to disclose appropriately in any oral or written format, is unacceptable.

Often there is a gap between what residents believe they need to know to develop as surgeons and what the faculty believe trainees need to know. For example, in a case cohort survey residents reported that focused, skill-based training in higher-level operations was their key learning objective, whereas attending surgeons identified the need for more fundamental skill sets and operative experience.[5]

The Resident Work and Learning Environment

As the learning environment continues to change, surgeons must embrace change if surgery is to continue to thrive as a profession and attract medical students. The ACS issued a "Statement on Surgical Residencies and the Educational Environment" in 1994, which is still relevant today. The statement, developed by the Graduate Medical Education Committee of the ACS, put forth the following recommendations regarding the resident work environment:[6]

- The relationship of resident and attending staff faculty should be mutually supportive.
- The balance of time worked, and time off must be carefully structured so that residents assume increasing responsibility for patient care during the course of the program.
- Residency programs must provide for appropriate supervision for all residents.
- Support services must be adequate so that residents do not spend an unreasonable amount of time in noneducational activities.
- Efforts should be made to eliminate the excessive and uncoordinated use of the paging system by minimizing calls of a nonessential nature.

- The personal needs of residents for adequate, private, and convenient sleeping quarters while on call; food facilities for nutritious meals, study areas, and a lounge; and a safe physical environment are essential to the working environment.
- Medical liability insurance should be provided to all residents.
- A maternal leave policy should be specified at the time of the resident's employment.
- The institution should be strongly encouraged to provide adequate day-care services for all residents' families.
- Programs should facilitate access to appropriate and confidential counseling and psychological support services.
- The educational environment should be enhanced with a library of current textbooks and journals that are readily accessible at all hours to residents.
- Residents should be fairly compensated for their work, and every resident should be salaried and provided with reasonable annual paid vacations and educational and personal leave.
- Initiatives to provide relief for student-incurred debt should be explored and developed.
- The curriculum should include formal preparation for the practice of surgery, including education in the ethics of practice and the profession.
- A policy regarding sexual harassment that is consistent with the policies of the institution should be in place in each department and should be strictly enforced with safe reporting structures.

Wellness, Quality of Life, and a Secure Learning Environment

These recommendations are meant to provide a supportive learning environment in which all residents should be able to thrive. Important areas of emphasis in the list of ACS recommendations are personal well-being, quality of life, and professionalism. Creating a positive learning environment in surgery is essential to the future of our profession.

Recent studies, however, suggest that stress and burnout are more prevalent among surgical residents and practicing surgeons than once thought.[7-9] Surgical residents and faculty may be subjected to sexual harassment and discrimination—factors that also contribute to burnout, as research shows.[10-12]

"Microaggression" is a term that is increasingly used to categorize a specific type of harassment or discrimination consisting of unintentional or intentional actions or statements that denigrate a person on the basis of gender, race, ethnicity, sexual orientation, or other characteristics. The victim often suppresses these actions out of fear of retaliation, and the offender, therefore, believes what has been stated is acceptable. For example, a faculty surgeon might introduce a group of female residents as "my gals" in a conversation with a patient while referring to males as "my residents." Similarly, patients may assume women residents are nurses rather than physicians. Research shows that residents may encounter such mistreatment, which the AAMC defines as events that "occur when behavior shows disrespect for the dignity of others and unreasonably interferes with the learning process."[13]

An optimal learning environment is free from mistreatment and microaggressions. Mistreatment falls into several categories, including sexual harassment or physical punishment/threats; discrimination or harassment based on gender, race, ethnicity, religion, sexual orientation, or disability; and public humiliation or intimidation. Faculty and trainees should acknowledge that it is impossible to learn in an environment in which harassment or discrimination is accepted. Studies indicate that these fears lead to high rates of faculty and learner stress, turnover, and attrition.[14] The PD and program faculty can eliminate mistreatment by creating a supportive learning environment that emphasizes excellence, introspection, tolerance, inclusion, and the immediate recognition and remediation of inappropriate behaviors. Specific interventions in residency training to address stressors that may lead to burnout and discriminatory behaviors include formal training in emotional intelligence and focused discussion groups for faculty and residents (separately and together) in which these topics are openly discussed and pathways to improvement are identified. Having trained educators or mental health professionals serve as moderators of these discussions can facilitate improvement.

Following the expanded national discussion regarding diversity, equity, inclusion, and anti-racism, many organizations, including the ACS and the ACGME, are exploring new tools and best practices to address these important issues, and many new programs will be forthcoming. A formal discussion created through a learning collaborative sponsored by the ACGME titled "Equity Matters" has an aggressive timeline to define and implement these practices. In addition, a multi-institutional study sponsored by the the ACS, ACGME, ABS, and Northwestern University Feinberg School of Medicine's department of surgery (the SECOND Trial) is designed to evaluate the mitigation of stress, burnout, and harassment during surgical training.[15]

Finally, there should be a clear understanding that if residents experience any mistreatment or microaggressions, they should feel comfortable coming forward to program leadership. The imbalance in power between learners and faculty can deter reporting despite assurances that retaliation will not occur. For that reason a secure anonymous reporting system and a structured process, which may include an ombudsman, need to be available to ensure reporting reaches leadership. All reports should be investigated; if mistreatment is found, appropriate actions should be taken. This responsibility falls on the Designated Institutional Official (DIO), who is an invaluable resource in resolving these concerns. Furthermore, concerns need to be escalated to department leaders who are empowered to effectively transform the culture as necessary.

In addition to a learning environment free from mistreatment and microaggressions, there must be an emphasis on resident well-being, including easy access to an array of health services and an expectation that time is available to pursue needed health services, including primary care, dental, and mental health services, as well as the general acceptance that occasional time off may be required for important health matters. Access to mental health services is particularly important for residents and faculty members as stress and anxiety are part of their daily lives. In the last two years during the Coronavirus Disease 2019 (COVID-19) pandemic, the need and use of mental health services has increased significantly. Increasingly, behavioral health services can be accessed via telehealth options and low-cost institutional subscriptions are now available. Remote counselors and behavioral health providers are often better accepted and used among learners, who may prefer to avoid the undeserved stigma that may come from seeking mental health help.

Residents should have access to meet other basic needs, such as food, essential personal protective equipment (PPE),[16] rest areas, and special accommodations for learners with disabilities. Adequate workspaces and computer access should be provided to trainees, especially if they are assigned to work on electronic health records. Additionally, surgery-specific educational materials in readily available digital formats must be accessible to residents, including relevant and updated medical literature. Finally, learners from other programs or advanced practice providers must not impede or impinge on surgical resident learning.

Surgeons can be stereotyped in the media as brash, intolerant, and impatient; these impressions may lead patients, students, and others to expect aggressive and discriminatory behaviors from surgeons. Although such characterizations are fading away, this perception continues to mar our profession. The PD and teaching faculty should formally recognize these behaviors in our surgical culture and work to eliminate them. Readers are encouraged to review additional discussions of these topics in Chapter 7 of this manual.

Regulations

Within any residency program, certain regulations must be addressed and followed. Several organizations set these rules, including the ACGME, ABS, and AAMC.

Accreditation Council for Graduate Medical Education

The ACGME sets strict qualification for residency program directors (PDs).[2] A single faculty member must be designated as the PD, with overall program accountability to meet requirements. PDs should have at least three years of educational and administrative experience and must be approved by the Graduate Medical Education Committee. They should be board-certified, have a current medical license, be clinically active, and possess a track record of engaging in and fostering scholarly activity in the program. Because the PD is critical to residency program stability, frequent changes in leadership should be avoided; in fact, the ACGME encourages PDs to be appointed for at least six years to ensure program stability. Because the PD role is critical to the success of the residency program, salary support for the PD is required to compensate their time. For general surgery residency programs, the ACGME requires 30 percent full-time equivalent, or 1 1/2 days per week. Different requirements are set forth for residency programs based on their size and the amount of administration required. The PD is a role model for the learners in the program and as such must demonstrate professionalism. The PD also must approve core program faculty and should ensure that residents have appropriate learning environments while working with faculty members.

Faculty members have the privilege of teaching residents how to care for patients, develop their procedural skills, and foster their professional development. Faculty members must be role models of professionalism and provide high-quality patient care. They must demonstrate a strong interest in resident education and should participate in educational activities such as grand rounds, journal clubs, and morbidity and mortality conferences. Like the PD, faculty must be board-certified and hold appropriate institutional appointments. Core faculty are designated by the PD and must have a significant role in the education and supervision of residents, including teaching, evaluation, and providing feedback to residents.

American Board of Surgery

The operative experience, one of many components necessary to train residents, is often considered central to any surgical training program. Faculty must engage residents in the OR so that they may participate in operations, acquire and hone surgical skills and techniques, and eventually reach competency in independent performance. The ABS requires that residents perform 850 operations over five clinical years, including at least 200 during the chief resident year. There is an implicit understanding that graduated responsibility will lead to progressive autonomy over the five years. In return for participation opportunities, faculty expect residents to assist in the care of patients, including preoperative and postoperative care, as of the 2019-2020 published guidelines.

There is a movement toward competency-based education in training residents. Historically, after a designated time in training, trainees graduated from a surgical program and moved into independent practice. More recently, readiness for practice has been brought into question by reports that graduates entering fellowship programs did not meet fellowship directors' expectations.[17,18] A subsequent survey conducted by the ACS explored this issue further and showed that 94 percent of young surgeons felt they were ready to practice; however, only 59 percent of older surgeons believed residents were adequately prepared for transition to the attending role.[19] This dichotomy may be due, in part, to changes in the training environment over time, including work-hour restrictions, workplace efficiency pressures, and liability threats.

As a result, interest in competency-based education has grown over the past few decades.[20] One such way to move competency-based education forward is by implementing Entrustable Professional Activities (EPAs), which are the core procedures and skills required for independent practice.[21,22] EPAs integrate competencies across multiple domains to gauge progression through residency training. The ABS recently introduced the following EPAs: the evaluation and management of patients with right lower quadrant pain, biliary disease, inguinal hernias, and trauma. Residents also should be prepared to provide surgical consultation to other specialists. These EPAs are now being piloted across several residency programs.[23]

Association of American Medical Colleges

One expression of expectations between residents and their faculty is the AAMC Compact Between Resident Physicians and Their Teachers.[24] Originally published in 2006, this pledge remains relevant and delineates the expectations for both the faculty and trainees and defines conduct specific to fulfill their obligations to one another. The core tenets of this compact are excellence in medical education, highest-quality patient care and safety, and respect for residents' well-being. Commitments of faculty and commitments of residents are shown to the right:

AAMC Commitments of Faculty

- As role models for our residents, we will maintain the highest standards of care, respect the needs and expectations of patients, and embrace the contributions of all members of the health care team.
- We pledge our utmost effort to ensure that all components of the educational program for resident physicians are of high quality, including our own contributions as teachers.
- In fulfilling our responsibility to nurture both the intellectual and the personal development of residents, we commit to fostering academic excellence, exemplary professionalism, cultural sensitivity, and a commitment to maintaining competence through life-long learning.
- We will demonstrate respect for all residents as individuals, without regard to gender, race, national origin, religion, disability or sexual orientation; and we will cultivate a culture of tolerance among the entire staff.
- We will do our utmost to ensure that resident physicians have opportunities to participate in patient care activities of sufficient variety and with sufficient frequency to achieve the competencies required by their chosen discipline. We also will do our utmost to ensure that residents are not assigned excessive clinical responsibilities and are not overburdened with services of little or no educational value.
- We will provide resident physicians with opportunities to exercise graded, progressive responsibility for the care of patients, so that they can learn how to practice their specialty and recognize when, and under what circumstances, they should seek assistance from colleagues. We will do our utmost to prepare residents to function effectively as members of health care teams.
- In fulfilling the essential responsibility we have to our patients, we will ensure that residents receive appropriate supervision for all of the care they provide during their training.
- We will evaluate each resident's performance on a regular basis, provide appropriate verbal and written feedback, and document achievement of the competencies required to meet all educational objectives.
- We will ensure that resident physicians have opportunities to partake in required conferences, seminars, and other non-patient care learning experiences and that they have sufficient time to pursue the independent, self-directed learning essential for acquiring the knowledge, skills, attitudes, and behaviors required for practice.
- We will nurture and support residents in their role as teachers of other residents and of medical students.

AAMC Commitments of Residents

- We acknowledge our fundamental obligation as physicians—to place our patients' welfare uppermost; quality health care and patient safety will always be our prime objectives.
- We pledge our utmost effort to acquire the knowledge, clinical skills, attitudes, and behaviors required to fulfill all objectives of the educational program and to achieve the competencies deemed appropriate for our chosen discipline.
- We embrace the professional values of honesty, compassion, integrity, and dependability.
- We will adhere to the highest standards of the medical profession and pledge to conduct ourselves accordingly in all of our interactions. We will demonstrate respect for all patients and members of the health care team without regard to gender, race, national origin, religion, economic status, disability, or sexual orientation.
- As physicians in training, we learn most from being involved in the direct care of patients and from the guidance of faculty and other members of the health care team. We understand the need for faculty to supervise all of our interactions with patients.
- We accept our obligation to secure direct assistance from faculty or appropriately experienced residents whenever we are confronted with high-risk situations or with clinical decisions that exceed our confidence or skill to handle alone.
- We welcome candid and constructive feedback from faculty and all others who observe our performance, recognizing that objective assessments are indispensable guides to improving our skills as physicians.
- We also will provide candid and constructive feedback on the performance of our fellow residents, of students, and of faculty, recognizing our life-long obligation as physicians to participate in peer evaluation and quality improvement.
- We recognize the rapid pace of change in medical knowledge and the consequent need to prepare ourselves to maintain our expertise and competency throughout our professional lifetimes.
- In fulfilling our own obligations as professionals, we pledge to assist both medical students and fellow residents in meeting their professional obligations by serving as their teachers and role models.

Essential Leadership and Faculty Resources

Role of Leadership in Supporting the Educational Mission

Despite these laudable expectations and agreed-upon processes to produce a new surgeon, many potential pitfalls lurk along the way. Some pitfalls relate to inadequate access to financial and physical resources, including financial investment in educational technology, simulation labs, access to space and clinical environment technologies, adequate salary support to trainees, and the infrastructure for education. Other pitfalls relate to the rising pressure for clinical productivity for individual faculty and departments, potentially stressing the sense of value and reward that comes from serving as a trainer to a young surgeon. To deliver on this essential mission requires the investment and expectations set by the leaders of the institution.

The significance of any mission is reflected in the related financial investment. In the case of educating residents, at most training institutions the department chair is responsible for delivering the required financial support. The greatest investment is in salary support for essential functions: program and associate PDs, laboratory skills personnel, core curriculum faculty support, and administrative support. The chair must cover these investments or partner with institutional leadership to secure adequate financial resources. Financial support that enhances the learning environment also is important, including food at essential conferences, social gathering support, the hosting of journal clubs, special events around visiting professors, events that highlight the accomplishments of residents and faculty, graduations, and the sharing of good news of life events for members of the surgical education community. These investments demonstrate the value the department places on balancing educational experience with essential social interaction.

The department chair also is responsible for establishing a positive learning environment. The chair must model high standards of professionalism in interactions with faculty, residents, and staff and must be willing to address breaches in professionalism. Surgeon educators should view the participation of residents in their practice as a privilege even though it may sometimes feel like a burden. Faculty who do not respect this privilege must be counseled or even removed from the teaching service. Residents, similarly, must be held to achievable standards of engagement and participation. The chair must be available to the residency PD both to offer guidance and to assist in corrective measures when needed. As a complex human system, full of intense life moments, a department is somewhat similar to a family, requiring leaders to demonstrate wisdom, empathy, and responsible execution of one's responsibilities to ensure a cohesive, high-performing unit—no easy task.

Role of Faculty in Supporting the Educational Mission
Faculty are invaluable leaders in the department and serve as daily role models for surgeons in training. Yet most of these individuals have little formal training as educators. Surgeons in particular often forego institutional training programs to enhance their roles as educators, citing conflict with clinical activities. Chairs and educational institutions need to create incentives for surgeons to participate in educational training opportunities both locally and through national organizations, either financially or through accolades and advancement. Educational scholarship and contributions must be acknowledged as important elements of academic advancement for clinical faculty.

The ACS Academy of Master Surgeon Educators™ has placed a national emphasis on the value of scholarship in education. Members are generally preeminent surgical educators who exemplify the standards for residency education and innovation by maintaining the highest standard of surgical education at all levels. This effort both defines the importance of education scholarship and offers a recognized credential, much like those conferred on the traditional research community.

The ACS offers a Surgeons as Educators course for surgeons who will have educational responsibilities in their institutions. The Society of American Gastrointestinal and Endoscopic Surgeons has developed the Train the Trainer program, based on the U.K. University Health Service program created to foster national dissemination of laparoscopic colectomy about a decade ago. This simulation-based educational program teaches surgeons how to optimize their teaching skills in the OR, one of the most complex learning environments in the hospital.[25-27] The simple steps of (1) setting learning and technical educational goals for a case right before the operation at the scrub sink sets agreed-upon understanding of the trainee's personal experience with the teaching attending; (2) agreeing upon a plan to pause and address falters in the operation resulting from a lack of trainee technical experience or familiarity with a step; (3) learning how to have a structured discussion during a misstep in execution of the case to allow resumption of progress without the dreaded "walk to the other side of the table," which is demoralizing for faculty and trainee; and (4) using a postoperative debriefing to identify takeaway points learned during the case. This structured, simulation-based training program for faculty can improve educational performance of faculty and learners alike. Similarly, academic institutions across the U.S. and the AAMC host faculty development opportunities throughout the year. Chairs are encouraged to invest in these faculty development initiatives.

The chairs and the faculty set the expectations for valuing education as a core mission. The participation of leadership in educational conferences, the tone of didactic conferences, and the expectations that faculty and trainees will be present for conferences all help to create a successful learning environment. A mandatory annual faculty retreat and separate annual resident retreat also demonstrate the importance of the educational mission. The evolution of that mission to allow for innovation can enhance educational performance. Annual faculty reviews by chairs and chiefs that include an assessment of teaching efforts demonstrate that the department values education. If leaders, such as chairs, senior faculty, and division heads, are absent from these events, the message sent is that the educational mission is secondary and that training is not a priority. Only leadership can ensure that educational performance receives the value it deserves.

Leaders also must set the tone and enforce professionalism. They establish a culture of inclusion for all members of the surgical team that is nonpunitive, optimizes learning from errors and failures, and insists on truth and integrity. Leaders must create training pathways to welcome faculty and fellow residents to an environment that supports education and excellence. Leaders must ensure that faculty and staff are trained to be agents of an anti-racist, equitable, and inclusive practice environment. This includes training so that bystanders who witness targeted harm will step up in response (refer to Case Scenario 6 found later in this chapter for further discussion of the role and responsibilities of the bystander). Surgeons, as individuals and as a community, are only as good as what we tolerate in our presence.

Clearly Defined Expectations for Faculty and Residents
Program faculty enter a mutual commitment with their surgical residents. In return for the resident's time and service, faculty are required to supervise and guide resident education and ensure that trainees acquire the knowledge, clinical finesse, and technical skills required for surgical practice. As such, performance expectations should be explicitly described for both the trainee and faculty member.

Defined expectations should be set for faculty with respect to their role as educators, including educating residents and medical students as well as serving as role models for professionalism and delivering high-quality patient care. Similarly, faculty should model behavior consistent with respect for all aspects of resident and patient diversity. Lastly, faculty should provide appropriate and regular feedback to trainees, and trainees should be receptive to this feedback as they progress through the residency program.

For the trainee, the more granular the description of the expectations, the more likely the goals and progress will be achieved. It is helpful to describe expectations of the trainees by postgraduate year (PGY). These expectations should include goals for clinical care management, technical skills, decision-making, academic productivity, education of self and others, and professionalism. Surgical residents are expected to participate actively in educational activities and patient care in a graduated fashion such that they assume increasing levels of responsibility during their training. Further, they must demonstrate respect for patients and all members of the health care team. Residents also have a responsibility to the patients to seek faculty supervision, especially in complex situations that require advanced knowledge or skills. Residents also have responsibilities to educate fellow residents and medical students as appropriate.

What Does Success Look Like?

Below, we provide case scenarios of common educational experiences that can challenge the resident or the faculty. Suggestions are provided for addressing these scenarios in a positive, edifying way.

Case Scenario 1
A PGY2 resident is allowed to close the abdomen under direct observation and in tying the fascia under tension, the resident is deviating from basic technique of locking the knot, and an inconsistent approximation may occur. Although this resident is known to be knowledgeable about their patients and generally well prepared before an operation, a fundamental skill clearly has not been developed.

Q: What is the appropriate response?
A: In this case, the attending needs to ensure that the abdomen is closed correctly and may approximate the fascia to mitigate tying under tension. More importantly, the faculty member needs to talk to the resident after the operation and agree to teach the resident the appropriate technique to tie under tension (potentially meeting them in the simulation lab) with the expectation that they will practice, learn the technique, and subsequently demonstrate the skill. In this way, the resident will learn the value of critique and the opportunity to improve a skill set. Taking the time to point the deficiency and commit to teaching the resident the correct way to complete a task in a positive way will optimize the resident's learning, such as learning to ask for help when needed and to stop doing a technique they know is being done incorrectly.

Case Scenario 2
A PGY3 resident scrubs in on a case with a surgical oncology attending to perform a gastrectomy for a gastrointestinal malignancy. However, the resident did not read the patient's history or otherwise prepare for the case.

Q: What is the appropriate response?
A: While this lack of preparation may make an attending feel anger and disrespect and desire to dismiss the resident from the OR, some steps can turn this into a win-win. First, given the lack of preparation, the resident should only assist in the case and not be the primary surgeon. Trying to guide a resident through a case without preparation is an ineffective teaching method. Similarly, as the resident assists, the attending may ask graduated guiding questions to assess the resident's knowledge. Ideally, the attending should point out challenging aspects of the case to the trainee so that the next time they have a similar case together, this experience won't be wasted. The attending also should explain to the trainee why it is important to read the patient's history and the operative case in advance. The resident must understand the mutual commitment that the faculty and trainee have to one another. By reading in advance, the steps of the case and technical nuances experienced by the trainee will be retained to a greater extent. Finally, the attending may ask all residents to call and discuss the operative case the day before or at a preoperative conference. Another technique might be to assign the resident to give a case conference to demonstrate that they are prepared in the future. This scenario is a great opportunity for the attending to set expectations for the resident in advance of the case.

If a resident is chronically ill prepared, the PD should be informed to determine remedial steps. If this event is isolated, it may be appropriate to ask why it happened. If this represents a new pattern of behavior for the resident, a discussion regarding why this is happening can determine if an exceptional personal stressor has developed that may require assistance or if there is a systemic issue in the work expectations of which the PD should be aware.

Case Scenario 3
A second-year resident covers clinic with Dr. Smith, a busy breast surgeon. The clinic has five patients scheduled every hour, with 20 patients to be seen from 8 am to noon. As the resident sees patients, she tries to ask the attending questions about management, clinical trials, and so on, but the attending is too busy to teach.

Q: Ideally, what should the resident do?
A: This is a challenging situation for the resident and the attending. Ideally, clinics would accommodate the time for questions beyond the specific patient decisions. However, 20 patients in a half-day leaves little time for in-depth education. Having some insight regarding the challenges of a busy clinic will serve this resident well. Ideally, the resident would come to clinic armed with the fundamental principles of breast care and breast surgical oncology acquired through

independent reading and didactic conferences. While ideally residents should prepare for all clinics with prescreening of the patients, such prereview is often infeasible during work hours given their commitments during their 80-hour workweek. Efficient, focused examinations and assessments by the resident appropriate to their postgraduate year during the clinic will help the clinic go smoothly and stay on time, allowing more time for education and higher-level dialogue regarding management decisions and clinical trials.

Obviously, this adjustment is dependent upon the resident's emotional intelligence and situational awareness. If there is time pressure in clinic and there is a lukewarm response to inquiries regarding patient management decisions, it may be best for the resident to explicitly state: "Wow, this is a really busy clinic! I have several follow-up questions regarding management and possible clinical trials. Would you have some time after clinic to discuss these questions?" The attending should enthusiastically accept that request, particularly if clinic notes are to be completed efficiently and accurately by the resident. With this more thoughtful approach, the working and learning environment will be improved.

Case Scenario 4
A senior trauma attending is scheduled to give the intern lecture on the acute abdomen. The interns were told to read the material in the *Surgical Council on Resident Education* (SCORE) curriculum in advance of the lecture, and the attending was asked to make this presentation interactive without slides, as the interns were to be prepared. The attending shows up and asked how many interns read the material. Only three hands went up.

Q: How should the attending respond?
A: All faculty will likely have had this experience at some time or another. Unfortunately, a very normal human response is to be a bit angry and disappointed.

Although the attending could simply leave the conference and return once the residents had met their end of the educational bargain, rescheduling is often difficult in structured schedules of residencies for both the attending and the residents. In this case, the attending should continue with the interactive session, engaging with the interns who did complete the reading assignment; the attending should move forward with presenting the information that was in the reading materials. This approach is fair to those interns who did complete the assignment; those residents who did not read it may be left behind, but this response may serve as a stimulus for them to prepare fully for the next didactic session. The three interns who did read the material will, in essence, lead the way and demonstrate how their reading of the material resulted in improved education.

Case Scenario 5
A fourth-year resident is well prepared for a laparoscopic colon resection. When he shows up for the case, the resident is relegated to holding the camera. This seems to be a pattern for this attending surgeon.

Q: What should the resident and program leadership do?
A: There are always things to be learned even when holding the camera. However, this is certainly not an ideal situation for resident training, particularly for residents who have the level of training and skill set to perform portions or all of a procedure under supervision. This situation occurs less frequently when the faculty understand and are committed to their roles as trainers. At the end of the procedure, the resident should talk to the attending about goals and preparations for the next procedure, specifically including which portions of the case the resident would like to perform and what type of feedback to receive. The resident should also describe previous experience with similar cases to indicate where they are on the learning curve. Prior to the next procedure, the resident should again touch base with the attending to discuss the case specifics and goals for the procedure. This approach demonstrates preparation and commitment to the attending and provides an opportunity for open dialogue. The Train the Trainer program fosters this sort of give-and-take in setting expectations.

However, if attending makes this practice chronic, the PD, supported by the chair, needs to intervene. A discussion regarding the attending's role as a teaching surgeon is needed. The resident will most certainly be unable to remedy this problem alone, nor should leadership place that burden on the resident. To ensure that all facts are considered, the PD first should gather information by speaking directly to residents who have worked with this attending, as well as the attending. Effective use of annual confidential resident evaluations of the faculty and the program will likely have identified this concern more broadly and can help a PD address the issue. If there is a clear pattern of not allowing residents to participate appropriately in procedures, a candid discussion with the attending should occur. For example, it may be related to the challenging nature of specific cases or being relatively new in practice. The expectations for resident participation should be discussed as it is every attending's responsibility to train surgical residents at the institution. The attending may benefit from participation in a Train the Trainer teaching course. On occasion, however, this pattern of using residents only as assistants remains persistent. If this pattern of lack of engagement in the teaching program extends to participation in didactic sessions, and to the perioperative period (clinics, wards), this faculty member may need to be removed from the teaching service. It is also important to ensure that the attending is not discriminating against certain cohorts based on gender, race, ethnicity, or other characteristics in the residency program regarding whom they are willing to train.

Case Scenario 6
An attending meets up with the resident team in the work room before heading off to rounds. The attending sees an intern of Asian descent eating noodles with a pair of chopsticks and says, "You should eat that with a fork, you are in the United States after all."

Q: How should the resident respond?
A: This is harassment based on ethnicity and represents a form of mistreatment. There is a power differential between faculty and trainees, and therefore, the resident, fearing retribution, is unlikely to point out to the attending that this comment is inappropriate. This event should be reported to the PD or chair. What may be one person's notion of microaggression may feel like outright racism to another.

A rare resident may feel comfortable directly addressing the statement, for example, by asking a clarifying question: "I am not sure I heard you correctly. Can you clarify what you said to me?" A second statement may help to explain to the attending why this statement was unacceptable: "When I hear statements like that, it makes me feel undervalued and singled out for my background." The use of "I" statements to focus on observations and thoughts/feelings avoids accusatory-sounding statements towards the attending. However, in the imbalanced power dynamic of this setting, such a direct approach is rare.

This scenario also highlights the need for bystander training and application, as there is an essential role that observer colleagues need to play in this situation. They may do so by speaking to the harmed resident after the fact, acknowledging the insult and thereby providing important emotional support. Failure to reach out further exacerbates the harm. If they are senior residents who have a solid relationship with the attending, a direct discussion may be offered. However, this response also is challenging in the imbalanced power status of our hierarchical surgical culture.

This group of observers also need to escalate their observations to the program leadership. Department-wide education in bystander roles for faculty, residents, and staff can be helpful to mitigate the impact of harassment on certain cohorts. However, direct conversation from leadership to the offending attending (or resident or staff in other cases), including discussion of possible penalties, is often the only durable solution to stop these behaviors.

Conclusion

Education is a core mission of any college or school of medicine and the affiliated medical institutions that host surgical training programs. To successfully execute this mission, it is critical to clearly define the expectations of faculty to educate the next generation as well as participate in their own continuing education and development as teachers. It is also imperative to define the expectations of the learners toward their own education and how they can develop into a surgeon capable of independent practice. Trainees and faculty must maintain the highest level of professionalism and foster a learning environment free of harassment, mistreatment, or microaggressions so that optimal learning can occur. Lastly, both trainees and faculty must be prepared for the inevitable situations that will develop to challenge learning and training experiences. Education is a lifelong pursuit. Just as learners eventually become educators, educators become learners, learning from the younger generations. All must be open to these experiences to advance their own development, attain the highest level of professional performance, and fulfill their commitment to their patients and their profession.

References

1. American College of Surgeons. Statements on Principles: Medical Education. Available at: https://www.facs.org/about-acs/statements/stonprin. Accessed September 25, 2020.
2. Accreditation Council for Graduate Medical Education. ACGME Program Requirements for Graduate Medical Education in General Surgery. Available at: https://www.acgme.org/Portals/0/PFAssets/ProgramRequirements/440_GeneralSurgery_2020.pdf?ver=2020-06-22-085958-260. Accessed September 28, 2020.
3. Dickinson KJ, Bass BL, Graviss EA, Nguyen DT, Pei KY. How learning preferences and teaching styles influence effectiveness of surgical educators. *Am J Surg*. 2021;221(2):256-260.
4. American Board of Surgery. About us. Available at: https://www.absurgery.org/default.jsp?abouthome. Accessed October 15, 2020.
5. Purnell SM, Bass BL, Benavides B, Martinez S, McNeil S, Dickinson K. Template for a program tailored ACS/APDS Phase I curriculum: from needs assessment to implementation. [published online ahead of print, March 2021]. *Am J Surg*. 2021;S0002-9610(21)00170-7.
6. American College of Surgeons. Statement on Surgical Residencies and the Educational Environment. Available at: https://www.facs.org/about-acs/statements/16-surgical-residencies. Accessed September 28, 2020.

7. Lebares CC, Guvva EV, Ascher NL, O'Sullivan PS, Harris HW, Epel ES. Burnout and stress among US surgery residents: psychological distress and resilience. *J Am Coll Surg.* 2018;226(1):80-90.
8. Balch CM, Freischlag JA, Shanafelt TD. Stress and burnout among surgeons: understanding and managing the syndrome and avoiding the adverse consequences. *Arch Surg.* 2009;144(4):371-376.
9. Shanafelt TD, Balch CM, Bechamps GJ, et al. Burnout and career satisfaction among American surgeons. *Ann Surg.* 2009;250(3):463-471.
10. Ceppa DP, Dolejs SC, Boden N, et al. Sexual harassment and cardiothoracic surgery: #UsToo? *Ann Thorac Surg.* 2020;109(4):1283-1288.
11. Hu YY, Ellis RJ, Hewitt DB, et al. Discrimination, abuse, harassment, and burnout in surgical residency training. *N Engl J Med.* 2019;381(18):1741-1752.
12. Nukala M, Freedman-Weiss M, Yoo P, Smeds MR. Sexual harassment in vascular surgery training programs. *Ann Vasc Surg.* 2020;62:92-97.
13. Mavis B. Measuring mistreatment: honing questions about abuse on the Association of American Medical Colleges Graduation Questionnaire. *Virtual Mentor.* 2014;16(3):196-199.
14. Ellis RJ, Hewitt DB, Hu YY, et al. An empirical national assessment of the learning environment and factors associated with program culture. *Ann Surg.* 2019;270(4):585-592.
15. U.S. National Library of Medicine. The Surgical Education Culture Optimization Through Targeted Interventions Based on National Comparative Data - "The SECOND Trial" (SECOND). Available at: https://clinicaltrials.gov/ct2/show/NCT03739723. Accessed October 11, 2021.
16. American College of Surgeons. American College of Surgeons Statement on Resident Access to Personal Protective Equipment. Available at: https://www.facs.org/about-acs/statements/resident-access-to-ppe. Accessed August 24, 2021.
17. McKenna DT, Mattar SG. What is wrong with the training of general surgery? *Adv Surg.* 2014;48:201-210.
18. Mattar SG, Alseidi AA, Jones DB, et al. General surgery residency inadequately prepares trainees for fellowship: results of a survey of fellowship program directors. *Ann Surg.* 2013;258(3):440-449.
19. Napolitano LM, Savarise M, Paramo JC, et al. Are general surgery residents ready to practice? A survey of the American College of Surgeons Board of Governors and Young Fellows Association. *J Am Coll Surg.* 2014;218(5):1063-1072. e1031.
20. American Board of Surgery. American Board of Surgery Statement Regarding Residency Redesign. Available at: https://vascular.org/sites/default/files/ABS%20Statement%20on%20 Residency%20Redesign%20-%20 04%2016.pdf. Accessed September 23, 2020.
21. Brasel KJ, Klingensmith ME, Englander R, et al. Entrustable professional activities in general surgery: development and implementation. *J Surg Educ.* 2019;76(5):1174-1186.
22. Greenberg JA, Minter RM. Entrustable professional activities: the future of competency-based education in surgery may already be here. *Ann Surg.* 2019;269(3):407-408.
23. Stahl CC, Jung SA, Rosser AA, et al. Entrustable professional activities in general surgery: trends in resident self-assessment. *J Surg Educ.* 2020;77(6):1562-1567.
24. Association of American Medical Colleges. Compact Between Resident Physicians and Their Teachers. Available at: https://www.aamc.org/ media/24276/download. Accessed September 23, 2020.
25. Wyles SM, Schwarz E, Dort J, et al. SAGE(S) advice: application of a standardized train the trainer model for faculty involved in a Society of American Gastrointestinal and Endoscopic Surgeons (SAGES) hands-on course. *Surg Endosc.* 2017;31(5):2017-2022.
26. Mackenzie H, Cuming T, Miskovic D, et al. Design, delivery, and validation of a trainer curriculum for the national laparoscopic colorectal training program in England. *Ann Surg.* 2015;261(1):149-156.
27. Wyles SM, Miskovic D, Ni Z, et al. Development and implementation of the Structured Training Trainer Assessment Report (STTAR) in the English National Training Programme for laparoscopic colorectal surgery. *Surg Endosc.* 2016;30(3):993-1003.

AMERICAN C
SURGEONS A
OF SURGEON
COLLEGE OF
AMERICAN C
SURGEONS A
OF SURGEON
COLLEGE OF
AMERICAN C
SURGEONS

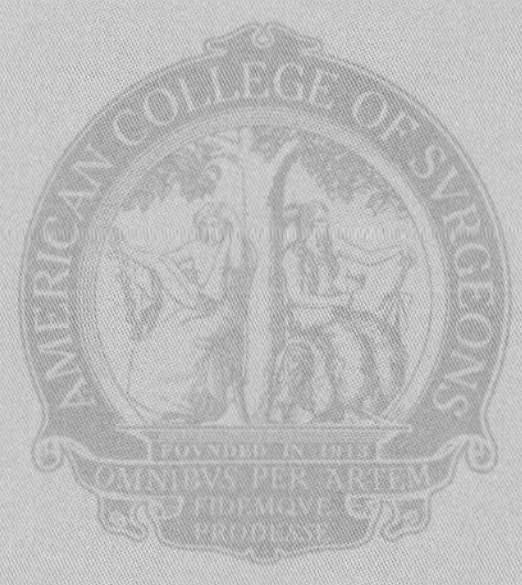

AMERICAN COLLEGE OF SVRGEONS
OMNIBVS PER ARTEM
FIDEMQVE
PRODESSE

INDEX

Index

Page locators in *italics* indicate figures and tables.

A

B

C

D

M

N

O

P

Q

R

S

T

Z